Narrative Medicine

"Lewis Mehl-Madrona is an extraordinarily gifted physician and healer. I saw him transform the lives of profoundly affected patients. Mostly, he was sitting next to them, listening carefully and telling them stories. I was amazed."

David Servan-Schreiber, M.D., Ph.D., Clinical Professor of Psychiatry, University of Pittsburgh, author of *The Instinct to Heal*

"Dr. Mehl-Madrona's work with Narrative Medicine is both powerful and exciting. He meets each patient as a unique individual instead of a diagnosis. He provides story after story of successes that are not within the normal spectrum of modern medicine, and breaks down narrative medicine into components so we may catch a glimpse of how it achieves its success. He brings the reader back to listening and compassion, the two human aspects of medicine that are crucial to the doctor-patient relationship. His view of medicine and healing expands how one looks at the illness, health, and community."

Ann Marie Chiasson, M.D., MPH, CCFP, Clinical Assistant Professor of Medicine, University of Arizona

"It is clear from Lewis Mehl-Madrona's work that healing is far too complex a process to entrust to the western medical profession. And in opening the door to indigenous voices from outside these professional doors, the present volume is both illuminating and invaluable. My hope is that this book will serve as a beacon and an inspiration for the broadest collaboration in defining and enriching our orientations to health, illness, and cure."

Kenneth J. Gergen, Mustin Professor of
Psychology, Swarthmore College

"Stanford Medical School trained Mehl-Madrona invokes the philosophy of his Cherokee and Lakota ancestors to remind us that the path to redemption for today's health care world is to honor the patient's life story with all of its elements of culture, community, family, health beliefs, spirituality, and individuality. Mehl-Madrona's narrative contribution is possibly the most inclusive philosophy ever proposed in medicine.

"After reading *Narrative Medicine,* when we come face-to-face with that terrible question, 'Doc, how long have I got to live?' we will know that the answer cannot be found in a statistic or the natural history of a disease, but depends upon your unique story—the one told up until this point and especially the one authored from this point onward."

Farrell Silverberg, Ph.D., author of *Make the Leap:*
A Practical Guide to Breaking the Patterns That Hold You Back

"Our stories bring us comfort and help us become acquainted with our unanticipated dreams and fears. *Narrative Medicine* helps us connect to this personal taproot enhancing our understanding of how we can find our way back to wellness in crisis."

Roberta Lee, Continuum Center for Health
and Healing, Beth Israel Medical Center, New York

Narrative Medicine

The Use of History and Story in the Healing Process

Lewis Mehl-Madrona, M.D., Ph.D.

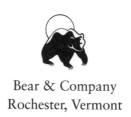

Bear & Company
Rochester, Vermont

Bear & Company
One Park Street
Rochester, Vermont 05767
www.BearandCompanyBooks.com

Bear & Company is a division of Inner Traditions International

Library of Congress Cataloging-in-Publication Data
Narrative medicine : the use of history and story in the healing process / Lewis Mehl-Madrona.
   p. ; cm.
Includes bibliographical references.
Summary: "Seeks to restore the pivotal role of the patient's own story in the healing process"—Provided by publisher.
ISBN-13: 978-1-59143-065-0 (pbk.)
ISBN-10: 1-59143-065-8 (pbk.)
1. Narrative medicine. I. Title.
[DNLM: 1. Medicine, Traditional. 2. Narration. 3. Indians, North American. 4. Professional-Patient Relations. WB 50.1 M498n 2007]

RC48.M44 2007
610.69'6—dc22
                                                    2007005985

Printed and bound in the United States by Lake Book Manufacturing

10 9 8 7 6 5 4 3 2 1

Text design and layout by Rachel Goldenberg
This book was typeset in Sabon with Bodega Serif as the display typeface

To send correspondence to the author of this book, mail a first-class letter to the author c/o Inner Traditions • Bear & Company, One Park Street, Rochester, VT 05767, and we will forward the communication, or e-mail him at narrativemedicine@gmail.com.

To my children and grandchildren,
for they are the future.

Contents

Foreword

We are surrounded by stories. At the largest level, our stories enfold, protect, and constrain us.

Every building you see started as an idea. The dimensions of the idea—should it be round or square, energy-intensive or energy-efficient, tall or short, brick or steel—emerged from the stories of the culture in which its architect lived. Planes, trains, automobiles, bicycles, pavement, sidewalks, canyons of buildings that are our big cities all started first as thoughts, all grounded in the stories of what is right and good and consistent with how people should live.

Every invention grew out of a story. Even the stories of the stories grew out of stories—consider Plato's story of the shadows on the walls of the cave, ancient notions of the perfect archetype, the search for the ultimate story from Gilgamesh to Genesis to Stephen Hawking.

In a similar way—but for those of us who grew up in modern Western culture a far less obvious way—our bodies are our stories. Not just our body decorations, like the way we wear our hair or our piercings or tattoos or makeup, but our bodies themselves.

There's a perhaps apocryphal story that Dale Carnegie related about Abraham Lincoln. One of Lincoln's advisors was recommending a man for inclusion in his cabinet, and Lincoln said no.

"I don't like his face," Lincoln reportedly said.

Horrified, his advisor said, "But he's not responsible for his face!"

Lincoln replied, "Every man over forty is responsible for his own face."

Lincoln understood that over the course of our lives, we create and re-create ourselves in a way consistent with our stories about ourselves and the world around us. And, just as Lincoln reportedly felt about a man's face, Lewis Mehl-Madrona suggests that each of us carries in our entire body the legacy of our stories.

Lewis's book is compelling, in large part because it rings so true. All of us, at one time or another, have managed to work ourselves into a sickness, a panic attack, or an exhaustion of one sort or another. And all of us have managed to push through illness—or push totally past and around illness when everybody around us was falling sick—when we knew we had to.

It should come as no surprise that our immune system cells are rich with receptor sites for neurochemicals like serotonin, which vary with mood and story, and that mining this relationship between mind and immune system is one of the richest and most fascinating fields in modern psychiatry. But we don't need to become completely Aristotelian about it all to grok its reality. Simply tell some stories and listen to hear if they sound true, look at their effect, check with your gut for their reality.

This book is rich with stories, some of which you will carry with you for the rest of your life and integrate into your own stories. Thus, it will not only inform you, the simple act of reading it will also heal you.

THOM HARTMANN
PORTLAND, OREGON
JANUARY 2007

Thom Hartmann is the award-winning, best-selling author of more than a dozen books, including *Walking Your Blues Away, Screwed: The Undeclared War Against the Middle Class, The Last Hours of Ancient Sunlight,* and *The Edison Gene*. His groundbreaking work in attention deficit hyperactivity disorder and psychotherapy has been featured in *TIME* magazine, the *New York Times,* and in media around the world.

Acknowledgments

I want to especially thank Jamaica Burns, my editor at Bear & Company, and Evelyn Leigh, my copy editor, for their amazing help in improving this book.

I am also grateful to my friends and colleagues at the First Nations University of Canada (particularly Janet Smylie and Willie Ermine) and at the University of Saskatchewan (especially Peter Butt, Keith Ogle, Raymond Tempier, Roland Dyck, James Waldram, Marie Battiste, William Albritton, and Anna Hunter) for some stimulating conversations that influenced this work.

I want to thank my students in Indigenous Knowledge 302 (spring semester 2006) for letting me test some of the material on them through lectures. I was especially grateful to Kimber Worme, whose ancestor was led across the winter prairies by a coyote, and who questioned everything I said.

I'm also grateful to the Discursive Therapies program at Massey University in New Zealand and to Andy Lock for creating the program that I found so helpful. I want to acknowledge my teachers there—particularly Tom Strong, Ken and Mary Gergen, Rom Harré, and Susanna Chamberlain—for influencing my thinking about health and medicine toward a narrative direction. This book arose from a class assignment in narrative therapeutics by Dr. Vincent Hevern for which I gave twelve lectures (one for each chapter of this book) at the University of Saskatchewan and reflected upon what those present thought about the material. Vinnie kept losing the material and I'm hoping he'll eventually get around to reading it, but his agreement to this assignment (somewhat altered from his original plan) gave me a structure for writing this book. I kept working and reworking the material based upon participant responses in my seminar until Jamaica and Evelyn got hold of the manuscript and could really shape it.

Without these people who have invited me to share their stories and their personal healing journeys, none of this work would be possible. To protect their privacy, all names have been changed.

I'm especially grateful to our local elders for our many discussions about what is indigenous, what is culture, what is traditional, what is contemporary, and what is story.

I use stories in most of my clinical encounters. I try to choose stories from my client's own culture. I take the concept of indigenous knowledge and rights seriously. In this book, I have used only stories that I have heard orally, but that are also available from multiple written sources. I freely change the stories to fit the needs of the clinical situation and the people with whom I am working. Perhaps that is the nature of cultural change, to take what is available from the past and to revise it to meet the needs of the present.

INTRODUCTION
Awakening to Narrative Medicine

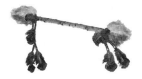

Diseases cannot be reduced to pathological facts, they constitute other worlds.

OLIVER SACKS[1]

Despite areas in which modern medicine shines, the prognosis for some illnesses is little better today than it was one hundred years ago. The incidence of some illnesses seems to be increasing. The U.S. Department of Health and Human Services calculated 1028 patient-episodes of mental illness per 100,000 people in 1955 and 3806 in the year 2000.[2] New illnesses such as AIDS, avian flu, fibromyalgia, and chronic fatigue syndrome seem to appear as quickly as old ones are eradicated. Once we have reached age five, we have no greater life expectancy today than we did in 1905.[3]

This state of affairs is reflected in the relationships between doctors and patients. Both are increasingly unhappy. Managed care in the United States and time pressure in other countries has led to the ten-minute office visit with the family doctor. Specialists are sometimes allotted fifteen minutes. In the United States, people have little opportunity to tell their stories to their doctors, and doctors have no venue for listening to patients. Taking a careful history is no longer cost effective. Television commercials inform patients what drugs to request during their brief visit with the doctor. Diagnoses are made in fifteen minutes or less after a succession of rapid-fire, yes-or-no questions. Doctors increasingly rely on answers to these questions to guide their decisions about what laboratory tests to order, and then let the results of those tests make the diagnosis. Illnesses that fall outside the realm of what the lab can diagnose are relegated to the confusing, the psychosomatic, the ridiculous, and the unimportant.

In a seeming rush to separate itself from culture and tradition, conventional medicine has eliminated much of the art of healing—those elements of doctoring that may be more important than the specific medicines provided. In its rush toward technological solutions (part of a broader social movement stretching across the twentieth century), medicine has progressively diminished the importance of the doctor-patient relationship, and of caring, compassion, and intent, in favor of diagnostic imaging and technical procedures. Discarding these long-standing, common aspects of healing practices has been to our detriment. Many of these arts can only be found now in the practices of the world's indigenous cultures. Recovering these lost arts could infuse medicine with renewed vitality and effectiveness. We need to hear new and different voices. *Narrative Medicine* is about revising our concept of medicine to enable the incorporation of these voices into modern medicine.

Ethicist Daniel Callahan writes that medicine needs to abandon the quest for immortality as its project and begin to consider quality of life.[4] Immortality is unattainable; the quest for longevity is expensive and draws from the resources available for the many to serve a privileged few. When we focus upon quality of life, we find other compelling stories that draw our attention away from conventional medicine as the only option. My favorite competing stories come from North American Native culture, since this is my heritage. Had I been born Chinese, however, I would now be comparing and contrasting the traditional Chinese story about health and healing with the conventional biomedical story. Circumstances of birth and later life experiences led me to where I am today. That is my context.

I was born in the Appalachian Mountains of southern Kentucky to a family of mixed Scottish and Cherokee ancestry. We didn't have much in the way of medical care and largely relied on local healing practices and folk medicine. I never met my father, though, through process of elimination I traced him through the U.S. Air Force to the Pine Ridge area of South Dakota. He was apparently part French Canadian and part Oglala. He and my mother met at a USO dance, but I think they were both too proud and stubborn to get together once I was conceived. My grandparents raised me while my mother worked her way through college and began her teaching career. They raised me in a complex mix of Cherokee heritage and modified Christianity—how modified I only came to understand later when I studied what regular Christians believed.

My mother eventually married a German farmer/milking parlor serviceman, and we moved to southeastern Ohio where I finished high school. I really didn't have much appreciation for my heritage and culture, except to know that the Cherokee identity—those principles and stories instilled by my grandparents—saved my life in my difficult battles with my stepfather. I supposed I was the chosen one, since my half-brothers and -sisters were not given these teachings.

Medical school made me aware of the value of my heritage. A famous and intimidating professor stood ponderously before us on the first day of pharmacology class. His glasses were perched on the end of his nose. With virtual papal authority, he removed his lecture notes from the inside pocket of his suit coat. He surveyed the room in pregnant silence. "Boys," he announced (he apparently could not acknowledge the women in our class), "life is a relentless progression toward death, disease, and decay. The job of the physician is to slow the rate of decline." I felt a lump in my throat. This was not how I wanted to see myself or be seen. His teachings so conflicted with those of my grandparents and great-grandmother that, by the next weekend, I had found a Cherokee healer with whom to study.

This sparked a journey that has continued for over thirty years of studying traditional healers and collecting stories about their work and their patients. I have sat in ceremony with healers in such diverse places as Arizona, New Mexico, Wisconsin, New York, Vermont, Hawai'i,

California, Canada, and even France, Germany, Austria, and the former Yugoslavia. I have felt the power of the many prayers embedded in sacred land in North America and in thousand-year-old churches in Europe.

I have also been immersed in conventional medicine for over thirty years. I graduated from medical school in 1975. I completed residencies in family medicine and in psychiatry at the University of Vermont. I earned added qualifications in geriatrics. I completed a Ph.D. in clinical psychology, though from a somewhat innovative graduate school that emphasized cross-cultural psychology. I did a postdoctoral fellowship in alcohol research at the U.C. Berkeley School of Public Health. I worked for twenty-seven years in emergency medicine. In 2004, I stopped my E.R. work, but I continue to practice mainstream family medicine and psychiatry.

Throughout this time, I have tried to bridge cultures and to develop an approach that will allow the patient and his or her family to be active collaborators in the healing process, recognizing the wisdom of indigenous cultures—that relationship matters, that people have to believe in the treatment and the doctor, that the support of family and community are necessary to make treatments work, and that far more than biology and pharmacology determine the success or failure of each medical encounter. I have traveled the world in search of healers. I have felt the sadness when treatment fails and people die. I have seen the limitations of narrow points of view on the part of many cultures.

I have traveled through a variety of United States institutions, longing for that place where I could develop a truly integrated program that was inclusive of the world's cultures and especially of the Native cultures of North America, since that is where we are located. For many reasons, I couldn't find that place. Two years ago, I moved from the University of Arizona to the University of Saskatchewan in Canada, where I have been working with aboriginal communities in rural and remote areas and developing a training program in cross-cultural health and mental health. Saskatchewan is the environment in which this book was written. As I write this, the snow is blowing outside and the cars are hardly moving in the –20°C weather. Nevertheless, sweatlodges are happening this afternoon, and I will be going to one with two Cree healers from Meadow Lake.

In my work, I have come to understand that integration, while desirable, is not necessary. Respect and tolerance are what is actually required. The world's traditional healing methods will persist above ground or underground, despite what mainstream people do. This has been the experience of Native people in the United States and Canada.[5] Cultures persist and evolve despite what is done to destroy them. I discovered the narrative philosophy and practice to be the best means of allowing diverse stories to coexist and interact, so I present it as a framework in this book for the restoration of traditional healing systems into a valid position within world cultures.

I propose that medicine must reinvent itself to include the voices and visions of indigenous peoples. Those of us within medicine must discover how to get from where we are today to a paradigm (or a story) that is more conducive to health and well-being. We need to think differently about medicine, psychotherapy, and healing. What we have are collections of stories that make sense to members of the cultures who tell them. The world's indigenous medical systems deserve appreciation for their wisdom. These traditional methods of healing include North American Native, traditional Chinese medicine, ayurveda from India, and African medicine, to name but a few. They hold many useful stories about health and disease, as valid in their own right as the stories told by conventional medicine.

As doctors, we serve our patients best when we exercise judgment and match stories to particular people, cultures, and circumstances to achieve the best possible outcome. However, in our increasingly global, modern culture, conventional medicine claims to be the truth, rather than one of many truths. Studies of indigenous knowledge from around the world teach us that many other valid ways of perceiving and learning about the world exist, beyond the European American scientific model. When we reconsider our models of medicine and psychology from the standpoint of other cultures, we begin to see that it also is an anthology of stories, not necessarily superior to the world's many other healing traditions.

In *Coyote Medicine*, I wrote about a traditional elder who told me that health and disease evolved from the way we answered four simple questions: Who are you? Where did you come from? Why are you here? Where are you going? This wisdom is common in indigenous knowledge systems about health and illness. Kim Anderson[6] wrote that her elders asked four similar questions: Who are you? Where did you come from? What are your responsibilities? Where are you going? These questions are powerful because they force us to tell a story about ourselves. That story becomes our identity. Medicine and psychology must also answer these four questions. The answers become stories about the profession's identity.

We did not always have trauma surgery. This has emerged as a modern story about how to save lives. We can say we prefer it for healing damage caused by accidents and war, even though our preference doesn't mean that it always works, or that it can't be augmented by prayer, distant energy healing, or visualization. The worldviews behind different stories about healing do not necessarily conflict with one another. We can be multicultural, using several different anthologies of belief. When we compare and contrast different knowledge systems, we learn what we prefer and how practical a given approach is for our particular context.

Within any healing art, whatever else we do, we treat by telling a story. The term *narrative medicine* arises from the impossibility of separating treatment from the stories told about the treatment, the audience hearing the stories, and the context in which the stories are told. This is as true for the conventional medical approach as it is for any other healing modality.

First we weave a time-sequenced narrative that includes what we have been told about the course of the various symptoms. This is called the "history of the illness." We combine this history with evidence from laboratory and imaging studies to form an interpretive story that tells the patient and family what caused the problem (from evil spirits to mercury amalgams to viral infections). We use this story rhetorically to position ourselves as trustworthy experts who can be believed. Then we offer a prescription (do an exorcism, remove mercury fillings, prescribe an antibiotic) to eliminate the ailment.

We build patient confidence through our use of all the tools language and communication provide. We use what psychologist Michael Bamberg of Clark University calls "small stories"[7] (short vignettes that barely qualify as tales in the classic sense) to position ourselves as caring, compassionate, knowledgeable, and believable. To the extent we are perceived this way, to the extent we are believed, we create an expected outcome and our treatment works. First and foremost, medical treatment is a story that we instantiate upon others.

When our preferred story about sickness and cure differs too much from those of our patients, their families, and their cultures, they may choose their more familiar stories, perhaps searching for healers who are more similar to them. How many patients come to us and then go home to their local healers when our story emerges as unsatisfying? When people don't believe our stories, they won't follow our treatments. Instead of using terms such as *noncompliance* or *lack of adherence,* we could just say the story we told didn't go over well. We weren't sufficiently convincing.

Patients who do not follow our instructions are exercising their functional autonomy to disagree with our story when it contradicts their preferred stories. To our chagrin, they are free to do something different than what we want them to do.

As much as medicine operates from stories about the world, patients operate from stories about their encounters with doctors. If we listened to all these stories and could hold them in our minds simultaneously, we could grasp our culture's concept of doctors' roles, of all that people think doctors are supposed to be and do.

We would hear stories that define good doctors, bad doctors, mean doctors, addicted doctors, incompetent doctors, heroic doctors, caring doctors—all manner of doctors. An oft-repeated story is about the doctor who picks up a life-threatening illness in its early stages, when it is still a confusing collection of symptoms, permitting an early intervention that saves the patient's life. This doctor is a hero, which all doctors want to be. The flip version of this story is about the doctor who misses the illness, allowing the patient to die, and is then sued for malpractice. From these stories we can see that many people hold doctors responsible for their health and

well-being—blaming them if death occurs, charging them with preventing death at all costs.*

We doctors have an especially rich investment in wanting to be the
main character in a medical hero tale, wrenching lives from the jaws
of death and making diagnoses from obscure facts that would stump
even Sherlock Holmes. We are drawn to medicine as a career to become
this hero. This story about who we are supposed to be—our medical
identity—torments and tortures us. What if we make a mistake and someone dies? Then we fall from heroic grace and become the main character
in a tale of disgrace and failure. We may even turn to drugs, alcohol, or
suicide. We become tragic antiheroes in stories of lost potential and good
people gone bad. This fear keeps us awake at night, constantly studying
and worrying about things we might have missed and mistakes we may
have made. This is not necessarily bad, as taxing as it may be when driven
by fear. Nevertheless, the stories that we doctors tell ourselves about our
role are important determining factors in our behavior and approach
to treating patients. Our stories about ourselves interface with patients'
stories about us and merge into the unfolding treatment story, which the
patient may or may not accept. This story is what is efficacious, not the
various treatment modalities mentioned in the story. Healing rises or
falls on the quality of the story, not the modalities chosen.

---

*Paradoxically, it is not the incompetent or bad doctors who are usually sued, but the
doctors who are arrogant and don't listen, whether they are correct or not. Medical
researcher Wendy Levinson recorded hundreds of conversations between physicians and
their patients.[8] Half of the selected doctors had never been sued, while the other half
had been sued at least twice. On the basis of those conversations, she found clear differences between the two groups. The surgeons who had not been sued spent three minutes
longer with their patients than those who had. They were more likely to make orienting
statements to prepare the patient for what to expect. They were more likely to encourage
further dialogue and to demonstrate active listening, and they were more likely to laugh
and be funny during the visit. They did not, however, appear to provide better medical
care. The difference was in how they talked to their patients. Next, psychologist Nalini
Ambady took these tape recordings, edited out the actual words, and presented the gar-
ble—which preserved intonation, pitch, and rhythm—to lay people, who were still able
to predict which doctors had been sued and which hadn't.[9] These lay people knew absolutely nothing about the physicians. They correctly realized that the doctors who sounded
dominant and arrogant were sued, and those who sounded concerned were not.

When we actually listen carefully to the amazing stories people tell about how they got well from serious, life-threatening diseases, we realize that no culture's stories or belief system can explain everyone's healing. Sometimes healing defies a rational explanation. Healing stories are often unique, lying outside the diagnostic and treatment stories of the world's medical systems. This observation puts us on a collision course with rational positivism, the basis for declaring medicine scientific, based upon discoverable facts and principles. Treatment becomes effective (or more effective) through how it is presented as part of an over-arching story inclusive of everything.

An example will further this discussion. A mother brought her five-week-old daughter to the family medicine clinic for an urgent visit. The mother began calling the clinic when her daughter was three weeks old, and had been doing so with increasing urgency ever since. This was her second child, who had been seen several times in the office and once in pediatric emergency. When I saw this child, she was five weeks old and had been without bowel movements for the past ten days. She was sleeping poorly and was fussy and irritable all day. She vomited after nursing. For the past thirty-six hours, she had had what is called projectile vomiting, in which the vomit actually projects well beyond the baby.

When we examined the baby, her abdomen was mildly distended. Poking and prodding upon it increased her irritability and fussiness. Her cheeks, trunk, legs, and arms held a fine, faint rash that had been present for the past week, not seeming to bother her. One eardrum was mildly red.

Most of us with conventional medical training would approach this child similarly. This is because we share a certain story about health and disease. Without question, our approach does save lives, but it isn't the only possible approach, and not even the only one that can save lives, or even always the best one. Within our story, we start by imagining the worst. Our story focuses upon the mechanical things that can go wrong and become life threatening. People come to us fearing the worst, and are relieved and reassured when the worst does not come to pass.

The resident (a physician in training) and I approached this baby, contemplating emergent conditions like pyloric stenosis (blockage of the end of the stomach), volvulus (twisting of the intestine upon itself), intussusception, (telescoping of the intestine into itself), other causes of intestinal blockage, Hirschsprung's disease (a condition in which the nerves that coordinate the movement of food through the intestines are congenitally lacking), and congenital hypothyroidism, to name a few possibilities. When an X-ray of the abdomen returned normal, we ordered an ultrasound. We drew blood for thyroid studies, electrolytes, and calcium, and obtained urine to rule out a bladder infection. What were we to do when the ultrasound was normal? Luckily, when the baby returned from the diagnostic imaging department, her abdominal exam was also now normal. She slept through our poking on her belly. Based upon the rash, pink ears, fussiness, and other symptoms, we felt justified in making a diagnosis of "viral syndrome."

Making a diagnosis is synonymous with constructing a story. It is an act of making meaning from isolated observations. It is a social activity in that everyone has to agree with the diagnosis (the story) for it to be a good one. Part of selling a diagnostic story is telling it in such a way that the involved lay people (family, patient, and friends) will believe it. Our diagnostic stories are prescriptive in that they provide a rationale for people to do what we tell them. When people don't share our rationale, they don't follow "doctor's orders." We have to build a good story to get people's cooperation. This was as true in the days of leech bleeding and bloodletting as it is today. When people reject our story, they seek out others, such as those told by alternative medicine doctors, Chinese medical practitioners, shamans, witchdoctors, faith healers, and more. These people do just what we do—tell a story to build a rationale for a different kind of treatment.

For our case with the five-week-old baby, once we leave the highly correlated world of diagnostic imaging with structural gut abnormalities, we enter a jungle of possibilities, including the realization that we don't actually have certainty about what to do. Some physicians would interpret the pinkish-red ear as otitis media and give antibiotics, "just in case," which would probably be treatment more for the physician than the child. Other physicians would offer Tylenol or Advil for symptom relief, while each would build a story about what they thought was wrong and how what was offered would treat the cause. Another practitioner might try some tincture of belladonna.

The resident and I convinced ourselves that we could diagnose a viral illness. We created a story of a viral process, only partially expressed because of the conferred immunity from breastfeeding. We marshaled our supporting evidence—pinkish-red ears, rash, fussiness, irritability. We reasoned that the lack of stools, which is common among breastfed babies, could relate to a higher-than-average metabolic rate due to the virus. We decided to congratulate the mother on the power of her breast milk to keep her baby relatively healthy in the face of a viral illness, thereby making diagnosis more difficult for us. I prefer to call this an explanatory story rather than fact, because it reminds me that there are other ways to put together the same observations and even better stories could emerge over time. The interaction and dialogue through which shared stories are generated has only just begun.

In my experience, people who come to the doctor want more than just a good explanation. They want more than reassurance. I wanted to give this mother something, but something potentially empowering, not requiring the continued surveillance of a medical professional. I made the intuitive leap that this mother could handle a simple prescription for chamomile and peppermint tea. I told her the story of Peter Rabbit and how his mother had given him chamomile and peppermint tea to calm his stomach and make him sleep after his antics in Mr. MacGregor's garden. "If it worked for Peter Rabbit, probably it will work for your child," I said, with some humor. She smiled and agreed with a nod. Then we discussed how to prepare and administer the tea. I asked her to return the next day in case my story wasn't as good a map for this territory as I had hoped.

When mother and baby returned the next day for follow-up, mom stated with pleasure that the tea "had worked." The baby's bowels moved, the vomiting stopped, the child slept for six hours straight, and the irritation and fussiness resolved. Was it the tea or the story in which the tea was embedded? Add to this brew the mother's sense of relief when she was reassured that nothing terrible was wrong with her baby, possibly related to my ability to make rapport and tell convincing stories or to the fact that the virus had already run its course. Did we heal the mother sufficiently for her to heal her child? We don't know; but to the chagrin of evidence-based medicine advocates, we know that the tea cannot be considered apart from the story containing everything that happened.

Stories like this illustrate why I often place "heal" in quotation marks, to call attention to the possibility, as suspected by many aboriginal healers, that healing arises mysteriously through dialogue—in this case, the interaction of mother, baby, resident, nurses, imaging technicians, phlebotomists, receptionists, and me. Awareness of the storied nature of medical practice allows us to bring back the importance of relationship to healing, a story often told by indigenous healers.[10] The power of reassurance and having tea to serve as a vehicle for the expression of maternal love and caring may have been sufficient to initiate a healing dialogue between mother and baby after they left the office.

Would you be surprised to learn, as I did when they returned, that this woman's husband had lost his job when the child was two weeks old, multiplying the stress within the family? Mom's stomach was in knots. This new information prompted me to further congratulate the woman for managing as well as she had in the face of adversity. At every visit, we open new drawers and cabinets and doors within the person's house, always learning something new. We can now imagine a richer story in which the infant experienced the increasingly stressful ambience of the family and had physiological consequences. We could invoke the extensive literature on the gut-brain connection to help us explain this. However, one of the advantages of a "narrative approach" over logical positivism is that we can accept this narrative on its own merits. We can declare its validity without reference to a normative sample. We don't have to extract any principles about the correlation of paternal job loss and infant vomiting. People are richer and more idiosyncratic than one simple correlation. Many different stories could be told about paternal job loss at two weeks of age. Now we are more aligned with aboriginal knowledge and practice, in which we can entertain with interest a connection between life events and the events experienced without having to explain, generalize, or interpret. We don't have to find the "right" story to explain what happened. It is enough simply to add this story to an archive of stories, which we can then explore more holistically—without having to dissect the underlying elements of the stories and make specific correlations.

Consistent with indigenous approaches, a narrative approach allows us to accept the validity of people's stories without reference to correlations or large population studies. The underlying principle is the connectedness of all things, but this manifests in different ways in different families and cultures. A narrative approach does not seek to make a specific correlation of family stress with infantile vomiting. If the next ten cases of infantile vomiting do not resemble this story in the slightest, that does not invalidate the story. It can and does stand alone. People and their situations, families, cultures, and biological responses are all different.

There is no doubt that experimental science and observational epidemiology are useful. Science can tell us amazing stories about the world. My current favorite scientific story comes from Wade Davis's book *The Clouded Leopard*.[11] Davis tells us a story about the behavior of the giant lily from the Amazon, which opens its white blossoms briefly at dusk. The flower buds rise above the surface of the water and rapidly open, releasing an intense fragrance that has been building in strength all afternoon. The metabolic processes that generate the odor raise the temperature of the central cavity of the blossom by about 20°F (11°C) over the outside temperature. The color, smell, and heat attract a swarm of beetles, which converge on the center of the flower. As night falls and temperatures drop, the flower closes, trapping the beetles inside the carpel of the flower with a single night's supply of starch and sugar. The next day, just before dusk, the anthers (male parts) of the flower release pollen and the sticky beetles are allowed to go. In their mad dash to find more food, they are covered with pollen, which they carry to the stigma of another flower, thus accomplishing pollination.

This description is scientific, but not explanatory in the way of most diagnosis–treatment stories, which rely on a cause-and-effect understanding of how things work. The story of the giant lily is more like the stories of spontaneous healings that inspire awe and wonder, making us think, "Wow, that's amazing. How in the world did that happen?" We realize that healing is a great mystery, perhaps even defiant of explanation. This is where myths, legends, and spiritual narrative enter the picture.

The correlations that have been made between abdominal X-ray patterns and anatomical conditions are helpful. From the recording of trial and error experience since the dawn of X-ray photographs, we have good ideas about the signs that indicate an actual anatomical diagnosis of volvulus, intussusception, and malrotation. We have developed similar correlative understandings for ultrasound patterns and anatomical conditions of the abdomen. We know from collecting data that these conditions are often fatal without surgical intervention. Here is where population studies shine. We have developed risk–benefit analyses to convince ourselves (easily) that surgery is better than near certain death. So, the recording of observational data is useful.

What we forget is that our observations and correlations can be put together in myriad ways when it comes to developing a larger story about what's going on. Have we let ourselves become arrogant based upon our successes with the life-threatening structural diseases—intussusception, volvulus, and the like? We generalize that arrogance to myriad other areas where our performance is not so great—cardiovascular diseases, schizophrenia, diabetes, and children's unexplained vomiting. In keeping with that, the improvement in lifespan that has occurred over the last one hundred years has been largely the result of changes in the treatment of childhood diseases.

Our Western medical story is not necessarily privileged over the traditional Chinese story, the ayurvedic story, or the spiritual healing story. Indigenous cultures have also been recording observational data in the form of stories for as long as humans have had language, and are emphasizing that their stories are as valid as the European scientific story. For example, Edward Jenner is credited with discovering that cowpox infections conferred immunity against smallpox infections. In fact, he learned this as a story told by milkmaids. They knew that they couldn't get the smallpox once they'd had the cowpox. Jenner merely publicized what the dairy community already knew. He took the idea further by intentionally inoculating people so that they would come down with cowpox to prevent smallpox, but the idea came from stories already circulating in his environment. He just expanded it to large populations outside the dairy world. He built upon an indigenous, local story.

Similarly, many of the indigenous people of Thailand and surrounding areas survived the tsunami that hit in 2004 because of their stories.

A number of stories informed the people to run for the hills when the water receded and fish were stranded on the newly uncovered beach. Anthropologist Kathryn Coe of the University of Arizona tells a similar story about an event that occurred in Africa at the turn of the century.[12] The native people of an equatorial lake had stories that informed them never to build houses below a certain altitude above the lake. Though no scientific justification was provided, they followed these stories, unlike the Europeans, who thought such ideas were poppycock. When a large carbon monoxide bubble rose out of the lake, as it did every several hundred years, the Europeans were killed, while the indigenous people lived high enough from the surface of the lake to survive. For centuries, stories have contained perspicacious observational wisdom. These stories don't provide what biomedicine would consider a satisfactory scientific explanation, but neither did the milkmaids' cowpox story. It just told how things worked.

Most disturbing is the tendency of physicians to tell a story that dictates a specific ending, as in telling a person when she will die. We get numbers from the median or mode of a population of people with cancer, for example, and then tell everyone that the mean is how long each individual will live. Leon Gordis describes the conventional wisdom well: "A patient asks his physician, 'How long do I have to live, doctor?' and the doctor replies, 'Six months to a year.'"[13] The fallacy of this approach lies in the inability of population studies to predict where an individual person will fall on an actual survival curve, which is generally bell shaped. For example, in one case conference I attended at the University of Saskatchewan, a researcher presented a study from the provincial SaskHealth database showing that the median survival for women with metastatic breast cancer was 3.4 years. In almost a footnote, he mentioned that he discarded 2.5 percent of women from the analysis because they were outliers, living an average of forty-three years after diagnosis.[14] In actuality, only a small proportion lived 3.4 years. That number was just an average.

We use survival curves and statistics to talk about disease as if it were independent of the people who have it and their stories. This so-called natural history approach is grounded in the idea that the patient and her family and culture have no relevance to survival. It usually ignores the stories of the 3 percent at the far end of the survival curve who live much longer than the mean. Those of us who record and save the stories of people like this—those who have supposedly lethal diseases but outlive their doctors and their doctors' predictions—fear that telling patients how long they should expect to live sets up a self-fulfilling prophecy. Indeed, psychologist and immunologist Alastair Cunningham of the University of Toronto showed that the best predictor of how long a patient lives in the presence of metastatic cancer is how long the person thinks they will live.[15] Similarly, in one of my studies the best predictor of response to an AIDS treatment that was later shown to be statistically ineffective was how strongly the patient believed that it would work.[16] I observed similar findings with a treatment for autism that was later shown to be biologically inactive—the best predictor of success was the parents' enthusiasm for the treatment.[17]

Here is where the conventional medical story about the "natural history" of a disease—which, according to this thinking, is supposed to progress in an orderly fashion regardless of the acts of the person who has the disease—diverges from indigenous stories of healing. These stories accept that healing is always possible, though not producible on command. In some contexts, like vodou (voodoo) or boning practices from Africa, telling people they are going to die is as good as killing them.

Some children spontaneously resolve malrotations, volvulus conditions, or intussusceptions without surgery. We can't explain this. Our medical story relegates these events to the realm of spontaneous remissions. Other cultures tell stories that attribute these healings to acts of God, Divine Grace, or the power of prayer. We actually have no knowledge about how spontaneous the healings were, just that they happened without our providing any mechanical treatment (for example, drugs or surgery). Unlike the stories of healing told by indigenous cultures, the medical stories preferred by mainstream culture generally exclude actions by supernatural beings (God, angels, spirits). I prefer to call such healing stories mysteries instead of spontaneous remissions. It seems better to admit our uncertainty than to use empty words that make us sound more knowledgeable than we are, at least to the uninformed.

My accounts of so-called miraculous cures have generated criticism in academic and medical circles. In academic circles, speaking of terms such as *cures, healing, spirits,* or *medicine powers*—can bring down rain upon the head of one who uses them. Anthropologist William Lyon of the University of Missouri at Kansas City has agreed with me that today's academic standards automatically question the scholarship (or sanity) of anyone who believes in spirits or in people's ability to cultivate relationships of power with them. Lyon is one of the few courageous anthropologists who has written about his actual observations of medicine ceremonies, and he has personally experienced some of the effects of academic skepticism and ridicule.* Nevertheless, he has continued to report what he saw and experienced in healing ceremonies, as I too have done.

My vision in approaching this work is similar to what Black Elk is reported to have said of his biographer, John G. Neihardt. Just as Black Elk said that he believed Neihardt had been sent "to save his [Black Elk's] great vision" and that he (Black Elk) had been waiting for him to arrive, healing elders have told me that they expect me to share their wisdom with mainstream culture. Black Elk said, "What I know was given to me for men and it is true and it is beautiful. Soon I shall be under the grass and it will be lost. You were sent to save it, and you must come back so that I can teach you."[18] My goal, like Neihardt's and William Lyon's, is to save and promote the visions and wisdom of aboriginal cultures for health and healing—because we desperately need this perspective and their stories.

It's not too late to acknowledge the merit of indigenous perspectives for the modern world. In the indigenous worldview, for example, each person is the sum of all the stories that have ever been (or ever will be) told about him; the idea that our identity is formed from telling ourselves these stories leads us to realize that each person is unique and

---

*I had the privilege of reading Lyon's amazing book on medicine powers and spirits that his academic publisher actually dropped, presumably for reasons related to Lyon's acceptance of medicine powers and their descriptions by traditional informants as real. Since he didn't interpret these stories as fictional, he couldn't be acceptable to an academic press. I look forward to the day when this important work becomes publicly accessible. For now, throughout the book, references to his work will be from my personal correspondence with him and from his unpublished manuscript.

must be approached individually to discover how he will heal. No two people with the same diagnosis are narratively alike. All the stories are different. Treatments can't work if the stories we live have no place for healing.

We physicians would serve our patients better if we could learn how to listen to people tell their own valid renditions of their realities and the worlds in which they dwell. If we wish for people to "comply" with our medical prescriptive stories, what we say must resonate with the stories of the health decision-makers within families (often wise grandmothers in aboriginal or Hispanic culture), and with family and cultural stories about how to live and what is meaningful or valid. (For example, taking medications that reduce sexual potency may not be compatible with a culture's stories about what it means to be a man.) If we can respect other stories or worldviews that differ from our own and entertain the possibility that these stories and views might work as well as (or even better than) our own, we will be more capable of and open to cross-cultural collaboration. We might begin to "speak so that we can listen" instead of lecturing the world from our position of superiority. We might be better able to form collaborative partnerships to reach desired goals.

Our world needs more multicultural, collaborative partnerships with its diverse cultures. We doctors need to practice in a style that is respectful of the world's many different stories about health, sickness, meaning, purpose, and life. A narrative approach to medicine can help us, as can an understanding of collaborative language and learning systems. In listening to others' perspectives with equal respect as to our own, we develop shared language and eventually shared stories about the meaning and purpose that we forge in common. When we work from shared stories that respect all involved families and cultures, we eliminate patient noncompliance since we all work from the same shared map showing how to get from a state of sickness to greater health.

We also need cross-cultural research programs, which by nature will require us to collect stories. They will require collaborative partnerships with the knowledge holders of other traditions, and the development of collaborative language systems that will help us understand each other. They will require our listening very carefully to each other and learning how to translate our stories into each other's frameworks (the nascent field of knowledge translation). We might end up comparing the outcomes from the imposition of our biomedical paradigm (story) with traditional healing used within its own community of origin. We might learn that people's historical, local practices are more effective, within those communities, than externally imposed biomedical approaches. We might even learn that our expensive biomedical approaches to health and disease work, but can be equivalent to using a Gauguin painting to kindle a campfire.

I conclude with the story of a Latina woman I interviewed during a workshop in Los Angeles. In that sun-drenched environment, Alma presented a story to me that was logical, comprehensible, and beyond my medical understanding. She had healed from a relatively incurable illness. Alma clearly shows us how medical expectations can influence outcome and presents an example of resistance to being "programmed" to die on command. She shares with us the amazing healing power of love. She shows us a very unique path to healing that can inspire us, but is not a formula for getting well. It was just her path.

Alma had previously been diagnosed with Wegener's granulomatosis. Her symptoms had been severe. By the time of my interview, she was essentially well. When I asked her to what she attributed her healing, she said, "Love."

"How so?" I asked.

"I began by doing everything the doctors told me to do," she said, "but then I realized that they were looking at me as if I were dead. They were already at my funeral. I didn't like that. I didn't like feeling like a corpse when I walked into the office. That's when I decided to go to the spiritual healer."

Alma then described her meetings with the healer who extracted a curse from her, massaged her, rubbed herbs over her body, prayed to the saints and the spirits, and conducted various ceremonies for her. At the same time, she went to the *curanderos,* traditional Latin American folk healers, for herbs. Over time, she said, she learned to love herself with a fraction of the love that the angels had for her. She credited that as starting her improvement.

Next Alma met a man who loved her almost unconditionally. That feeling of being loved brought up memories and pain from previous bad relationships. To his credit, she said, this man stayed with her while she worked that out. She almost left him many times, but he insisted she stay with him while she went through her crises. "He told me I could only leave him when I was feeling good. That really helped and we're still together."

"What do you think of the doctors now?" I asked. We were sitting on a deck in Santa Monica, overlooking the Pacific Ocean, its blue deeper than the sky. A gentle wind passed over us, carrying the smell of the sea. Occasional clouds cast shadows upon the water.

"They're nice young people, but they're misguided." The wind picked up, swaying the tree branches. Cars and trucks clogged the Pacific Coast Highway below us. "They don't know God or Spirit or Love or plant medicine. They don't know how our people have healed for centuries. I guess you can't expect much of them, though if you want to die, they'll hold your hand and encourage you to do so." Surfers came and went on the shore.

"What advice do you have for others who are ill?"

"That's easy," she laughed. "Find people who can have the faith and hope for you that you don't have. It's contagious. Eventually you will feel it, too. And when you find love, for yourself and from anyone else, sink your teeth into it and hold on for dear life. Don't give up."

This story is valid in its own right. It doesn't have to lead to a study, to any particular prescriptive practice, or to any interpretation, except to say, "Wow, that's really something. I'm really happy to hear that."

That's what we will explore in the remainder of this book—a medicine based upon stories as a means to understanding and healing. I hope to further our sense of story as an intersection with the world's indigenous cultures, a bridge to connect us with people from around the world. We will explore the stories that emerge in dialogue with others, with nature, with God and the spirits, and with illnesses. These stories give us clues about healing—how it works, how to do it. They show us our connectedness to one another and teach us about the indigenous principle that we are never separate from our surroundings or from our culture.

1
The Roots of Narrative Medicine

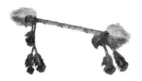

The Universe is vast. Nothing is more curious than the self-satisfied dogmatism with which mankind at each period of its history cherishes the delusion of the finality of its existing modes of knowledge. Skeptics and believers are all alike. At this moment, scientists and skeptics are the leading dogmatists. Advance in detail is admitted: fundamental novelty is barred. This dogmatic common sense is the death of philosophical adventure. The Universe is vast.

ALFRED NORTH WHITEHEAD[1]

The concept of narrative medicine offers a paradigm or perspective from which we can contemplate contemporary medicine and psychology. The narrative perspective offers a position outside of medicine from which medicine can be viewed and discussed. Though contemporary medicine engages in self-criticism, it rarely steps outside of itself to address the assumptions (stories) that define it. A narrative perspective allows us to identify these stories and to engage people outside of the field of medicine in discussing their desirability.

A storied approach to health and healing argues that our stories (or our series of interpretations about the world) are only as good as they are practical, and that it is impossible to determine their absolute "truth." Rather than argue truth, we settle for learning which stories are best for particular situations, people, times, and places. Contemporary biomedicine becomes just one of many stories about health and disease. A common indigenous story, for example, is that disease is a side effect of disharmony and imbalance. Imagine a healer from that tradition trying to talk to a medical practitioner who sees disease only in anatomical terms. The healer's discussion of sources of disharmony in a person's family and spiritual life seems irrelevant to the physician trying to categorize the type of tissue damage in an organ. Progress is being made, however, in recognizing that these stories also have validity.

A storied approach to health and healing situates itself well within the developing field of indigenous knowledge. Aboriginal groups throughout the world recognize that wisdom is contained in stories. Traditional elders answer questions by telling stories. It is up to the listener to determine what they mean.

Indigenous knowledge systems usually recognize that we humans are integrated upon the Earth, and that we already share land, food, and air. Social justice emerges when we consider the importance of maintaining diversity and autonomy for the world's people. Awareness of difference can be a reason for celebration and learning, or it can provoke a response in which the "other" is eliminated. A contemporary example is provided by the hatred and stereotyping of Turks and Kurds along the Turkish-Iraqi border. From our perspective in North America, those differences that seem so enormous to them seem trivial to us.

The history of colonization has been about elimination through death and assimilation, apropos to the ongoing Turkish debate about whether to use their military against the Kurds. Indigenous people throughout the world are challenging the point of view that leads to conquest and colonization as they assert the primacy of their own precontact stories. A narrative approach to medicine allows their stories (traditional Chinese medicine, ayurvedic medicine, North American Native healing, Mayan healing, African healing, and more) to coexist with the stories produced by the dominant, mostly white culture that relies largely on pharmaceuticals. We discover that the conversation is more interesting when everyone is given a seat around the table.

Despite its claims of superiority, conventional medicine itself is the third leading cause of accidental death in the United States.[2] Similar to the stance taken by Galen in the first century BCE, medicine says that "what it cures, it cures, and what it cannot cure, cannot be cured." The examples of pharmaceutical companies withholding information on the dangers of drugs like Vioxx (which increases the risk of heart attacks and strokes[3]) shows that medicine's story (so closely linked to that of the pharmaceutical companies) is not always altruistic. Even as I completed this book, new scandals were emerging about the drug Paxil.[4]

The multibillion-dollar U.S. complementary and alternative medicine industry competes with conventional medicine to fill its gaps, but does it succeed? The many available alternative therapies are confusing to sort out. New fields and experts rise and fall yearly. Today's popular cure for autism, for example, is forgotten next year.[5] How is a person to decide what to do? Even holistic medicine* case conferences often present the same bland collection of recommendations for everyone—eat more fruits and vegetables, take some vitamins (but not too many), get reiki, have hypnosis, try acupuncture, take some herbs. Is this enough? In any city in America, we can emerge from a holistic doctor's office with a shopping bag full of supplements and other products, but does this make us healthier? Does it work?

My criticism of alternative and holistic medicine resembles my thoughts about conventional medicine—that it constructs experts who are supposed to know more about the person and her condition than she does, that it purports to fix people from a position outside of them, that it fails to respect and elicit people's local knowledge about how to heal themselves. In short, holistic medicine can also take away people's sense of power and agency, just as conventional medicine does, but with theoretically more natural substances. This is not a real change, just an improvement by substitution that also does not work all the time.

A plethora of mysterious illnesses, including fibromyalgia, chronic

---

*I am using the term *holistic medicine* to refer to treatment that takes into account the whole person, body-mind-spirit, and which preferentially relies on less toxic treatments prior to more toxic treatments; as in herbs first, surgery second.

fatigue syndrome, and Lyme disease, defies medicine's ability to diagnose and treat. Illnesses related to lifestyle—diabetes, heart disease, chronic obstructive lung disease—are becoming the major causes of death. Conventional medicine has a dismal record at helping people change lifestyle. Less than 10 percent of people, for example, make lifestyle changes after a heart attack,[6] despite Dean Ornish's having shown that these changes can prevent the next heart attack and actually reverse atherosclerosis, the inflammatory process within arteries that leads to heart attacks.[7] Drugs or procedures do not change lifestyle. I frequently point out to doctors in training that psychiatric drugs do not cure poverty, homelessness, isolation, or loneliness. They merely take the edge off the pain caused by these conditions. So what do we do with these limitations of conventional and holistic medicine?

To begin exploring this question, I want to tell a story told to me by Norman, a Haida physician from British Columbia. This story has a "phoenix rising" quality. It inspired me to think that we can rise above our circumstances regardless of our origins, and, through diligence, persistence, and courage, overcome all odds to reach our goal. It struck me that narrative medicine is emerging this way too. We are struggling against the binds and fetters of conventional medicine to bring a different perspective to health care, one that is more sustainable and nurturing than the conventional model. To do this, we must overcome obstacles the way Namasingit does in this story, as he rescues his wife from Killer Whale. Like all stories, this one may mean something different to each reader, but this is what it meant to me. Its spirit will work on each person who encounters it, and it will do with that person what it wishes. That is the nature of traditional stories.

Our story begins with a child who lived alone with his grandmother and a great blue heron in a shack of brush at the edge of a village.[8] The rest of his family, including his mother, had gone to the spirit world. His father remained unknown. The great blue heron suffered from a cracked beak and, in gratitude for the family taking him in, he taught the child all he knew, which was enough to lead the youth to become a great hunter, able to find game when no one else could. He could catch large salmon when others' hooks remained empty. By the time he reached adulthood, he had built a big house for himself and his grandmother, as large as any in the village.

We can let this young man represent marginalized people, like those of us on the outskirts of medicine, who are bridging cultures. He is an indigenous version of a Horatio Alger character, though he makes good through his relationship with and respect for an animal as well as his hard work. In this indigenous culture it is not just hard work that allows one to succeed; spiritual power is also required. When I tell this story in my practice, I ask my audience to recognize those who have inspired and uplifted them—whether animal, grandparent, great-uncle, or aunt. Suffering people often have sources of inspiration in their lives who they may forget. I recently told this story to a Dene woman who was able to overcome her depression by reconnecting to the spirit of her grandmother. She did this by performing a daily ceremony that her grandmother had done with her as a child to protect her from abusive parents. The ceremony reinvoked that feeling of protection and comfort, which was enough to pull her out of her depression (a story in which nobody loved her).

When his house was finished, the young man wanted a wife. Unfortunately for them, none of the girls in the village caught his eye, perhaps because they had treated him badly when he was still very poor, teasing, mocking, and spurning him. He decided to take the great blue heron's advice and seek a wife from the sea. He laid up a supply of smoked fish, oil, and wood for his grandmother's winter survival and then disappeared in his canoe over the smooth, glasslike surface of the summer sea, in search of a wife.

I take this to mean that we don't have to "get hitched" to conventional medicine, but can make our own way, carving out our own territory. We're not stuck with the resources and characters with whom we grew up. We can go outside of our limited and narrow confines to seek our healing from other people, cultures, and experiences.

One year later, an impressive canoe arrived at the village. Its design was unlike any the people had ever seen. It was decorated with haunting and provocative images. The young man sat in the bow. Exotic foods, carved chests, copper, jewelry, blankets, and hides spilled over the sides. A small cloud seemed to float amidst this bounty. The people gathered, curious. They asked the young man where he had been. He didn't answer, and proceeded to the house to get his grandmother. "Come meet my wife," he said to her. She came down to the canoe, but all she could see was a little cloud. "This is my wife," he said, pointing toward the cloud. His grandmother stood next to the cloud and invited her to come into the house in the manner appropriate for a grandmother to address a grandson's new wife. The young man returned to the shore to push the canoe farther up onto the beach.

Mainstream culture has yet to dream of the potential resources available for healing. The young man in our story found them beneath the sea. Magic was presumably required to allow him to breathe and live underwater for an extended period of time. In this case, the great blue heron held the key to this transformation and shared it with the young man in gratitude for his family's kindness.

The curious villagers followed the young man to his house and milled around outside. Inside, the young man asked the cloud to take off her hat. A small voice from inside the cloud said, "You do it." He touched the top of the cloud, picked it up, and set it behind him. Then everyone could see his wife. The people were breathless at the sight of her beauty. After she had settled into the house, the young man prepared to go fishing.

Once we show our riches—cultivated by authentically practicing the wisdom and traditions of our communities—people around us will get curious. We must hold faith in the past and practice our magic until the forthcoming results cannot be disputed.

Just as he was going down to his canoe, his grandmother asked if it could be snowing in the kelp bed. He looked and saw a snow-white form bobbing up and down in the waves. Recognizing a white sea otter, he chased it in his canoe for the entire day. After a grueling day at sea, he finally speared it under its tail so that the pelt would be perfect. He brought it home for his grandmother to skin but, despite her care, one drop of blood spilled onto the pure, white fur. His wife offered to clean that spot off in the sea. She walked out to the rocky point where clear tide pools lie free of sand. When she slipped on a wet stone, the pelt fell into the sea. She dove into the ocean to get it, but Killer Whale rose beneath her and lifted her clear of the waves. She clung to his dorsal fin for safety as he carried her away. The young man saw this happening from a distance and ran to the shore. He jumped into his canoe and paddled to the spot where the whale had dived, but could find nothing.

We will have challenges and opposition. I often use this part of the story as a template for an illness that has grabbed the person. An illness is similar to a kidnapping whale in the way that it can suddenly take away your happiness. Action is required. The young man did not lie down and pine, giving up on ever finding his wife. He was self-empowered to take action, which is how healing begins.

The young man returned to the village for a four-day fast. Afterward he drank devil's club juice and ate corn lily leaves until the wind blew through him. On the fifth day, he bathed in aged urine and gathered the supplies he needed. On his fast, he had received a vision for how to proceed. He had been told what supplies to take, which included a mussel shell knife, twisted cedar limbs, goat hair, a whetstone, a comb, some goosegrass, and some dried bearberry leaves.

Our visions and the spirits will show us how to overcome the challenges we face. The contemplative and purifying part of the preparation cannot be skipped. We are all too tempted to do this in Western culture. We want to jump into action headfirst without letting the spirits tell us what to do. Patience is required in the early phases of the healing journey.

The young hunter returned to the spot where Killer Whale had dived. He tied his canoe to the kelp, and then dived deep into the sea. He found a trail on the sea floor. The first animals he encountered on this trail were four blind geese. They smelled him and named him Namasingit, which referred to his capacity to make things which were broken whole again, and which conveyed to him an important healing ability. With his mussel shell knife, he opened the eyes of three of the geese. He fed them goosegrass. When the eyes of the geese were open, they gratefully told him which way his wife had gone, and he proceeded down the trail in that direction.

Helpers along the way—family, spirits, friends—will give us needed guidance and show us where to go. They require something from us, however. Rarely in stories is help freely given. We must earn it through our own merits and preparedness. The young man was able to do this because of his help from the spirits prior to his journey. He came prepared.

Armed with his new name, Namasingit was surprised upon his path by a great blue heron who was repairing a cracked canoe. This was not a common sight anywhere, least of all under the sea. He felt a great affinity toward the bird based upon memories of his childhood teacher, so he tossed some of the bearberry leaves he had into Heron's mouth, remembering how much the other heron had enjoyed them. While Heron chewed them, Namasingit gave him some cedar planks for his canoe. Then, they heard footsteps. "It's the killer whale's sentry," exclaimed Heron. "Quick. Hide under my wing."

We must show these helpers our appreciation and respect and offer them gifts. When we do, they will protect us like Heron protected Namasingit.

Namasingit squirmed under the wing just in time to avoid detection by the watchman, who lumbered along on wooden legs.

"I heard something," said the watchman. "And I smell a human! Where did you get that cedar? What have you seen here?"

"Nothing," retorted Heron. "You are wrong. Your nose is playing tricks on you. You are smelling things that aren't there. I got this cedar

from around here. Maybe once it was dropped into the water by people, but that must have been some time ago."

"Fine," the watchman grumbled and prepared to lumber off. Then he saw the bearberry leaves and grabbed a handful to eat. That seemed to satisfy him and he left. Namasingit then offered more bearberry leaves to Heron. In exchange for his help, Heron told Namasingit that his wife had been taken to the home of Killer Whale, who wanted to marry her, but only after she was given a fin.

"Go further up the trail," Heron said. "Help the slave who is making the preparations for attaching the fin, and maybe he will be of assistance to you." Namasingit thanked Heron and headed up the trail.

Not too far along the trail, he came upon a slave who was using a red snapper tail to split kindling. When that red snapper tail broke, the slave cried out in alarm. "Master will beat me," he sobbed. Namasingit had power now that he had a name. He offered to help the slave.

When we help others, we are sometimes rewarded with help in return. In most journeys, we must perform tasks to demonstrate our resolve.

"Here," Namasingit said, offering to take the snapper tail. "I will fix this for you." He sucked on the end of the broken wedge and it became whole again. Then he gave the slave some bearberry leaves to eat. The slave was very grateful.

"Your wife is in Killer Whale's house," the slave said. "She's tied up there. I am building a fire to steam a fin for her. You have been kind to me, so I will help you. When the fire is built, I will take water into the house to heat over the fire. I am known to be clumsy. I will trip and spill the water into the fire. When the room fills with steam, you take her. She sits on the other side of the room from where you will enter. I can puff up like a blowfish and am known to do so when I'm upset. They'll not suspect anything because they'll know I'll be upset and fearing a beating, so they'll expect me to puff up. This will make it harder for them to run after you."

Through kindness and healing, we can find allies in the camp of our enemies as Namasingit did. Accomplishing each task on our healing journey gets us that much closer to our goal.

The slave was true to his word. Namasingit crept close behind him. Just as the slave was about to put the water down, he spilled it into the fire. In the thick steam that rose, Namasingit ran straight to where his wife was tied, cut her bonds loose with his knife, and led her by the hand out the door amid the chaos of steam and shouts. The slave swelled up like a bulging bullfrog so no one could get past him for quite some time, giving our hero time to escape.

Namasingit ran with his wife past Heron, past the geese, and back to where he had dived into the sea. Killer Whale and his troops were closing in. They were getting closer and closer. When the whale was almost on top of them, Namasingit threw down the goat hair he had brought with him, and a great kelp forest sprang up. He and his wife climbed up the kelp to the canoe. By then Killer Whale had broken through the kelp forest and was again closing on them. Namasingit threw down the whetstone and an island formed between them and Killer Whale. This bought them a little more time, but again Killer Whale swam around the island and began closing the gulf between them. Namasingit threw down the comb and a reef formed. This allowed them to reach the beach. His grandmother was there waiting for them, smiling to herself and tanning the snow-white pelt.

The goal is reached. I think of narrative medicine as stealing back from killer whales the art of healing, the essence of doctoring, the powerful medicine of caring, the stories that make us well. Without this, the technology is empty and often destructive. We need the healing arts to make use of healing technology, which is what indigenous cultures can teach us.

Within what I am calling narrative medicine, I am seeking new ways to conceptualize and integrate the wisdom of indigenous cultures, the insights of holistic medical practitioners, contemporary social sciences, and our developing understanding of the importance of story in behavior and even biological science. Within this new synthesis, medical doctors invite other voices to join in creating the explanatory story of the illness. We see that most of our explanations are culturally driven and that we cannot separate biology from culture.

We have two very different potential scenarios—the viewpoint of modern medicine and what we would achieve if we succeed in integrating conventional and indigenous worldviews. The table summarizes the differences between the two, which we will review in detail. I want to show that these principles of narrative medicine are very similar to the common principles of indigenous knowledge systems and provide a bridge between cultures that has never before been so accessible.

Narrative Medicine	Conventional Medicine
Multiple causality	Unilateral causality
Systemic explanations	Mechanistic explanations
Entanglement; interdependence; circularity; relationship to quantum physics	Independent variables; linearity; cause and effect; randomized controlled trials; classical mechanics
Community focus (disease is seen as originating through relationships within a community)	Individual focus (disease is seen as originating within the individual)
Solutions do not necessarily relate to causes	Solutions arise from understanding cause, and grow logically out of one cause
Healing focuses upon restoring harmony and balance	Healing focuses upon finding a specific biological or genetic cause and fixing that
Disease arises from dysfunction; it occurs through susceptibility, which relates to imbalance and disharmony in relationship	Disease is defined by structural suffering and anomalies; caused by biological factors or genetics (cause and defect paradigm)
Relational self	Individual self
Cooperate; win–win	Compete; win–lose
Disease is found within relationships	Disease is found within individuals and specifically within organs

Illnesses Have Multiple Causes

Indigenous people have recognized from time immemorial that simple ideas of cause and effect are rarely useful. One elder told me, "If you think you know what's going on, you're wrong. If you know what's going on, it's trivial. It's always much more complicated than you could ever understand. The spirits don't even let us know why things happen, so whatever explanation you can think of isn't right."

On the forefront of modern epidemiology—the study of how diseases originate and spread—is the idea that all conditions have multiple causes. These multiple causes have been primarily seen as part of a linear approach, but the new science of complexity is transforming the concept of "cause" into sets of networks of nonlinear distributed interactions where new and old things combine and new orders of self-organized complexity emerge.[9] What this means is that simple explanations become less and less possible. Conventional medicine remains largely locked in the idea that we should be able to identify one cause of every disease. Within this multiple, interlocking causality approach, new paths emerge through internal local interactions of interlacing networks. This is the opposite of reductionism.

Maria's story illustrates the impossibility of isolating single causes. I inherited Maria from a psychiatrist who believed wholeheartedly (and single-mindedly) in the biological model of mental illness. Maria was on more medication than I could fathom. Whenever Maria or a family member complained about an old symptom or the appearance of a new symptom, this doctor either added a medication or increased the dosage. When I saw Maria, she was shaking from her high doses of medication.

I slowly began decreasing Maria's medication levels. As we decreased the dosages, Maria stopped shaking and began to make more sense. We finally reached a low dose beyond which she thought her problems were worse. Regardless of the dosage of medication, she still believed people were out to get her. Her prior psychiatrist had tried unsuccessfully to make this go away with medication, which it wouldn't. Instead I listened to Maria's story about what was going on. Part of this story involved her awareness that she had smoked way too much marijuana. That fit, since too much marijuana tends to make people paranoid. But beyond that, her story was that women who didn't like her (they had fought over boyfriends) had recorded her voice on an iPod device and used a special machine to broadcast those voices to the inside of her brain. She recognized that the voices were making negative comments that she had previously heard others make about her. She reasoned that someone had to have recorded these comments and were now broadcasting them to her. When asked what would help, Maria was sure that a psychic could stop the broadcast. She believed that it was pointless to find the machine and break it, because they could just buy another.

I found a traditional healer who people said was psychic, and Maria accepted her. They made a good relationship; the healer performed a treatment that resembled reiki and then did a ceremony to stop the broadcast. The voices in Maria's head stopped for a week. After that, they started coming back but at much reduced volume. Another session and ceremony eliminated them again. This was much more effective than her previous high-dose medication had been, and illustrates the idea of treating the story.

Thinking in a one-dimensional way about Maria proved counterproductive. Maria was raised in poverty in a family that revolved around alcohol and drug use and domestic violence. She had been involved in heavy drug use herself. Her current boyfriend beat her regularly. Her life was miserable. To blame all of her troubles on biology is shortsighted, but this is our current, dominant paradigm, the one that narrative approaches are opposing.

We Need Systemic Explanations and Solutions for Problems

Explanations and understanding should be sought in the relationships among interconnected entities, rather than through a mechanistic model in which events can easily be traced through a chain of effects, like the infamous mousetrap game.

This became apparent to me when I visited Teresa in a remote northern community. Teresa was what I had been trained to call "floridly manic." The conventional explanation is linear, linking the cause to defective genes, and, according to this model, the proper treatment is

pharmacological. Since Teresa's mania had reached psychotic proportions, I offered her some medication. I wanted to prevent her from being
hospitalized, which I thought would be even more traumatic for her
than any side effects of medication. Teresa refused. "My family will take
care of me," she said. I was skeptical, but she was adamant, so I offered
the support I could.

I visited Teresa every month for nine months and watched her family take care of her as she said they would. Counter to what my training led me to believe, their love and her continued embeddedness in a
social network kept her grounded, and her psychosis and mania slowly
disappeared. A traditional healer "doctored" her several times with the
full support of her community, and the priest exorcised evil and prayed
over her regularly. At the end of nine months, Teresa had fully recovered
without medication, hospitalization, embarrassment, or residual shame
within the community. How did this happen? I can't say. It was a systemic solution. The entire system within which she lived responded, and
something new emerged that is impossible to predict from the perspective
of a linear, cause-and-effect model.

Traditional Healing Is Defined by Entanglement, Interdependence, and Circularity

More than any other concept I can think of, the idea of interdependence most clearly defines the difference between indigenous healing
approaches and Anglo-European culture. It is precisely this aspect of
healing that story or history is uniquely able to capture and convey.

When we feel connected to nature through ceremony and in daily
life, we cannot easily destroy nature. We cannot easily strip mine, leave
uranium tailings as radioactive mining waste, or ignore global warming. We personally feel the plight of the plants and animals. We feel the
effects of rainforest decimation.

Before moving to Saskatchewan, I worked at the University of
Arizona in a primarily involuntary psychiatric hospital. The patients we
admitted included the most impoverished, severely mentally ill people in
the community. They included people who chronically misused drugs,
often several at a time. They included the retarded and the developmen-

tally disabled. In southern Arizona society, these people had been taken out of families and relegated to agencies that "cared" for them. Typical outpatient care consisted largely of medication and case management. The seriously mentally ill were lucky to see a psychiatrist quarterly to have their medication adjusted. All too infrequently, they had no housing. Each case manager had up to one hundred and twenty souls to look after. That made it impossible to see some people very often. These people remained isolated, alone, unsupported, and living in relative poverty. Is this better, I wondered, than the situation in developing nations, is which seriously mentally ill people are kept in the community and tolerated?

Carl Bell, professor of psychiatry at the University of Illinois College of Medicine said, "This thing called psychiatry—it is a European American invention, and it largely has no respect for nonwhite philosophies of mental health and how people function."*

A silver-haired colleague raised the possibility that psychotic people simply die in the third world. In fact, their mortality rates are lower than in the developed world.[16] I wondered if they could ever become as severely ill as some of our patients did. Isn't community required for the regulation of emotions, I wondered? Don't we need other people to soothe and comfort us and help us to maintain our moods on an even

---

*As an example of conventional psychiatry's lack of focus on non-whites, a recent UCLA meta-analysis of the best available studies on psychiatric drugs for depression, anxiety, schizophrenia, and bipolar disorder considered 9,327 patients, of whom none were Native American.[10] Of 3,980 patients in antidepressant trials, only two were Hispanic. Of 2,865 schizophrenia patients, only three were Asian. Among 825 patients with bipolar disorder, none were Hispanic or Asian. Culture has long been known to have a profound effect on the development of what we call mental illness and upon how it is expressed.[11] Americans of Mexican descent have twice the risk of disorders such as depression and anxiety and four times the risk of drug abuse, compared with recent immigrants from Mexico. Assimilation is associated with higher rates of psychiatric diagnoses.[12] Black and Hispanic patients are more than three times as likely to be diagnosed with schizophrenia than white patients, even though the rates of the disorder is the same in all groups in careful diagnostic studies.[13] White women in the United States are three times as likely to commit suicide as black and Hispanic women, possibly related to the strength of social networks among black and Hispanic women.[14] Maria Oquendo, a psychiatrist at Columbia University, points out that anorexia is astonishingly rare in nonindustrialized countries, reflecting the cultural underpinnings of what psychiatry assumes to be biological.[15]

keel? In a traditional culture in which consciousness-altering substances are sacred, could anyone ever misuse drugs as severely as in mainstream North American culture? We had already been debating the many diagnoses of bipolar disorder, the new national epidemic, which seemed to us to stand for emotional instability primarily related to the misuse of drugs (cocaine, crystal methamphetamine, marijuana, alcohol, opiates, and more). Each person with a drug problem was treated as an isolated individual. No community came together to care for them.

I came to appreciate that we psychiatrists were in charge of the flotsam and jetsam of rampant capitalism. The side effects of the severe competition characteristic of American life were the "losers." These were the families who fell apart, the isolated, the homeless, the "have-nots." While the great American myth told us that even the poorest of the poor could grow up to be president, this was mostly fiction. People born into fragmentation and isolation tend to grow up to live in fragmentation and isolation. They learn this story about life and enact it. Children surrounded by drug and alcohol addiction learn to be drug- and alcohol-addicted. This is the dominant experiential story and stands in sharp, painful contrast to the television stories played out on prime time each evening. These are the dramas of the "haves," or the police dramas where attractive cops take ugly, scuzzy, bad people off the streets to lock them up and throw away the key.

In the United States, the impossibility of rising out of poverty and isolation to match the television role models allows another way to be a hero—that of the gang member or criminal. To be a good criminal, drug addict, schizophrenic, or gang member is often more accessible than achieving the American dream. Just as in theater, people adhere to roles or positions in which they become overwhelmingly engrossed.[17] They become completely absorbed in the performance of the part, much like a violin virtuoso. These roles are not played out at a distance by detached actors. Rather, people become lost in them.

People play roles that are inherently and overwhelmingly social. These roles feed back to generate personal identity; the roles do not arise from intrinsic, internal identities. No one is isolated. We must all enact one or many roles and may be evaluated for how appropriately and convincingly we carry out these roles. Skilled role-taking requires many different abilities, and multiple role enactments form a kind of repertoire. People function more adequately in daily life if they have more roles (options) available to enact.

People can become completely immersed in their particular roles, which is what makes the enactment believable. People who have little involvement in the roles they enact are considered shallow, superficial, or unbelievable. High levels of absorption result in identity being equated with the role, the expenditure of great effort in playing the role, and the involvement of the entire body in the role. Roles range from the scripted "casual encounters" of flight attendants on airplanes to the dramatic, even fatal reactions of individuals put under curse by sorcerers in traditional cultures. High levels of involvement echo the concepts of Mihaly Csikszentmihalyi (pronounced *chick-sent-me-high-ee*) set forth in his flow theory, in which people experience a deep engagement in activities in which absorption is maximized (e.g., playing improvisational jazz music).[18]

Highly absorbing roles (mother, father, schizophrenic, chronically ill) may be demanding enough to preempt other roles. Other roles, such as doctor or police officer, may contain specific but wide time boundaries, which may be extended by emergencies. For example, physicians on holiday may be called upon to render aid in medical crises on airplanes, and off-duty police officers may respond to crimes committed in their presence (as when an off-duty police officer happens to be standing in a bank line when the bank is robbed).

All roles come with expectations, which are "the rights and privileges, duties and obligations, of any occupant of a social position in relation to persons occupying other positions in the social structure."[19] California psychologist Theodore Sarbin wrote about how these expectations form a bridge between society and the actual behavior of individuals. He wrote that social expectations comprise a large set of beliefs, knowledge, and judgments that inform people how to play their various roles.

Sarbin distinguished between general, specific, formal, and informal expectations. For example, we physicians are generally expected to do more good than harm and specifically expected to perform the procedures relegated to our specialty. General surgeons are expected to know how to remove diseased gallbladders. Emergency physicians are expected to know how to repair lacerations. The medical role is formal, requiring licensure, an office, and even hospital privileges. Informal roles include being the black sheep of a family or the "responsible daughter." These roles do not require licensure or a special environment in which to perform. Roles are more or less clear and the social consensus about how a role should be enacted may vary among different subcultures. For example, the role of mother is played somewhat differently in Jewish culture in Williamsburg, Brooklyn than in Native American culture in Wounded Knee, South Dakota. People can even disagree about what constitutes an adequate performance of a role. One student may love a particular teacher, while another files a complaint with the university about the same teacher.

My conclusion from my foray into American institutional psychiatry was that treatment rarely worked. Instead of seeing the "mentally ill" as bad children who wouldn't take their medication, I saw them as optimizing adults who didn't find the benefits worth the side effects. Hallucinations and grandiosity were preferable to the stark reality of living homeless in poverty and isolation. So were cocaine and crystal methamphetamine. These observations are borne out by studies of the healing power of social networks for people with schizophrenia in developing countries. In this story, *Washington Post* staff writer Shankar Vedantam tells the story of Krishna Devi, a woman that psychiatrist Naren Wig had seen years previously for schizophrenia.[20]

> [She] sat in a courtyard surrounded by religious pictures, exposed brick walls and drying laundry. Devi had stopped taking medication long ago, but her articulate speech and easy smile were eloquent testimony that she had recovered from the debilitating disease.

> Few schizophrenics in the United States are so lucky, even after years of treatment. But Devi had hidden assets: a doting family and an embracing village that never excluded her from social events, family obligations, or work.

> Devi is a living reminder of a three-decade-long study by the World

Health Organization (WHO)—one that many Western doctors initially refused to believe: People with schizophrenia typically do far better in poorer nations such as India, Nigeria, and Colombia than in Denmark, England, and the United States.

Conventional physicians were so shocked by this study from the 1970s that they repeated it and produced the same results, resulting in the conclusion that stronger family ties in poorer countries have a profound impact on recovery from schizophrenia.

Most people with schizophrenia in India live with their families or within other social networks. This is in sharp contrast to the situation in the United States, where most patients are homeless or live alone, in group homes, psychiatric facilities, or increasingly, jail. Indian patients are given low-stress jobs in a culture that values social connectedness over productivity, while patients in the United States are excluded from working and penalized with loss of benefits if they try to work. Indian families sit in on doctor-patient visits, because families are considered central to the problem and the solution, unlike the United States, where private, individual appointments are the norm.

The director of this study, Norman Sartorius of the WHO, recommended that developed countries should help provide financial support to families to help them take care of their relatives, which would save money on hospitalizations and incarcerations. Caregivers could be given time off from work. Doctors could enlist recreational and religious groups to replace the social networks that patients lose. Sartorius said, "Social factors play a major and important role in the outcome of disease. Very few solutions are medical in medicine."[21]

José Bertolote, a psychiatrist with WHO, said, "Pharmaceutical companies, which control the scientific production of research at universities, are not interested in saying, 'Social factors are more important than my drug.'"[22] He noted that Indian psychiatrists dispense more than drugs, including spiritual advice, family counseling, and even matchmaking services. For example, when psychiatrist Shantha Kamath in the southern Indian city of Chennai was asked for help in arranging a marriage for a family's schizophrenic daughter, Kamath's written instructions told the parents how to interact with their daughter and listed the skills the young woman needed to learn before the doctor would arrange a match.

This WHO study tracked 3,300 patients over thirty years in twelve countries. Patients in poorer countries spent fewer days in hospitals, were more likely to be employed, and were more socially connected. Between one-half and two-thirds became symptom free, compared to one-third of patients in richer countries. Nigerian, Colombian, and Indian patients were less likely to suffer relapses and had longer periods of health between relapses. Doctors in poorer countries stopped medications when patients became better, unlike doctors in richer countries who demanded that patients take medications for their entire lives. A separate study in rural China revealed that low doses of medications could be as effective as high doses and virtually eliminated side effects.[23] Also in this study, older, cheaper medications were as effective as newer, more expensive antipsychotic drugs.

In country after country, the WHO study found that strong social and family ties trumped high-tech medical facilities. In the northern Indian city of Chandigarh, for example, there are no nurses, so family members stay with patients when they are hospitalized and take care of them. Psychiatrist Naren Wig found that family members were more effective than strangers in calming agitated patients.

Washington Post journalist Shankar Vendantam tells the story of Lakshmi Ramachandran of Detroit, who took her son Raj back to Chennai, India, when he was diagnosed with schizophrenia. While he had to be forced to socialize in Detroit, the neighbors in Chennai would come seek him out. The Schizophrenia Research Foundation (SCARF) in Chennai has independently confirmed the WHO findings.[24] SCARF treats 1,200 patients per year on an annual budget of $67,000, which includes the costs of dispensing free drugs, running three residential facilities for one hundred and fifty patients, and offering vocational training for one hundred patients per day.

They consider social connectedness so important that families are told to secretly give money to employers so that patients can be given fake jobs, work regular hours, and have the satisfaction of getting paid—practices that would be considered illegal and unethical in the United States.

The WHO study found that in richer countries, 52 percent of patients were in full or partial remission five years after diagnosis, compared with 73 percent in poorer countries. When the percentages of patients with acute psychotic symptoms more than 75 percent of the time five years after diagnosis were compared, the percentages were 22 percent in London, 25 percent in Washington, D.C., 15 percent in Agra, India, and 13 percent in Ibadan, Nigeria.[25]

A Community Focus Is Essential to Understanding Individual Illness

Indigenous cultures focus upon the community when one person is sick. The community is only as strong as its weakest link. The sick person is seen as serving the community by offering himself or herself to demonstrate the imbalance and disharmony that has ensued. The ill person is appreciated for having performed that function. When one person is ill, the entire community is ill. My sickness is your sickness, for we are connected. I cannot separate your suffering from my suffering. We are in this together.

Conventional medicine discourages us from seeing each other as connected. French Philosopher Michel Foucault linked this idea to the militaristic notion of quarantine.[26] In times of illness or epidemic, each individual family was isolated in the house and counted. Police measures ensured that people did not leave their houses.

For conventional medicine, the community is largely irrelevant to the disease of the individual, except in the sense of epidemics or the role of social medicine in keeping the poor (long recognized as having a much heavier burden of disease) away from the rich, so as to protect the health of the rich, a concept that emerged in western Europe at about the same time as the autopsy.

The indigenous idea that the intent, beliefs, and prayers of the community can heal the sick person has a correspondence in the ideas of early and charismatic Christianity, but not so much in the Protestant "good works" approach so characteristic of modern culture, in which God helps the doctors and the scientists who help the people get well. The notion of sitting in ceremony and praying has a Christian equivalent in prayer circles and the Roman Catholic mass, but has largely disappeared from serious consideration by conventional medicine.

Indigenous cultures also recognize the importance of the entire community holding the belief that the person can get well. A solid unified intent is recognized as crucial to successful ceremony. The beliefs of the community are unimportant in the view of conventional medicine, compared to the science of the illness, or its natural history as it is called. The illness unfolds according to its own essential properties and it is considered magical thinking to believe that the wishes of the community surrounding the sick person can influence the illness.

Another example serves to illustrate this. Cheryl was the scourge of her community. She would walk topless down the streets. She was hypersexual, hallucinating, and delusional. She talked regularly to Elvis Presley (which perhaps she did, but this couldn't be confirmed), claimed to be the wife of Tom Cruise (which could be confirmed as untrue), and had special, magical powers. Her seductiveness made people very uncomfortable. The Roman Catholic influence in the community was strong with widespread and intense disapproval of Cheryl's behavior. Community members wanted her removed and sent somewhere to be fixed.

Cheryl was sent south to a psychiatric hospital and was put on a boatload of drugs. The drugs didn't seem to change her thinking or her outrageousness behavior, but her speech was now slurred, she shook and often didn't make sense. Cheryl believed that her problems had started with heavy marijuana use, which she had stopped sometime before.

When I started seeing Cheryl, we agreed that her medication should be reduced. We started slowly reducing it and, to my surprise, she got better with each reduction. When a healer from Manitoba came to town, Cheryl went with him and let him doctor her for several days. She believed that he had cured her. She continued to progressively reduce her medication.

One year later, Cheryl is living happily in a community that has apparently forgotten her former indiscretions. With community support and within her social network, Cheryl shows no signs of psychosis, delusions, hypersexuality, or any of the other psychiatric descriptions that had previously been applied to her case. Because of their strong belief in healing and miracles (from both the traditional aboriginal and the Roman Catholic points of view), the community members have faith that Cheryl has been irreversibly healed. They can forgive and forget the past, for it is inherent in their worldview to do so.

Cheryl is now living with a boyfriend and helping her sisters care for their children. She feels fine. She wonders why I still come see her each month. I tell her it's because I miss her and just want to say hello.

Solutions Do Not Necessarily Relate to Causes

Indigenous cultures give us different platforms from which to recognize our hidden assumptions. Growing up in a non-mainstream, minority culture gave me awareness from which to see what modern medicine was missing.

Colin Saunders manages a teen program for drug misuse in Vancouver, British Columbia. In his public talks, he discusses "the identity of substance abuse," describing his program as a "collaborative adventure intent upon dissolving the impoverishment that occurs when people are oppressed or overwhelmed by difficulties, dilemmas, and discord within their lives."[27] He believes that therapeutic practices should not be imposed upon people by experts, but should arrive from those seeking the services. Services are best designed by those who use them. These people have more knowledge about what's needed and what works than the abstract theories of experts. In his workshops, Saunders teaches that the problem of substance misuse can disappear when young people, together with their families and other concerned persons, join in creating solutions.[28] Solutions emerge when people join together, which in itself helps eliminate the isolation and alienation that encourage substance misuse.

The medical model argues for a genetic defect within the substance misuser that facilitates or encourages this use. Even the alternative medicine model argues for an inborn allergy to the substance, which leads to the "addiction." What I have observed in indigenous North America is an attitude that it doesn't matter how the problem got here. When we join together to oppose it and do ceremony about it, and dialogue about how we can support each other to resist it, the problem can go away. I have seen that work for cancer, heart disease, substance misuse, depression, bipolar disorder, and numerous other conditions. The "cause" is relatively unimportant in generating the solution. Additionally, the spiritual world contributes substantially to whatever the solution turns out to be.

Giselle's story illustrates this principle. Giselle was a young woman who apparently had a psychotic break during church camp. I wondered about sex or drugs or abuse, but she simply remembered nothing about the incident. I would have called her experience a brief psychotic episode, but the hospital doctor called it schizophrenia. A third consultant called her bipolar. Against her will, Giselle was placed on Seroquel, an antipsychotic drug, and experienced every possible side effect. I agreed with her and her mother that the drug could be eliminated. Why shouldn't we see what Giselle was like off medication?

When the last of her Seroquel was gone, Giselle was not psychotic. She was irritable. She lacked motivation. She was apathetic, and she could occasionally be mean. Within the realm of my conventional psychiatric training and because I had to give her a label, I called her problem "mood disorder not otherwise specified"—placing her somewhere in the spectrum of bipolar disorders. But what really helped her was charismatic Christian healing. Giselle became the center of prayer meetings. The pastor led services for her. Lay healers participated in a laying on of hands. She was anointed with oil. People gave testimony for her. Through this approach, her negative symptoms disappeared and she resumed an active engagement with life. We never knew what caused her problem, nor did we have to.

Healing Focuses upon Restoring Harmony and Balance

Across Indian country in North America, poorly educated healers (by mainstream cultural standards) are sitting with sick people, tortured people, and suffering people and helping them find solace. They are not sufficiently educated to address specific defects in biological or genetic factors. They engage with herbs and plant medicines, but in a rather different way from our naturopathic colleagues. The traditional healers know fewer herbs than do the naturopaths and medical botanists. They know the herbs that live around them. They have spent years with these herbs, eating them, cooking with them, smoking them, drying them, protecting them, harvesting them, making tinctures and infusions with them, sleeping with them, meditating in groves where the herbs grow. They have ingested and encountered the spirit of each herb, and that is what they offer the people who come to them. The spirit of the herb comes to the people to restore harmony and imbalance.

This notion of balance is crucial to indigenous thought about health and disease and appears to be largely missing from the dominant culture. Traditional healers across North America sit in trance and meditate on the source of imbalance and disharmony in the relationships of a person's life. They dialogue with the person and the family. They dialogue with members of the community. I've even seen them ask family dogs about what's out of kilter. They communicate with the family ancestors and the spirits of the place where the family lives. They ask the plants for an opinion. They gather all this information and then offer suggestions through the thoughtful use of story and the enactment of ceremony for how to restore the balance. Sometimes they give direct commands for action, but almost always couched in the traditions of the community—for example, return to traditional behavior and eschew modernism—or because it was a direct command from an ancestral or geographic spirit. These commands, too, are almost always directed at restoring a traditional lifestyle.

Their efforts are often successful, though usually ignored by the dominant medical culture. When they do not cure, when people continue to suffer or to die, the community still feels better. Meaning and purpose has been restored to the situation. Some deaths feel more complete and meaningful than others. Healing can sometimes just take the form of facilitating a good crossover, and can involve the community as well as the sick person.

Disease Arises from Dysfunction

Disease occurs through susceptibility, which relates to imbalance and disharmony in relationship. I still remember reading with awe descriptions of the black plague in Europe and learning how members of the same family with equal exposure to infection had very different outcomes. Some lived and some died. There were famous nuns during that time who spent their entire days with the sick and dying and did not die. More recently, in the history of Native North America, when all the members of a tribe received the same smallpox-infested blankets, not all died. There is a mystery of susceptibility and resilience that biomedicine has largely ignored in its epidemiological modeling. Even with AIDS, I have met people with astronomical potential exposure to the virus—more than twenty sexual partners per day for years during the height of the AIDS transmission epidemic—who did not become HIV positive. How does this happen?

I am not arguing against the infectious disease hypothesis. Long before Pasteur, the Lakota knew that there were invisible spirits, called the *minne watu,* who would make stagnant water and exposed food turn bad. Methods of public hygiene and food preservation far exceeded those of Europe at the same time period. The same was true for wound care. Long before the Austrian physician Ignatz Simmelweis championed the idea of handwashing between attending autopsies and childbirths to prevent infection, the people of Native North America knew about wound infections and had devised effective ways to prevent and treat them.

Perhaps based on observation, indigenous healing systems stress susceptibility and resilience, concepts that refer back to disharmony and imbalance. When we are out of balance, we loose our resiliency. Resiliency is a property that seems connected with the idea that we stand in a certain central location in reference to all the relationships of our lives. Elders say, "when you step off the good red road, then comes sickness and disease." The good red road is the road from wisdom to compassion, the road of connecting to all of life from the center of your being, from your heart. It is a road of forgiveness, compassion, and love. It is a road from which we even look our enemies in the eye and shake their hands for making us stronger.

This concept that disease arises from disharmony and imbalance leads us to realize that health and disease are inseparable from culture, geography, geology, and spirituality. In our healing practices, we begin by acknowledging the spirits of the land upon which we stand. We ask their permission to proceed. We address the mountains and valleys.

These are bona fide entities that must be acknowledged. Their permission is crucial.

Modern psychiatry and its *Diagnostic and Statistical Manual of Mental Disorders,* Fourth Edition (DSM-IV) calls this magical thinking, a potential sign of psychosis. I do remind my colleagues in conventional medicine that these practices make us stronger and more syntonic in our lives (better able to adapt to our surroundings), which mitigates the DSM-IV labeling, since the experiences of psychosis are supposed to be dysphoric (outside of the realm of "normal mood"). Nevertheless, many aboriginal people feel a deep oppression from the largely white, dominant culture when our understanding of our relatedness to nature is labeled psychotic or primitive.

Similar concerns relate to our understanding of spirituality in healing. The spirits are everywhere, conversing with us, helping us. We need their help. In ceremony, we respectfully honor them and ask for help. Through our requests and our willingness to honor our commitments, help comes. Again, this is seen as potentially psychotic thinking by DSM and by conventional psychiatry.

I am in awe of how the mainstream world has stripped nature of its power. I can't understand why so many humans insist on being so isolated and alone. Perhaps it makes them feel powerful. In our ceremonies, we continually talk about how we are only little people who are lacking in ability to do very much for ourselves and each other, about how desperately we need the help of the spirit world. Perhaps people don't want to feel so small and humble. Indeed, it would appear that much of Anglo-European culture is designed to make the privileged few feel powerful at the expense of the less-privileged many. This is certainly true in economics, where a privileged few hold the vast majority of the wealth, while the remainder serve them.

Nevertheless, in indigenous healing efforts, we honor the stories and the spirits of the people (culture). We honor the spirits of the land and the place where we live (geography and geology). We honor our ancestors and the higher spirits and the Creator and respectfully request their help. We believe this works, and we feel oppressed when told that we are psychotic, stupid, primitive, or childish to think so.

The Relational Self
Supersedes the Individual Self

In lectures, I often ask my audience to imagine what it would be like to have no individual self. This is hard for a person raised in modern culture to contemplate. From an early age, we are caught up in constructing stories of who we are, independent from everyone else. The New Age movement and popular psychology supports this approach. Self-actualization is supposed to be the discovery of our essential self, regardless of the rest of society.

Various contemporary philosophers, including Ron Shotter, Rom Harré, and Kenneth and Mary Gergen, have pointed out the absurdity of the search for the individual self. Indigenous observers also point to this obsession with the self and its needs as part of the explanation for many of our modern dilemmas. In indigenous culture, we are our relationships. If you ask a person, "Who are you?" they will respond with a list of relationships: "I am the daughter of Milly. I am the son of Chris. I am the brother of Lisa," and so on. How can one become deeply depressed if one has no individual self?

Depression is a shared phenomenon of a community and must be addressed by the whole community. From my indigenous vantage point, I suspect that the extremes of mood and affect that we encounter in modern culture would not be possible in tribal culture. I have written about the adoption of bipolar and schizophrenic people by elders into tribes and the subsequent disappearance over time of their symptoms through their participation in the life of the group.[29] I suspect this is true for each of us.

In North America, Native people greet each other by describing their ancestors and their relationships. Substantial time is spent learning who is related to whom and if the two strangers share any relatives. In Anglo-European cultures, introductions take the form of statements about one's position in the world and the declaration of status. These contrasts show the difference between living a relational self and living an individual self. Relational selves are easier to heal. Individual selves are hard to reach.

Cooperation Is Essential for Healing

I suspect that the Judeo-Christian metaphors of domination over nature and the ensuing attitude of separation from nature is necessary for our current ecological practices. Native people cannot understand how corporate man can separate himself from the environment and make decisions from which everyone suffers. How can short-term profit justify long-term environmental ruin?

The ramifications of ignoring potential environmental consequences is especially obvious in the far north, where the permafrost is melting and whole towns are sinking into the mud. Polar bears are venturing farther south to find food. Winter hunting has become more dangerous because the ice is not as strong as it used to be and people can fall into cold water; once upon a time, this could never have happened until spring. Lakes are appearing in the polar ice cap. If we cannot cooperate with nature, how can we cooperate among ourselves?

Perhaps the greatest invention of the Enlightenment and the Renaissance was individuality. When I construct myself as separate and unrelated to you, I can act for my benefit at your expense. In traditional culture, when we are connected, your loss is my loss and my gain is your gain. In ceremony, the leader always tells the spirits, "Hear their prayers, for their prayers are my prayers and my prayers are their prayers." This is apparently a primitive, tribal attitude.

In my previous work at the locked psychiatric ward, I was expected to deal with the dispossessed, the homeless, the abused, and the neglected. From the indigenous viewpoint, a family is never expected to stand alone, isolated from community. This is, however, the individualist, capitalist orientation, which holds true insofar as wealth permits the purchase of services that allow a family to exist in isolation from community. Those who are not wealthy cannot purchase these services, and so they suffer.

American culture has become punitive rather than reconciliatory. One of every twelve citizens has been in prison.[30] We dream up progressively harsher mandatory sentences for crimes so that first offenders are forced into the ranks of the hardened criminals and really taught well how to do their new job. I have often wondered about the purpose of this, but it seems to me that it serves to separate the privileged few from the masses. It is still the case that the privileged are not charged. I don't know how the United States will ever become more cooperative, or tribal. In some ways, I perceive Canada as a kinder, gentler culture than the United States. Canada has the most guns and the fewest murders per capita of any country, though it does have its own brand of rampant racism. Nevertheless, the justice system is not so punitive, and creative alternatives are used, such as restorative justice programs in aboriginal communities.

In the United States, and to a lesser extent in Canada, Native people have been placed in the most adverse locations—land that no one else wanted for any purpose. Economic opportunities in these remote, rural areas are limited. People's capacity to rise out of poverty prior to the introduction of casinos was minimal. Even with casinos, there is a potential ethical dilemma about capitalizing on other people's greed and addictions (gambling) to succeed, even if the cost is largely at the expense of the dominant culture (though many Indian casinos are full of Native people losing their money). A local joke says that Native America is taking the United States back "one quarter at a time."

Cooperation is crucial to healing. Perhaps this is why the American population is so ill (the most ill of all developed nations, despite spending the most money on health care). The United States is a showcase for the best and the worst of capitalism, and illness is one of the worst results.

Disease Is Found Within Relationships

In the view of conventional medicine, disease is found within organs. Autopsies with microscopic confirmation are the ultimate form of diagnosis. When we look for disease, we look for structural and enzymatic changes within individual organs. Aboriginal elders tell me that what we are seeking is only the footprint of the disease. Looking as we do, we only find the tracks and traces of disease, which, they say, is long gone by the time the person dies. Look for the disease within the relationships, they say. That is where it is found. The rest is consequences and effects of the disease. This leads us to a consideration of the logic behind spiritual healing, for it addresses what lies between people, or between people and spirits, or people and earth energies.

Is some of the potential value of conventional medicine that it offers us a break from being accountable for our own health as people? If it's all random and biological and genetic, then it's best left up to the experts. We can relax. We don't have to change anything. We're not responsible. We can just do what the experts tell us and let the chips fall where they may. For Europeans, modern medicine also broke the tight-fisted hold of the church. In that context, illness had been seen as punishment from God. Illness was not supposed to be cured because doing so interfered with God's divine will to punish. Healers were burned at the stake in thirteenth century France and Spain. Conventional medicine freed Europeans from this terrible burden, from this belief that illness was justified punishment. If it was merely random and genetic, and people weren't responsible, then the Church had to stop vilifying the sick. Clearly this was a step forward.

What must be pointed out, however, is that indigenous cultures didn't need this liberation. While the conventional medical story may have liberated Europeans who had been held captive by the Roman Catholic Church, it was not so beneficial to aboriginal people who did not have the same need for liberation. An Assiniboine elder put it bluntly:

> From the treaty, they took everything away, the diet, the way of life; all that was put on the earth by the Great Spirit. The new diet made the people weaker. It was too much change, too quickly. . . . [The old people] say that they brought sickness over from across the water; sickness like typhoid fever. And after they got rid of the Indian medicine and the people had to take white medicine, and some of it made us real sick. They kind of damaged our bodies through pills and their side effects. They were experimenting on us. It was the tame food, too. We were used to eating wild game. That's why they figured our bodies lacked the strength they had before.[31]

Thus, narrative medicine represents a search for a storied understanding of health and disease that works for all the world's peoples, and not just Europeans. It is as compatible with indigenous knowledge and healing as it is with European-derived approaches. It is not compatible with a position, like that taken by much of medicine, which restricts truth to only one story—that of biology and genetics. Conventional medicine has served people by freeing them from the bondage of Old World religions and giving them permission to not heal, address change, or restore balance and harmony—to just relax and be passive. Some need this, and we can be thankful that it is available for them. But not everyone wants this approach, which is why we need diversity and a more narrative approach to medicine.

Those of us who attempt to bridge the Native world and the world of conventional medicine are trying to conceptualize and integrate the wisdom of indigenous cultures with biological medicine. We believe that current medical explanations for health and disease are culturally driven, and that we cannot separate biology from culture.[32]

To summarize, a narrative approach to healing means:

1. We interpret our sensory experiences of the world by creating stories that simulate an unbroken chain of experience, connecting past events to the present—as well as to an imagined or desired future. These stories "summarize" our experiences to make them manageable to remember, tell others, and tell ourselves. Without these stories, life would resemble Joyce's novel *Ulysses*—an unbroken stream of sensory impressions without separation, organization, or editing. We have to make stories to organize experience into discrete packets—vignettes, chapters, and the like—that we can handle.

2. We tell stories about ourselves on every level of organization. Individuals tell stories to show others "who I am." Families tell stories that define their family. This manifests at weddings and funerals as stories that begin with "Remember the time when . . . " Communities tell stories to construct identity, as in the stories about a town's founder, or stories from Native communities about the great chief for whom the reserve was named (Poundmaker, Yellowquill, or White Bear, for example). Countries tell stories that come to be known as the history of that country

(Paul Revere's ride, George Washington's cherry tree, Lincoln's Gettysburg address, Teddy Roosevelt's charge up San Juan Hill). These stories are positioned in interaction to simulate identity for each conversation in which they are told.

3. The stories we tell (about ourselves and others) pull together observations, experiences, sensations, and perceptions into a unified whole that has plot, characters, meaning, action, beginning, and end.

4. These stories tell us what we need to know to interpret our world. They tell us what we need to know to classify and interpret new experiences. They tell us how to make sense out of what is happening around us. Without these stories, we'd be lost (or psychotic).

5. Culture arises from the synthesis of all the stories lived by a group of people in a particular time and place.

6. Stories offer us a way to speak eloquently and directly about concepts that are otherwise hard to define and communicate, like self and identity. Stories give us a fluidity of expression, an opportunity for improvisation, and a way to design alternatives.[33]

7. The stories we (at any level) tell inform our audience of how we want to be understood.

Throughout this book, we will consider the power of history, culture, and both traditional and contemporary stories to transform people, to inspire and motivate change and healing. In our fragmented, postmodern society, the mode of transmission of stories has been broken; most of us have lost our connection with our traditional stories. Our lives and work will be enhanced when we are able to integrate the voices and stories of multiple cultures, because we are beings of diversity. When we celebrate that diversity and recognize that we communicate through story, then we can begin to truly enjoy and respect each others' stories for the many truths that they contain.

2
Transcending Limitations

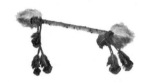

An old sensitivity had descended in her, surviving thousands of years from the oldest times, when the people shared a single clan name and they told each other who they were; they recounted the actions and words each of their clan had taken, and would take; from before they were born and long after they died, the people shared the same consciousness. The people had known, with the simple certainty of the world they saw, how everything should be.

But the Fifth World had become entangled with European names: the names of the rivers, the hills, the names of the animals and plants—all of creation suddenly had two names: an Indian name and a white name. Christianity separated the people from themselves; it tried to crush the single clan name, encouraging each person to stand alone, because Jesus Christ would save only the individual soul; Jesus Christ was not like the Mother who loved and cared for them as her children, as her family.

The sensitivity remained: the ability to feel what the others were feeling in the belly and chest; words were not necessary, but the messages the people felt were confused now. . . .

LESLIE MARMON SILKO[1]

The idea of transcending limitations is a truly rich concept that lies close to the heart of the idea of narrative medicine. In this chapter, we will hear stories about healers working through ceremony and trance states (transcending their own limitations) to help the people overcome their limitations (ordinary consciousness, the constraints of culture, illness). We will consider the power of ceremony (which is itself a story that we cocreate), the shaman's role, and the role for altered states of consciousness—including the trance state—as important aspects of transcending limitations. We will consider the story of one Native physician who, like me, is struggling to bridge cultures and to bring this idea of transcending limitations alive. Like me, he is struggling to overcome limitations imposed by culture and conventional medicine in order to become an effective healer.

Ceremony is an important part of how I work to help people transcend limitations. Like healing, ceremony should be seen as a verb that submits us to a process of transformation and not something that has efficacy in the way of a drug or a surgery. Ceremony provides the context from which we dialogue with the Universe, with angels, spirits, ancestors, and the Divine. It guides us into the world of the soul and its healing—providing a road for personal and spiritual transformation as well as community revitalization. Ceremony gives us a path to follow away from our limitations.

Indigenous knowledge teaches that we can't actually fix people. This is the Creator's job, most elders say, or "that is up to the spirits." The eminent medieval European physician Paracelsus, often considered the father of modern surgery and definitely the first physician to conduct a comparative study of surgical methods, held similar beliefs, saying that he "saw the essence of disease as spiritual." He always felt that "he had dressed the wound but God had healed the patient."[2] We lose power and effectiveness if we ignore a people's local knowledge for how to live well and how to heal when sick. External cures don't tend to work, whether they involve changing lifestyle, changing relationships, changing personality, or changing culture. People still suffer. We need to consider different ways of approaching illness, arising from multiple perspectives. These perspectives must include local knowledge from the people's own cultures about how to heal. We must discover how to collaborate with others to create healing stories, the roots of which must originate in the people who are being healed.

If we wish to transcend the limitations that some of medicine's contemporary stories impose upon us, we need to understand the situations in which the conventional medical story is useful and the situations in which other stories may be equally or more helpful. In order to do this, those of us within the profession need to become more humble about what we can do and what we can't do.

Just as personal stories are told to construct our identities, professions tell stories to define themselves. The dominant story that is medicine proclaims itself to be in pursuit of the one truth that will cure all disease and make everyone healthy, or as Daniel Callahan points out, immortal. The tremendous growth of holistic medicine and the persistence of the world's traditional medicines show that, like the Indians in North America, the other stories have not died out.[3] They are also needed. The biological or genetic story is interesting and sometimes useful, but it is not the only story. The stories of traditional elders who have never left their local communities and speak no mainstream languages are often more useful for healing than those of mainstream medicine.[4]

Conventional and holistic medicine tend to ignore the social determinants of disease, which are powerful and readily part of nonmedical stories. For example, Harvey Brenner's large-scale studies from 1973 on the effects of unemployment in America showed that a 1 percent rise in unemployment was followed by 6 percent more first admissions to psychiatric hospitals, a 4 percent rise in suicides, a 4 percent increase in admissions to state prisons, and 6 percent more homicides.[5] Brenner later found similar results in England and Wales.[6] These matters lie outside the conventional story about health and disease and rarely influence how medicine and psychology are practiced, though they should. We need to elicit and hear new and ancient stories about health and disease that take into account politics, unemployment, social policies, and the distribution of wealth. Our narratives need to expand beyond biology.

In an important article from 1983, entitled "Housing Poverty in Japan," Kazuo Hayakawa, a Japanese professor of environmental planning, said, "It is not too much to say that housing is of the greatest importance because it affects the whole of our life in every way; for instance health, security, and culture. Children grow up there, family life goes on there, and the greatest part of human life is spent there. Housing is related to human life day in and day out, and is the most important basis for the development of the total human personality in society."[7]

I received no lectures on housing during my medical training. We were relatively unconcerned with where the people we treated actually lived and worked when they were not sitting in our offices. This is another story that can change and must change as we become more collaborative with each other. From their perspective in New Zealand, where they work for social justice, Charles Waldegrave and Rosalyn Coventry described the effects of growing urban poverty on psychological and physical ill health.[8] They show how the poor, including aboriginal people, bear the brunt of illness. In my meetings with families and practitioners to create shared understandings of how illnesses are to be addressed, it has been helpful to refer to some illnesses as "diseases of colonialism" or "diseases of poverty."

Many of the chronic inflammatory conditions I encounter are based in the modern lifestyle. But we focus upon the molecular biology of diabetes, for example, without considering the social and political situations that nurture the conditions that allow it to flourish—conditions of being sedentary, of loss of meaning and purpose, of a diet high in sugar and other simple carbohydrates that is cheap and accessible to the poor, even provided to aboriginal people by government food programs. Even in my city of Saskatoon, groceries in poor neighborhoods often offer no fruits or vegetables for the people to buy. Poverty prevents them from traveling to other, more distant stores to shop. No wonder modern medicine is so unsuccessful in treating these chronic ailments.

Norman's story provides a good illustration of the coexistence of stories in North America. I met Norman, a Haida family physician from British Columbia, in Tucson, Arizona, where he was living while completing his master's degree in public health. After this, he was planning to lead a teaching clinic on the west coast of Vancouver Island, north of Nanaimo, one of the rural sites of the family medicine program of the University of British Columbia (UBC). Norman grew up on the Queen Charlotte Islands off the coast of British Columbia. His early life was full of struggle: alcohol-related problems abounded in his family, he lived in relative poverty, his father was verbally and physically abusive, his mother was addicted to pain medications, and he struggled to get through school. He eventually did graduate from the University of Northern British Columbia and attended the medical school program operated there by UBC. He did his residency in family medicine in Prince George and saw his mission as working with aboriginal people but also bridging cultures, as many members of his family had married Anglo-Europeans, and all of his training took place within that context. Norman can teach us something about how stories can be used to build a bridge between indigenous cultures and mainstream Anglo-European culture.[9]

Norman had transcended many limitations and continued to do so each day. He credited Creator and the Spirits for allowing him to transcend his personal limitations and become a physician. His ceremonial life was a rich part of making that happen. He used prayer and meditation each day when he arrived at work to transcend his personal difficulties so that he could be more fully present and healing for his patients. He relied on local indigenous healers and his spiritual life to transcend the limitations he felt from the application of conventional medicine to the many difficulties experienced by the people who came to see him. Many of these difficulties had no solution. And when nothing else could be done, you could count on Norman to tell a story that would make people laugh or change the mood—creating a small but significant transformation.

Telling stories is natural to indigenous people. As a medical student, I took an option that existed then at Stanford University to see patients one day per week for an entire year at the General Medical Clinic. Within that context, when the drugs didn't work as well as our pharmacology course suggested they should, I found myself telling stories like the ones my grandmother told me. Norman had the same experience. When conventional medicine didn't work, Norman also told stories. These stories have a healing power that allows us to transcend our own limitations, just as ceremonies do.

On the day I met Norman, we were both at a conference where the public address system buzzed like flies on a hot summer day. Whatever the speaker was saying was drowned out by that constant buzz. I sat with Norman because he was sitting alone at a table in the corner of the room, which is where I usually sit. He looked sad. Later I learned that he felt perpetually empty. He'd been too shy to meet the speaker, a famous doctor from Los Angeles. He'd had the opportunity, but had taken too long to speak up. The famous doctor didn't know Indian customs and had moved on before Norman could open his mouth.

Large Indian women were bringing trays of fry bread to the tables. Those would be followed by bowls of ground meat and the makings of Navajo tacos. Norman mentioned that he was hungry, but said he'd tell me a story anyway, because it would keep him from eating before all the food was delivered to the tables.

"I'd really appreciate hearing a story," I said. I love stories and I'm always looking for new ones I can tell people for their benefit. Someday I might meet another Haida who would need a good story. Perhaps I sensed that Norman's inner pain was deeper than his hunger pangs.

We were talking despite the speaker's buzzing noises, which we couldn't understand. The topic was antianxiety drugs, which neither of us really cared about. Most of Norman's patients needed food more than they needed drugs. I had learned that Norman worked in an Indian Health Service clinic on the Tahono reservation outside of Tucson. I remembered feeling a little nauseous when I met him, most certainly from the vitamins I took on an empty stomach before rushing to the meeting.

"I'll tell you this story because it's about how knowledge comes to the people," Norman said. "It's about how we stopped fumbling around in the dark. It's a much better way to learn than being put to sleep in these conferences. If you really want something, you have to go get it. Let nothing stop you. Make it your single-minded purpose." Norman started his story in the usual way, saying,

Once upon a time, the world was entirely black. There was no light anywhere. Everyone just ran into things, and lots of heads had bumps on

them. Imagine living in perpetual darkness! I think you've probably felt that way before as I know I have; that sense of being completely befuddled, completely in the dark, like we were when we were children and too young to know what was really going on.

Light did exist, but one old man owned it. He lived beside a river with his daughter. He kept the light hidden inside a box within another box within a third box and so on and so on, in a seemingly infinite sequence of boxes within boxes. He didn't want the light to get out. He didn't want to know if his daughter was ugly as a mollusk or more beautiful than sunset over the waves. This is kind of interesting, because I wonder how he saw a Western sunset with everything so dark. I also wonder how he got so scared of ugly, since everyone has some inherent beauty that can be cultivated, but he did prefer to keep the light hidden and not take the chance of learning whether or not his daughter was ugly. I guess you've had that experience, too, haven't you—that experience of knowing that there are resources around, but nobody knows where they are. Everyone suffers when that happens. You've probably seen the same things as I have, where people are so afraid of what could happen that they hide their capacities and tools from themselves and each other.

Baskets of corn chips sat on the table, along with a bland salsa. Napkins, browner than the tablecloth, were strewn about the table, along with half-empty coffee cups. A candle burned inside a red glass next to a centerpiece of sagging mums and asters. I saw Norman struggling as hard as I was to keep from reaching for the corn chips, piled in strategically placed baskets. We were both fighting with our middles. Norman continued his story.

Raven is our version of what you call Coyote in the Southwest. Raven stirs things up and makes change happen. He catalyzes different interactions to occur. Whether you like it or not, Raven makes the people grow and change. In this story, Raven accidentally bumps into the dwelling place of the old man and his daughter. He hit his head so hard that he was knocked out cold. He came back to awareness on the ground where he had to sit for a spell to gather his wits. While he was sitting there still dazed, he heard the old man singing to himself from inside. Raven heard about the light that was kept inside the many boxes so that the man would not have to learn that his daughter was ugly. Raven wanted that light. He was tired of hitting his head and stubbing his toes on things that he couldn't see. He was starting to get angry. He was thinking, "how dare the old man keep that light to himself." Maybe that's how change starts—with someone getting angry enough to upset the apple cart, to initiate revolt, to cause trouble, like Raven did.

This mention of Raven grabbed my interest, because I've always been fascinated by trickster stories from the world's many cultures. The startling conclusion from all these tales is that people tend to become complacent, get stuck in routines and habits, and need to be shaken up from time to time. Many cultures share this idea that we need to be tricked into growing and changing. Coyote, Raven, Crow, and Rabbit do this in mythology, depending upon the culture. They are humorous characters who make us laugh—first at them, but as we gain increasing awareness of our similarity to them, at ourselves. These tricksters seem to have the role of bringing humor into the world, which is probably as important as light or fire—other commodities they have provided. We could say that indigenous cultures today serve as the tricksters for conventional medicine and psychology. These tricksters bring levity, relationship, and meaning into the now humorless pursuits of medicine and psychotherapy.

Raven sat there for a long time, listening to that old man sing to himself. Isn't it interesting how people always give away their secrets. Raven learned all the old man's secrets, but hard as he tried, he could not find a door into that house. It was like magic. No matter where he waited, the old man and his daughter left on the other side, though eventually Raven got to know the different sounds of their footsteps. He learned from listening that the daughter sometimes went by herself to the river to gather water, leading him to form a plan.

The next time the daughter went alone to the river, Raven was ready. He stood upstream, and when he heard her footsteps, he turned himself into a little pine needle to drift downstream into her bucket. He'd planned to float downstream into the bucket, get carried into the house, turn back into Raven, find the light, and flee. He didn't expect her to drink the pine needle, so when you hear what happened next, you might say that the trick was on him. The daughter took a long drink of that clear, cool water, and before Raven could change shapes, he was inside her. He had no clue how to get out of her. He knew from the smells that he couldn't just go with the flow or he'd be released into the out of doors. He knew he had to improvise, and so he invented birth and reincarnation all at the same time, so that he had another way out that would keep him inside the house still remembering what his purpose was. Raven traveled down inside the girl, eventually settling in her belly exactly where he needed to be. This set a precedent for people who later died to get put back inside of a mother so that they had a way to get back to Earth in case they needed something as badly as Raven wanted light.

Over time, Raven grew and grew and got bigger and bigger. If you could have seen anything (which you couldn't), you might have guessed that the woman was pregnant, but the old man couldn't see a thing, so he didn't have a clue until the baby was born. The old man only knew something had happened by the baby's cries. If you could have seen that baby, which you couldn't, you would have seen that it was most unusual. It had thick, jet-black hair and a few feathers hanging here and there. It had a long, beaklike nose. Since the old man couldn't see it, he didn't know any of that. He only knew about its strong and irritating cries.

Like most grandfathers, the old man eventually fell in love with his grandson. This was good, because Raven was fumbling around in the dark, looking for those boxes that contained the light. As he grew big enough to walk, he had to struggle to remember what he came for, because it seemed so much easier just to lie down forget about it. It seemed to take forever to get big enough to walk.

Eventually, he got old enough to do more than toddle, to actually walk, and he ran right into those boxes and knew exactly what he'd found. He was trying to open the first and most massive box when his grandfather caught him and chastised him for touching the boxes. Raven played it well. He begged grandfather to give him just one box, just one of his many boxes.

Eventually, as most grandfathers would do, the old man capitulated and gave Raven the box. Raven pretended to play with it through his growing impatience.

No one knows for sure how many times Raven and the old man repeated this scene. Eventually, Raven got almost all the boxes. When he finally saw light shining through cracks in the next box, he started crying for the light. That made the old man even more stubborn, but Raven wore him down and he eventually gave in, handing the sphere of light to the young man, whom he now saw for the first and last time. As soon as Raven held the light, he turned back into Raven and flew out of the dwelling through the smoke hole in the roof.

Raven was so amazed at the changes that being able to see had brought into the world. He was so overwhelmed by all the things to see, that he forgot to notice Eagle who could now also see and was looking for lunch. Eagle dived for Raven, intent on eating him. Raven saw Eagle at the last moment, barely in time to swerve and save himself, but causing him to drop the ball of light. When it hit the ground, it broke in half, and hundreds of little slivers flew all over. The half-ball of light and all the little slivers bounced back into the sky, where they remain to this day as the moon and the stars.

Raven collected the remains of the ball of light and reshaped them into a ball. He flew it into the sky and left it where it is now. That's how the sun came to be in the sky. There's another story about how it learned to move across the sky. Light had come to the world, and the old man saw that his daughter was truly beautiful. Like so many of us, he hadn't needed to keep the light hidden after all. His fears had no basis. So many of us never learn that our fears are groundless.

"Does that mean we're truly handsome and don't need to sit over here in the corner?" I asked. The temperature was almost objectionably hot.

"Nah," he groaned. "It means we're ugly as mollusks. That's why those pretty girls don't come over here to talk to us. We're not exactly pulling them over like flies to the sugar."

"So you Haida believe in reincarnation?" I asked.

"Absolutely," he said. "But you've got to really want to come back for some good reason like Raven did. We don't have that wheel of karma thing that says that you have to keep coming back until you're enlightened like the Buddhists. It's not a moral thing for us. Whoever wants to come back comes back. You don't have to keep coming until you get it right."

The speaker finished his talk. We could smell the last of the food arriving. I watched Norman catch the eye of the woman carrying the bowl of meat. Her long, dark lashes lay beneath deep blue eye shadow. Her brown face was framed by long, black hair. Norman smiled at her as she sat the bowl down. He blushed when she smiled back. He quickly lowered his eyes and she was gone. He watched her beaded earrings sway as she walked away. I wondered what he was thinking. Maybe just that she probably had a protective family. Maybe that he was as ugly as a mollusk.

Over Navajo tacos, I learned that Norman had a wife, who hadn't come with him to Tucson. She was angry at him, for reasons that seemed common and familiar. She had been sick for most of the years they had been married. This reminded me of my past situation and the heaviness I carried. Norman told me about trying to leave his wife three years previously. He had filed for divorce and had begun a relationship with a woman with whom he shared more interests. People (mostly Anglo friends) told him that he could simply divorce his wife. They clearly didn't understand the aboriginal world from which he came, in which people are so interconnected he found it difficult to leave. Hard as he tried, he wasn't able to carry through with the divorce. His children shamed him into withdrawing the papers. He didn't want to face the community. He'd rather be miserable. He'd felt too guilty to even enjoy his new relationship.

Since it was just the two of us at our table, Norman told me about how his wife was torturing him. He said she was still punishing him for his transgressions, which I read to mean his attempt to have a nurturing life. She was keeping him from seeing his son until he called everyone he knew to confess his past actual sins and others that he said he didn't remember committing. His anguish could not be fully appreciated by our Anglo-European friends, who had fewer family ties and entanglements. Nor could they appreciate that these family matters interwove into his struggles to bridge cultures and stories about healing.

The lunch wound down. Everyone was getting up to leave. As we were walking out the door, Norman invited me to come to a ceremony with him on the Pasqua Yaqui reserve. He worked part-time there to earn extra money to support the pursuit of his degree. Outside, thunderclouds were building and it was preparing to rain. Tucson's monsoon season had arrived. Conference flyers were blowing across the plaza as the wind whipped up. Pieces of the *Tucson Daily Star* were stuck to fences. I shook Norman's hand and promised to be at the ceremony. I wanted to see more about how he was negotiating the interface where we were all struggling. I've always been drawn to ceremony, trance states, and shamanism as pathways toward healing. It would be pleasurable to share ceremony with Norman.

Awareness is basic to human life and one of the defining characteristics of consciousness. Once we are aware, next comes the capacity to reflect. Reflection on awareness is meditation. Reflection leads to dialogue as we consider how things could have been different. We talk about "what might have been." Much of my work consists of helping people to be more flexible and imaginative, to be able to consider other possibilities. I use whatever will work—imagery, hypnosis, storytelling, discussion, large group meetings, ceremony. I'm aiming for a kind of looseness of consciousness containing the capacity to adapt.

Common to many stories about healing is the power of mind and the power of ceremony. Ceremony requires us to transcend our ordinary consciousness and enter a state in which healing is possible, in which we can ask for and receive the help of spirits.

Indigenous healers work within a different mode of thought than conventional medical practitioners. They are more intuitive than logical. They observe reality rather than think about it. They intuitively grasp the totality of the situation and follow the movement of energy. They use awareness instead of rational thought. Their mind-set is that of being fully absorbed, like we are when we are with our new love, watching an engrossing movie, playing music with others, or skiing at the peak of our abilities.

People in ancient cultures and intact indigenous cultures are usually more adept than contemporary people at entering altered states of consciousness and communicating with spirits. Today, we can find tribal people who are adept at this. It is no accident, perhaps, that spiritual healing seems to be more common in remote areas with less contact with modern civilization, since people in those areas have retained skills at altered states. Additionally, they are more isolated from modern cultural views that healing is impossible without drugs or surgery.

Throughout the world, indigenous peoples combine chanting, breathing, drumming, rhythmic dancing, fasting, social and sensory isolation, and even specific forms of physical pain to induce altered states. The native cultures of Africa and pre-Columbian America use them in shamanic procedures, healing ceremonies, and rites of passage. The cultures of Asia use them in various systems of yoga, Vipassana, Zen Buddhism, Tibetan Vajrayana, and Taoism. The Semitic cultures use them in Kabbalah. Islam has Sufism. Only Western industrial civilization fails to hold these altered states of mind in high esteem. Western cultures tend to discount the remarkable experiences people have when they enter such states.

When we enter an altered state, our connections to each other and our environment become more obvious. At these times, people tend to describe a loosening and melting of the typical body boundaries. We may experience merging with another person in a state of unity and oneness. We may report virtually complete identification involving body image, physical sensations, emotional reactions, attitudes, thought processes, memories, facial expression, typical gestures and mannerisms, postures, movements, and even voice inflections. These altered states of consciousness represent the realm from which we can dialogue with illnesses and communicate with non-ordinary entities (spirits), nature (mountains and rivers), or the universe itself.

The literature on altered states of consciousness is extensive. In 1901, progressive Canadian psychiatrist Richard Bucke called it "cosmic consciousness."[10] In 1911, mystic and British religious writer Evelyn Underhill called it "consciousness of the Absolute."[11] Altered states catalyze the experiencing of new modes of perception, which lead to what philosopher Ashok Gangadean calls "meditative logic."[12] Abraham

Maslow, one of the founders of humanistic psychology, believed that people who had peak spiritual experiences tended to become less selfish, more self-confident, more humble, more capable of awe, more reverent, less fearful, more accepting.[13] Things seem more self-evident. Intuition is boosted. We cultivate these qualities. Trance states give us access to information and beings and conversations not present or accessible in our ordinary waking states.

This spiritual thirst arises from within, from unknown and mysterious sources, from what biologist Dean Hamer called "the God gene."[14] We spend our lives questing after spirit, after these peak experiences. This is why we keep going to ceremony. Houston Smith said, "We seem to have an innate need to experience and celebrate the spiritual dimensions of life."[15]

Large group ceremonies can be quite ecstatic, similar to what anthropologist Mircea Eliade described in his studies of shamans from the 1930s. He defined shamanism as "techniques of ecstasy."[16] He saw shamanism as the manifestation of the sacred in a human being. Through the trance state, all participants in the group ceremony experience the sacred. The more access we have to these spiritual realms and the more we explore the deepest regions of the inner world, the more power can flow. This power is spirit derived. The spirits give it to us for our temporary use in ceremony and healing. It is not ours to keep. The spirit-calling songs bring beings that speak with us to help us. The results of these conversations are unpredictable. No one knows exactly what will happen. As in any dialogue, each participant reacts to the other, and change occurs. Spirits can also be changed. The goal is to connect with spirits and have a conversation, not to perfect a specific technique. The point is to get there and have the dialogue, however one needs to accomplish it.

Group ceremony offers us a way to change our view of reality. We are seeking the unseen world. We are looking for sources of healing power that can help those who need it. Ceremony represents an attempt to achieve an unusual circumstance that produces a major shift in a less traumatic way than, for example, electric shock, bodily trauma, extreme fatigue, or a near-death experience. What cannot be forgotten is how much ceremony depends upon the group conducting it for its efficacy. Fasting or purification often precedes ceremony. Several days of ceremony in a row may be necessary. (Dene or Navajo healers in Arizona and New Mexico often use twelve days.) We need focus. We need coherent consciousness and lots of it to facilitate a change in physical reality. Groups, and especially large groups, provide that greater amount of consciousness. For transformation or to transcend limitations, we need focus and concentration during the trance state.

Group identification and group consciousness are further extensions of altered states. Participation in these larger groups supports the development of an altered state that supports our change. People can become aware of being part of an entire group that is conscious of itself. The depth, scope, and intensity of this experience can reach extraordinary proportions. Through participation in the consciousness of the group, people can experience others' visions and dreams, the anguish of mothers who have lost children, or the love, tenderness and dedication of saints who tend to the sick and the suffering. The experience of an animal's consciousness, including body image, specific physiological sensations, instinctual drives, unique perceptions of its environment, and corresponding emotional reactions, can be authentic and convincing. We can have complex experiences of the consciousness inherent in plants and botanical processes, including becoming a tree, a wild prairie rose, seaweed, an orchid, or a giant lily blossoming at sunset in the Amazon. People have reported experiencing the consciousness of bacteria living within the human gut.

These consciousness experiences can expand to the Earth itself with all its life forms. From this perspective, the Earth becomes one very large group. The Earth as a whole could appear to be one complex organism, oriented toward its own evolution, integration, and self-actualization.[17] People have reported participating in the consciousness of the Pacific Ocean, a forest fire in the Catalina Mountains, and a mountain itself. They have also reported experiencing themselves within the conscious awareness of volcanoes, tsunamis, earthquakes, and other forces. People have gone the other way and experienced the consciousness of molecules and atoms, inter-atomic bonds, electromagnetic forces, and subatomic particles. All of these experiences are examples of larger group consciousness influencing the individual.

People have reported participating in the consciousness of celestial bodies and astronomical processes, traveling to the moon, sun, planets, stars, and galaxies. In the broadest (and comparatively rarest) form of this experience the person can sense the consciousness of the entire universe. All the processes of the universe can be experienced as part of the organism and psyche of the all-encompassing universe system. One insight reported by many people after trance states is that consciousness is everyone and everything, something indigenous elders have asserted for many years.

Other important experiences include traveling out of body, clairvoyance, clairaudience (hearing the future), and telepathy. We can be aware of past lives, embryonal and fetal experiences, and future times and lives. We can experience the consciousness and memories of ancestors, "racial and collective consciousness, or the collective consciousness of the entire human species."[18]

Perceptions and stories that emerge from experiences with altered states of consciousness influence indigenous knowledge and worldviews. We see that our divisions and boundaries of the universe are illusory and arbitrary. In the Gaia hypothesis (or story), for example, God is considered to be the largest possible consciousness—what emerges when everything is considered as the largest possible entity and we imagine this entity to be conscious.[19] Aboriginal elders sometimes say each of us is a small speck in the body of the Creator. Buddhists talk about universal consciousness, or say that the Universe (everything, the largest possible system) itself is conscious.[20]

In meditating on this concept, it strikes me that we could conceive of ourselves as elements of the body of God or Creator in the same way that a red blood cell might comprehend itself to be a member of our body. Carl Jung wrote about the emerging concept of nonlocality and the expansion of awareness beyond the physical realms of the human body,[21] expanding into what physicist Ervin Laszlo later called a continuous information-conserving and transmitting field.[22] Whatever it is called, this is where shamans go to contact spirits and access information.

In a number of discussions over the years, anthropologist William Lyon has told me that he thinks shamanism represents the original science. He believes that every shamanic ceremony is in essence a scientific experiment, crude as it may appear to our eyes. The primary piece of equipment is focused human consciousness, and it has to be used with great precision and a sustained will. He believes the existence of shamanism in every corner of the globe speaks to its effectiveness, as well as its persistence, despite great efforts to squelch it and its practitioners.[23]

Reflecting upon the shaman's mode of thought will take us to Native views of a spirit world and help us see why healers master the art of altering consciousness so they are able to view events in this other world. I like to think the healer guides us toward a preferred future world. He or she serves as a guide to help the person who is sick select a path (a parallel reality) toward wellness. Rituals divert us to different worlds with different conditions and outcomes. They serve as portals between universes. Rituals alter the course of ordinary reality. Perhaps all possible outcomes do happen somewhere, and the healer merely makes some of them more probable than others.

Prayer is the centerpiece of ritual. It represents one very important way in which we communicate with larger groups, including the universe. As with any form of communication, it is less effective if some of the members of the discussion don't believe that the other members are really there. They would tend to stop talking. This is why ceremony requires a community of believers.

A successful prayer has intention (direction) and will (force). It is sincere, as when people pray until tears come to their eyes. Lyon introduced me to the work of anthropologist Frank Speck, who studied healing among the Naskapi people of Labrador and Newfoundland and concluded that their healing included a combination of "dreaming, wishing, intention, and the exercise of will."[24] A Naskapi phrase for that state of mind, which I use in my guided imagery work and storytelling, translates as "spirit-power thinking." Desire, or what is commonly called intent in twenty-first century parlance, is crucial for attracting spirits and building the power to heal.[25] Prayers are always answered if we will only listen. (Even if it's to hear, "No, what you want is not possible, sorry.")

Some ceremonies require a great deal of preparation. Thought may be concentrated on the ceremony for weeks beforehand so it is compacted into a singular point in time that becomes sacred. This kind of thought activity represents what the Dene called "the power source of all creation, transformation, and regeneration."[26] Historically, in North America, when the amount of consciousness required for a ceremony was more than the capacity of the person leading the ceremony, additional spirit helpers were invited to augment the power of the shaman.[27] Lyon says that "each spirit helper comes with a particular power ability."[28]

Ceremony has been discounted by mainstream medicine and psychology as superstition or as working through placebo. What I am suggesting is that ceremony is a primary means through which we communicate to larger groups and these larger groups speak back to us. Ceremonies create portals for dialogue between radically different levels (human and divine, for instance). Ceremony provides a venue for these larger groups to shape and change us during our interaction with them.

Ceremony "is a process in which a collection of alternative realities is poised on the brink of coming into being. It is a vision of potentialities cascading from the depths of our own brain's quantum machinery or spilling from the turbid sea of atomic uncertainties suddenly coming into being through the action of observation, at once individual and universal, unbounded by limits of either space or time."[29]

In ceremony, repetition leads to success. Traditional healing in the American southwest has been seen as "ritualistic persuasion."[30] The salient features of Ojibway healing have been summarized as "endless and ceaseless repetition," "persistent fixation of attention," and "the power of complete absorption while at prayer."[31] The power of complete absorption in prayer is an individual's input of personal will, which shifts us into other realities. Through the healer's repetition of prayer and songs and the continued recurrence and repetition of ceremony and ritual, we slip through the cracks between universes to change the outcome to which we are currently headed. We shuffle the cosmic card deck in our favor. Altered states of consciousness aid us in this process of hitting the mark, getting where we want to go, letting the desired future pull us in that direction. Obviously, our words must be repeated in conversation to be heard. Prayers must be said many times.

"The chief purpose of the Chippewa healer was to work upon the mind of the sick person and by that means, to produce recovery."[32] We persuade with repetition. Anthropologist Sam Gill confirmed this in his study of Navajo prayer. "The message of the prayer is highly redundant," he wrote. The "extent of repetition" is greatly out of proportion to the extent of the message that is borne in the prayer texts.[33] We need to repeat the message so that we all believe it with sufficient strength and force to get it across to the spirits. Repetition builds power. We need to direct a continuous output of sincere, willful, repetitive consciousness in order for reality to shift. The more we do, the better the effect. But we also need to know when to walk away. If we work too hard, the spirits may get the message that we believe what we ask is impossible. We continue the ceremony and the work until it feels done, and then we walk away. The feast after the ceremony represents that walking away. We celebrate. We have some fun. We play with the spirits. It's important they know that we know anything is possible, and that it isn't necessarily hard work. The work lies in changing ourselves, in changing our minds.

Mind is a powerful force, and unfortunately modern technological culture often exploits that fact. We do this when we tell people what to expect based upon what we believe to be true instead of letting people come to their own expectations. Within a framework of indigenous knowledge (supported by narrative medicine), we are trying to change this by reanimating the world, by restoring magic through ceremony and ritual. Lyon says that "Prayers must be accompanied by a great deal of sincerity (your will), humbleness (heart mode), intense focus of consciousness (the nature of your wish), and continuous repetition (empowering the observer effect over time), all in the proper order and recited at the proper time."[34] He said this was what led Native Seneca anthropologist Arthur C. Parker to conclude that aboriginal healing was "merely formula." Lyon believes that all four of these prayer attributes are essential to the success of any sacred ceremony. He says,

> We are talking about a small localized change in the overall flow of reality. Besides intent in prayer, the long duration of most ceremonies is also a measure of intent. In fact, repetition and long duration are cross-cultural characteristics of all American Indian medicine power ceremonies. Prayers are simply their means of probability selection. If the ceremonial participants are unified in their conscious effort, then they will generate a unified "observation" in

the process that eventually turns probability into their "wish." No doubt, the power of their unified observation is increased by adding more observers (ceremonial participants). More "observations" mean more consciousness input, and, in turn, a more powerful observer effect. Thus it is that in difficult cases a shaman will normally call for additional "ceremonial helpers."[35]

A clear focus of consciousness is also critical to the success of any ceremony. This sets the content. Once in place, the desired intent must be kept intact throughout the entire ceremony. There can be no disruption in that desire or intent, or failure will most likely result. For that reason, no one is ever allowed to come and go during the course of a medicine power ceremony. They are expected to remain within the ceremony house and active (not sleeping) throughout the entire duration. The Onandoga locked the door when the ceremony began "to preserve solemnity and prevent interruption. None may enter or go out, or even fall asleep. Anything like this would spoil the medicine."[36]

Lyon believes that sincere prayers, prayers that come from one's heart, are words that have been imbued with power. These words are not like ordinary words that come from the everyday speech of the head mode. Prayer words are different than thought-generated words. They are viewed as being more like objects that have a reality of their own. In Black Elk's view a "voice sent" (or prayer) is different from words spoken in general conversation. Navajo Doc White Singer said that "prayer is not like you or me; it is like a Holy Person, it has a personality five times that of ours."[37]

Doubt and skepticism can prevent the full power of a ceremony from building and culminating. The problem of doubt is the negative side of ceremony. A "doubting Thomas" among the participants interferes with the absorption, intent, coherence, and singularity of focus. The doubter is out of sync with the intent of the remainder of the ceremony's participants, and can therefore weaken the accumulated power, causing the ceremony to fail. It is another form of interruption. Expelling doubters before a ceremony begins is not an act of superstition, as earlier anthropologists believed, but rather is an act designed to ensure success. For this reason, Lyon notes that indigenous healers often refused to perform ceremony in the presence of whites.[38] An old Kutenai woman once told anthropologist Olga Johnson that, "the medicine men could always tell when anyone present was not a believer, and would make them leave."[39] What we fail to recognize is how important the context of faith and belief surrounding any activity is for its success. "[A]ny scientific investigation of medicine powers automatically contributes to their failure, since the investigators are usually full of doubt. . . . [W]hen everyone has doubts, changing reality becomes difficult. As one Tlingit informant put it: 'They used to believe in all that [medicine powers]. Now they don't believe, so it kills all the power of that.'"[40]

Lyon told me how shamans exhibit some type of power display at the beginning of a ceremony, which matches my own observations. Healers may relate how their power was acquired, where it came from, and other important contextualizing information. From the beginning, they dispel doubts that may linger in the minds of the participants, using every conceivable technique to engender wholehearted belief in the participants that magic will actually occur at that particular place and point in time. They do whatever they must to build the confidence that healing will happen. Some anthropologists, even Native Seneca Arthur Parker, see this as "selling snake oil," or as trickery, when actually healers freely acknowledge that the building of faith is essential, but not what accomplishes the healing. They see the healing as requiring faith, but not being faith healing. The healing itself comes from the spirits.[41]

Shamans have always excelled in the art of calling and conversing with spirits. This is a skill and a story that we desperately need to recover, and is one of the great gifts of aboriginal medicine to contemporary Western society. It is a much more powerful gift than the herbs or other objects contributed or used in the healing ceremonies themselves.

Norman was actively using ceremony to transcend his limitations and restrictions. Focus on the sacred allows us to transcend our own personal situations and limitations. Through his prayer and ceremony, Norman (and all of us) could rise above his personal situation and problems to provide healing for others (and through these acts, for himself).

Two nights after we met at the conference, Norman and I went to sit in a sweatlodge ceremony with Grandfather Jake, the local Tohono healer.

It was monsoon season in Tucson, and there were scattered mud puddles. The rattlesnakes were active, looking for dry ground. Mosquitoes buzzed overhead, a phenomenon only seen during monsoons.

When we emerged from the heat of the sweatlodge, Norman told me he had seen my culture's White Buffalo Woman, standing in the South, smiling at me, telling us both to love and forgive ourselves. One of Norman's Native patients who suffered from panic attacks had been in the lodge. His mother had died from a rattlesnake bite, and he had never been the same afterward. Grandfather Jake was helping him find inner peace. He eventually learned to walk away from panic on the good red road. He said it was better than the pharmaceutical road he had tried before.

The next day I attended another ceremony with Norman. The afternoon and evening's activities would include an opportunity to "give flesh." In this part of the ceremony, people who wish to suffer on behalf of someone else (so that the other person suffers less) offer small squares of flesh that are taken from the upper arm after the area and the people are purified with sage and tobacco smoke. The small pieces of flesh are usually dried in a cloth and sometimes put into a gourd as rattle material. The practice is not as gruesome as it sounds. The offerings are sufficiently small that they do not leave scars and are not particularly painful to make. Often an eagle feather is pinned into the arm and worn for the duration of the ceremony until the end when it is torn free. This is a bit more intense, but also reserved for the strongest and the healthiest. No one is permanently disfigured or disabled in this powerful, symbolic gesture common to Plains cultures. Any blood released from the taking of flesh is considered a gift to the earth of the vital essence that brings forth life. Participating in this offering ceremony also helps the healers enter an altered state of consciousness, from which they can persuade the spirits and other participants that the healers are sincere.

The origins of this practice are unknown and may have been transmitted and altered from the ideas of sacrifice and offering common among the Aztecs and the Incans. The practice may also have Roman Catholic origins from the symbol of the crucifixion; or perhaps it predates Aztecs and missionaries by hundreds or thousands of years.

"It smells like dung around here," Norman whispered to me. I struggled to suppress a laugh. Grandfather Jake was kneeling before the altar. Fred Falcon Butte, a healer visiting from South Dakota, was bending over him, picking up the razor blade to cut flesh from Jake's arm for the offering. I would have been mortified to laugh at such a solemn moment. Norman wanted me to laugh, I guessed, to break the tension. We were participating in a spiritual tradition that reached back millennia. We were caught in the mystery of healing.

We healers find our own healing in ceremony as well. Norman spoke to me about how much he suffered from the alienation from his wife and the reduced contact with his children. He needed regular ceremony as a way to release that pain so that he could keep going. This has been true for me as well. Ceremony has helped me to function on a high level for the work of healing people, despite my own difficult circumstances and suffering.

Grandfather Jake was offering flesh for a young man who was comatose after a car accident. The sun was hot this April afternoon. As we stood outside, sweat was dripping off the tips of our ears and gathering everywhere. Some of the elders sat underneath the shade of an arbor. The air smelled terrible. Someone was spreading horse manure over the garden near the wash. The wind was blowing from there into the ceremonial area. I imagined little particles of horse manure assailing my nose. That's what odor is, I thought—tiny, wind-borne particles of dung.

When it was his turn, Norman winced as the first square of flesh was cut from his arm. He was offering flesh for one of his infertile patients, trying to conceive. Every medical treatment available through the Indian Health Service had failed. The small pieces of flesh would be laid on a white cloth for drying. When dry they would be placed in a gourd rattle for use during the sun dance ceremony. Fred cut again. A small stream of blood meandered down Norman's arm. He watched its slow progress toward the ground, waiting for that moment when dirt and blood would mingle in the holiness of blood fertilizing the ground. (Norman's patient did conceive two months later.)

Grandfather Jake was a stout man. Naked from the waist, his belly protruded over a large silver and turquoise belt buckle. His power was derived from what Davis calls "a culturally perceived capacity to intervene directly on the spiritual or nonmaterial plane. This ability to mediate personally between the ordinary world and other realms of spirits and supernatural forces lies at the heart of the art of shamanic healing."[42] When Davis says "a culturally perceived capacity," we could also say that Grandfather Jake was living out the healer role or story within his community. Elders would say he lived the story as it lived him. Because we were comfortable with this story, Norman perceived him as talking to spirits and enrolling their help. We were believers and this was as important to Norman's medical treatment as seeing patients in the office.

Grandfather Jake's skin was dark. His long, black hair was tied back in a single braid, dropping like a stone toward his belt. He had a perpetual tear tattooed to the corner of his eye. He was both Catholic and traditional. After this ceremony, the comatose person whom he had been doctoring did fully recover. Did the flesh offering help? Everyone there thought so, though modern medicine's story would reject this possibility as preposterous.

A fly tried to land on Norman's wound. Fred shooed it away. Fred's son held the white cotton cloth, which received the small squares of flesh. A jet plane streaked across the sky overhead from the nearby Air Force base. Ants marked a steady trail over Norman's boot. He stopped wincing. I could see that Grandfather Jake was proud of him.

Later, I made a flesh offering for a teenage patient who had been strung out on drugs. I had worked with her when I was living in Tucson and she had continued to work with Grandfather Jake and his helpers. She and her mother were coming into the sweatlodge that was to be held after the offerings. We would pray for them and the others there. Later in the month, Grandfather Jake would take the girl on a short vision quest. They had moved north because the mother thought it was harder to find crystal meth, her daughter's drug of choice, in Prescott, though I thought it was probably everywhere. I had heard the girl was still on and off drugs, but less than before. I wondered if we had done her any good. Who knows? The Creator works in strange ways. (Today, several years later, the girl is off drugs and is going to university, where she is studying social work.)

Then Grandfather Jake offered flesh for his granddaughter, who had gallbladder disease. Norman was her doctor. Norman had given her some herbs, which she hadn't taken. He'd suggested a low-fat diet, which had gone the way of fry bread, potato chips, and french fries. He once did a sweatlodge ceremony for her. She'd come to that and had sung beautifully—a peyote version of "Amazing Grace." Her father, Thomas, followed the peyote road, too. Norman had sat in the lodge with him also. He didn't really go for the peyote church himself, except to support the people for whom the meetings were being dedicated. He didn't like throwing up partially digested peyote buttons, he said. (Jake's granddaughter's gallstones never dissolved, and she eventually had gallbladder surgery.)

Fred switched to the other arm. I knew that Norman had supplied Fred with a few disposable scalpels. He didn't want anyone to get AIDS from sharing the same knife. I wondered why Fred was using a razor blade. What had happened to those nice, new scalpels with the white plastic handles and the green rubber over the blade?

Fred handed the razor blade to his son, Little Freddie. Fred put his hands up toward the sky and looked in that direction. He began a long prayer in Lakota. I understood a few words. He spoke Lakota much better than English. Fred had shown up one week ago from South Dakota. He had announced that he was a peyote road man and seemed sincere. Thomas gave him a place to stay in his house. Both Thomas and his father, Jake, had been looking for a road man to lead a meeting for Thomas's daughter with the gallstones. Fred had agreed to lead one the next time he visited. He said he'd just come for a short visit this time to see his friend Harry, a Yaqui man in the Pueblo. He had to get back to South Dakota to do some ceremonies. But then he'd come back and maybe stay a while, because there were plenty of sick people here who needed medicine. He'd bring medicine back from South Dakota and stay a good while, he said. Then he'd do that ceremony for Thomas's family. Fred was to leave that night after the ceremony for his trip back to South Dakota.

Before we had started the offering ceremony, the audience had obediently shuffled in and sat on the low benches around the fire. We were one part of a larger ceremony and people would come and go to watch various parts and later some would participate in the sweatlodge. Led by old Pablo, who used a walker to get around, they had come to watch the flesh offerings and to take medicine from Fred, who kept it in an old plastic thermos on the altar. When Fred finished the Lakota prayer, he said some words in broken English. Norman knew most of the people assembled across the fire from Fred. He had seen them in the local clinic where he worked part time. The reservation around Tucson was not all that large. The same faces cropped up over and over again. Medicine's view of the body as complex machine, waiting to be diagnosed, modified, and repaired, had little to offer these people to assuage their suffering. Norman said that all he had were his prayers and the ceremonies in which they were offered. As he said later that day, their suffering was global and pervasive with nothing specific to attack or cut out. They had conditions conventional medicine does not have good success with— arthritis, diabetes, loss of meaning and purpose, heart disease, and other chronic problems.

After Thomas also gave flesh for his daughter, Fred spoke. "Creator," he cried. "Thank you for this man here. This man. The one they call Thomas." Fred turned his eyes from the sky and looked down at Thomas, who still knelt before the altar, holding his sacred pipe, his *channupa*, in front of him. He held the bowl close to his heart, the stem pointed skyward. Thomas's head was bowed.

"He's a good man," said Fred. "He's got a good daughter, a good wife. He's got a good family. He really cares about his daughter. He really cares about his family, Creator. That's why he's suffering for them. Like your son Jesus suffered on the cross. Just like that. He loves them so much he's giving up his flesh for them. That's all he really has, Creator, in this life, is his body. And he's offering his body for these people over here and for his daughter. That really touches me, Creator. So I really want to pray hard for him," he said, trembling as he spoke. I wondered if he had studied with the Baptist preachers from my Kentucky homeland. I hoped we had smelling salts in case he passed out from all that enthusiasm. Fred spoke with tender sincerity. I could feel his words vibrating through my body. Even my knees shook to match Fred's vibrato voice, cracking strategically. He seemed to be crying, but with his words, not his eyes.

"Creator," Fred pleaded. "Please, I ask you, please, help this man. Help his family. Help that beautiful daughter of his. Help her to be well. Take that sickness away from her. And all these people here." Fred waved his arm toward the audience of old people opposite us, ending where Pablo sat with his aluminum walker.

Another jet roared overhead, breaking the sound barrier. It cut short the cry of a hawk, circling overhead. The fire smoldered in the pit east of the altar. In it, stones were warming for the sweatlodge, which would follow the flesh offering and medicine-drinking ceremony.

Thomas's wife, Tina, stood at the edge of the gathering. There was prejudice against her because she came from the Hupa tribe of Northern California. People grumbled about Thomas going off the reservation to find a wife. She weighed almost three hundred pounds, and her smoker's cough was filled with sound. Over the years various doctors and community members had tried to talk to her about her gallbladder, hypertension, and diabetes, but to no avail. Tina's pride was that she made the best fry bread on the reservation. She made money selling her fry bread outside the mission church on Sundays. Norman knew from sitting with her and Thomas that she ate a good portion of the profits. But that was how it was with family. Everyone sat around eating fry bread, and occasionally a tourist would buy some.

As the fighter plane disappeared, Fred turned his arms skyward again. The hawk was gone. "Creator," he said. "Help these people. They're hurting so bad. I care for them so much that I pierce myself for them. I want to hurt like they hurt. I want to take their pain into my body so they won't have to feel it." An old woman smiled toothlessly at Fred as he continued his prayers. She was hunched over a walker, gesturing at horseflies buzzing overhead.

When Fred finished, he picked up the scuffed red-and-white thermos. He poured the dark greenish-brown medicine into a tin cup to pass to each person. His son filled a bucket with coals from the fire. Fred sprinkled cedar over the coals and carried the bucket to old Pablo, standing before his walker. Fred fanned the smoke over Pablo's body with his eagle feather. He handed the bucket to Little Freddie, who moved down the row of people, fanning each one before big Fred offered them a drink from the tin medicine cup. Fred seemed to be swimming upstream against a river of smoke. They finished the side opposite Norman and then came around to repeat the process. Norman winced at the bitter medicine. The taste of peyote always made his stomach a little sick.

Fred returned to the altar, where Norman was still kneeling. "Get up, my fran', get up," said Fred. His hand was there for Norman to grab for help in standing. They shook hands. Norman tottered for an instant, but Fred held him in a firm grip. Small drips of blood had clotted around the site of the flesh offering. "Now help me," Thomas said. "All of you," he called out. "Help me. We've got to take these piercings out of our arms."

Eagle feathers hung from wooden pegs plunged through the skin of Fred, Norman, Grandfather Jake, and Thomas's upper arms. Fred motioned Jake and Little Freddie to get on either side of him. He showed them how to wrap rawhide around the pins. "You just pull really hard," he said, "and they'll tear out."

"Pray for me," Fred called out. "I've done my best for you. I've suffered all I can for you. This is the last part, where these two men here are going to pull out these pins." He told them to untie the eagle feathers first. Fred had a new expression on his face as he waited for them to pull out those plugs. It was pinched-in and puny, as if he'd just tasted the microscopic particles of horse manure floating in the air.

"Go ahead," said Fred, stiffening himself. His muscles stood taut beneath the sailor's tattoo on his upper arm. Thomas and Little Freddie both yanked. Fred's pin tore through the flesh. Blood flowed down his arm from the new wound. Thomas's pin broke; he picked out the broken pieces. Then Fred took sage and rubbed it in his wounds. Thomas watched carefully and did the same for his own wounds. Fred's visage was visibly pained. Norman and I were both moved by what Fred had done for Thomas and the assembled people. Grandfather Jake and Norman waited patiently for their own piercings to be pulled out.

Once Norman's wounds had been smeared with goldenseal, Fred called out, "It's over. I've done everything I can do for you. You can go home now. If you get better, I'm glad. If you don't, then it's my fault. Blame it on me. Say I wasn't good enough. Say I didn't suffer enough for you. And that would be true. That's all."

In any indigenous community, when health professionals participate in traditional life, it makes a tremendous difference to the people. Being indigenous, Norman knew to do that as soon as he started working part-time at the tribal clinic. I do the same when I work in Saskatchewan communities. We know that conventional medicine requires the traditional medicine to do its best work. The traditional medicine sustains the people in ways that conventional medicine cannot. Traditional spirituality (anyone's) allows people to transcend their suffering and their pain, to soar toward the heavens despite crippled joints and limited mobility, to find joy despite illness. By participating in the reenactment of the traditional stories through ceremony, we physicians create a better medicine, a stronger medicine than we could have ever had without this involvement. That is what I hope you take away from this chapter—the necessity of integrating diversity and multiple perspectives into the practice of medicine, thereby enabling it to transcend its current limitations. Regardless of what we can or can't offer the people from the standpoint of conventional medicine, our presence, our offerings and sacrifice, our praying with them, our sweating with and for them, and our involvement in their traditional healing practices comforts them as nothing else could. In that context, we offer hope for people with withering limbs, sadness, fears, worries, breathing difficulties, and chest pains.

I wanted to talk more with Fred, but nature's call eventually won. I left Norman waiting beside the fire and walked northeast, following the wash, looking for a private place. Around the corner, behind a broad creosote bush, I made craters and ravines in the ground, a miniature version of the Grand Canyon. After checking around to make sure no one had seen me in the empty desert, I stepped out of the wash and returned to the ceremonial area, alert for rattlesnakes looking for their twilight meal.

The sweatlodge stood behind and to the west of the altar. It had already been covered with a large canvas tarp. Fred was stripping to his boxer shorts. He wrapped a towel around his waist. You could see the scars from many piercings on his chest. The blood had dried on his arms.

"I'm ready," he said. "Let's go. Where are those other two?" Then they heard Thomas and Grandfather Jake walking toward the lodge, speaking quietly in Tahono. They were a massive pair walking together. Norman removed his clothes and wrapped himself in a towel like everyone else.

Little Freddie would tend the door and carry the rocks. He stood majestically beside the fire with his pitchfork. Fred Sr. stooped low to enter the lodge. "*Hau mitakuye Oyasin*," he called out as he entered. ("To all my relations.") Grandfather Jake entered next, followed by Norman, Thomas, and me. Fred had already loaded his pipe with tobacco outside the lodge. He was ready for the door to close and the stones to enter. Then Little Freddie asked from outside if someone else could enter. Fred Sr. said sure. Thomas's daughter's boyfriend came in. It was dark outside.

"Glad you could come," said Fred. Fred took charge convincingly. Few could top him for dignity and decorum in leading the sweatlodge. He impressed me, even though I have attended many sweatlodge ceremonies. The young boyfriend squeezed into a place between Norman and Thomas.

"I just wanted to tell you, boy," said Fred, "it'll get hot in here, so don't be afraid to humble yourself. Put yourself on the ground. Touch the earth. Cover yourself with your towel. We'll use forty-seven stones just like it's always done back home."

Fred thumped himself on the chest. "I always do it *that way,* the way it was showed to me, 'cause that's the right way to do it. I just thought to tell you that." Fred shook his finger at the boy, or perhaps at youth and its follies. "You know," he said. "I wouldn't let my daughter go with someone who couldn't sit through a sweatlodge."

I could sense the boy squirming. Fred said they would start with seventeen stones and bring ten more inside with each round. He told his boy to bring the first seven to be blessed by the pipe. After those seven entered, the pipe left the lodge and was placed back on the altar. Then ten more stones were brought in quick order to complete the needed seventeen.

As the ceremony proceeded, we became more than our ordinary selves. Through the prayers and the trance implicit in the ceremony, we became more than we are usually capable of being. For that length of time, we transcended our limitations. Some of that transcendence would remain with us afterward. This is why we keep going to ceremony, to keep lifting ourselves up a little higher toward the heavens each time. To improve our capacity to help others and to be loving, kind, and compassionate toward others. To be all we can be and then more.

Intercultural stories like Norman's show how we can incorporate more stories than the one we learned from contemporary science into a "performance" or praxis to help diseases that conventional medicine largely fails to treat. From my experience with Norman, we see one way that indigenous ceremonial methods are used in the modern setting. We also see the power of belief, prayer, and the trance state in overcoming the limitations of modern medicine. We see the strength of combining stories and of exploring stories beyond the one in which we were trained. We see the power of the group to facilitate healing for individuals in ways that are mysterious and difficult to grasp outside of the concepts of coherence and connectivity.

Later, sitting outside Thomas's house with Fred and Norman, talking and resting in spells, I thought of my grandfather. I was reminded of the two of us sitting on our haunches together in the Kentucky hills, watching rabbits hop by. Sometimes grandfather would smoke a cigar and pray. Sometimes he would talk to me about what the spirits were telling him.

An old dog lay with us, resting from the heat. The sun was as good as gone down, feeble glories of pinks and purples streaking the Western sky. Darkness would overtake it soon. My grandfather was a proud man who kept his traditions. I had liked watching the sun go down with him. Peacefulness had surrounded us as it did for me with this sunset. I missed him greatly since he died.

Grandfather could make a tractor run without tools. When all else failed, he would sit before it and pray. He'd sing an ancient song and blow tobacco smoke all over the engine. Sometimes it would start that way. Grandfather said you never know with spirits what they can do, especially when it came to machinery. He said they weren't always in the mood to fix things, and when they were, sometimes you'd get an old spirit that hadn't grown up in the machine age and didn't know how to doctor things like that. But sometimes you'd get one that would rev the tractor up real good so it'd run for days without any further attention.

Grandfather liked to tell the story of Old Bessie, who was one of the first to get a modern stove. He said she'd run it just fine with the help of spirits. Couldn't ever understand about that there LP gas. Just figured it was wood and it burned or it was magic and the spirits took care of it.

Weren't no place to burn wood in the stove, so she figured the spirits did it. Cooked with a good, hot flame, too, grandfather would chuckle.

Grandfather always said modern folks were too feeble and puny to get much help from the spirits. They didn't believe in anything, anyway. He couldn't figure 'em, he'd say, out there running like raccoons with rabies, never sitting still, covering the good Earth with houses, crushing truth in greedy fists like quail eggs.

Norman's three years at the Pasqua Yaqui reserve made a difference to the people whose lives he touched. His concern with the stories and lives of the people with whom he worked took him farther than he ever could have gone with conventional medicine alone. His participation in the life of the people was transcendent. We, like Norman, need to turn toward the people for participation, for knowledge, and for assistance when we reach our limitations, as we so often do in conventional medicine. We need to trust the power of local knowledge and practice to add to whatever we bring to the table from our medical science. This is what Norman did and continues to do. It is my goal as well.

"I'm gonna take you out and put you up on the mountain," Fred suddenly said.

"You mean for a vision?" Norman asked.

"Yeah, like that," Fred said. "We'll sweat again. Four times total. Then I'll put you up. One day. Two days. Three days. Four days. You decide."

"How will I know?"

"Listen. Spirit will tell you. Now wait here. I'll be back."

3
The Maps
That Define Our Reality

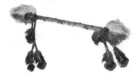

Everything should be made as simple as possible, but not simpler.

ALBERT EINSTEIN[1]

I remember thinking once that everything could be figured out, that formulas would be discovered to explain it all, that there were pristine and independent truths that transcended all cultures and stories. The person discovering those truths would certainly win prizes. Historically, in medicine, we have been driving toward certainty like Hannibal through the Alps or Patton into Italy, waging war with the darkness of ignorance, believing we can triumph. But what if health is a matter of equilibrium? What if disease and misfortune are related to disharmony? What if nature is pliable and plastic and molds to our intent and wishes? What if intent really does change material processes? What if it is all just story, and some stories no longer fit as well as they once did?

Narrative medicine helps us understand that everything we assume to be true about the world is just a story. The idea is simple—that it's all story and that we, as a culture, create our stories. This is not in a negative sense, as in lying or confabulation, but in the most positive sense as a creative act of meaning-making in which we produce a story or map that makes sense of our world and, to the extent it matches our environment, allows us to survive in that world. It even allows us to alter our world and even our physiology. What's different about the story of the person who is diagnosed with schizophrenia, for example, is the mismatch of his story with the environment. We can evaluate stories on the basis of how well they fit their context and environment.

Narrative medicine argues against the "natural history of disease" concept, which gives disease a predictable course regardless of the person, family, and culture. My goal is to overthrow this natural history in favor of individual stories that are embedded in families and cultures of which we need to make sense. Disease is embedded in a person, family, locality, and culture, and can only be understood through the many stories told that include the person and the illness. We cannot see an illness independent of the stories we tell about it. We cannot treat an illness without telling a story. We cannot position ourselves as healers or as experts, without telling stories. We cannot explain anything without telling stories, even if those stories are heavily laden with statistics.

Mainstream medicine teaches physicians to be skeptical about treatments that are not purely material or for which a palpable physical process cannot be invoked. Most of us are unwilling to consider that some of our beliefs might be inaccurate. We can only express doubt from within the shared beliefs of our peers. Narrative medicine helps us to understand that all is story, that we can believe everything and nothing, in the sense that we can work with those stories that seem helpful at the time without pledging allegiance to them for all time. Haitians practicing vodou or Amazonians ingesting ayahuasca believe in a story that includes spirits, souls, and potent magic. The shamanic or aboriginal story inseparably links mind and body. No one falls ill the day after falling in love, for example, but many of us do come down with colds after intense emotional distress.

Within a narrative framework, we are free to seek other stories about science and medicine to support our work. We can use these stories as bridges to indigenous medicines, which are based upon stories similar to those of the new physics that emphasize connectivity and the interrelatedness of all things. Unlike conventional medicine, narrative medicine is postmodern. It cannot be sure of itself. It relies upon diversity to sort out what works and what doesn't. It is forever a mixture of all the voices that sing it into being. New stories are evolving, but in the end, they too are just stories, with no hope of absolute certainty. Thus, regardless of how identified I may be with a particular aboriginal culture (Lakota or Cherokee, in my example), I have to admit, because I do live in a world of diversity, that my preferred story is only a story, after all, when it comes to truth. I live the story and it lives me, but it may be irrelevant to you. If you like it and pick it up, then it becomes meaningful. If you don't, it is useless. Its value consists in what you do with it. It is not intrinsically better than any other story.

A key notion behind the narrative approach is that we need to create a guiding story, a map that works and is pleasing, even as we recognize that the map is not the territory. Consider a story that Milwaukee, Wisconsin-based, Solutions Focused Therapist John Briggs told in a lecture at Massey University in New Zealand in 2005. During World War II, a platoon of soldiers was lost in the French Alps. They had no idea where to go. Their lieutenant found a map in the bottom of his pack. The soldiers examined the map, compared it to their terrain, and struck out in a verified direction, heading for safety. When they arrived, their Captain looked at the map. Without knowing it, they had a map of the Pyrenees Mountains in Spain—nowhere near their position in France. Nevertheless, the map had worked. It had helped them find their way back. Maps do not have to be correct to work.

The story shows that we need a map, regardless of its accuracy or point-to-point correspondence with our surroundings. We need structure to orient our perception or we are lost in what has been called pre-narrative awareness, or pure sensation without interpretation. This kind of experience presents as the confusion of psychosis, when the map has vanished and experience is overwhelming. The map interprets our experience in such a way that we can take action. The soldiers took the action of walking out of their position, following the map. Regardless of the accuracy of the map, it led them to take action, without which they would have surely died. It gave them the needed certainty to act.

For this chapter, I have a Dene* story about Coyote stealing fire.[2] All traditional cultures have stories about how the people obtained fire, which I take to represent knowledge. First the people appear (the subject of creation stories), and then they must gain knowledge (steal fire). Wisdom comes later, as we shall see, in stories about making rain and putting out fires. In the following story, Coyote shows how we can get knowledge that we don't know how to handle. A side effect of Coyote's stealing fire was that he set the grass and the bushes burning out of control.

Coyote's silent motivation for stealing fire was to benefit the people. Everyone in the Fifth World was cold. That had not been a problem in the Fourth World, since it had a ceiling and contained the heat quite nicely. But the Fifth World did not have a ceiling and the heat readily escaped, so the people huddled together in caves and against each other to stay warm. Perhaps Coyote felt a little guilty because it was his fault the people had to leave the Fourth World in such a rush, so he wanted to make amends.

So Coyote told the people about fire. Coyote, being a mythical being, had been present when Fire Man made Fire Mountain. Coyote knew firsthand about the healing properties and other benefits of fire (though his knowledge of its risks was sketchier). He begged First Woman to figure out a way to get fire, but she declined since the people didn't know how to handle it.

At first Coyote tricked Hosteen† Robin into flying to the top of Fire Mountain to check out fire and see how it might be captured. Robin flew too close to the flames and was almost consumed. He managed to return, but with his breast stained perpetually red. Robin was frighteningly pessimistic that the roaring flames could be captured or contained.

Next Coyote tricked Hosteen Owl to fly to the top of Fire Mountain, but to stay carefully away from the center of the mountain where the

---

*The Dene people live in a large reservation covering much of northern Arizona and northwestern New Mexico; they also live across northern Saskatchewan and Alberta and into the Northwest Territories. The Dene are also called Navajo in the United States.
†Hosteen is a Dene title of respect, similar to Honored Person.

flames flared unpredictably. Owl was to circle the mountain to gather information for Coyote about access. Unsuspecting Owl was set upon by two ferocious beings, monstrous guardians placed there by Fire Man to prevent anyone from stealing his fire. These guardians shot their fiery breath at Owl, making circles around his eyes and causing his head to come undone and spin all the way around on itself (which it still does to this day). Owl returned, convinced that these monstrous guardians could never be overcome.

After hearing from Robin and Owl, no one was willing to go but Hosteen Duck, and everyone thought he was a bit daffy. Duck agreed to cover himself with water and fly high around the mountain to gather more information on these monsters. Even he suffered, for the ashes turned many of his feathers black and gray, but he did return with important information—the monsters had lidless eyes and voracious appetites. When no threat was perceived, they sat around scratching themselves the way Hosteen Dog was wont to do, giving Coyote useful ideas.

Coyote tied a long cedar bough to his tail. When he shook it around, he looked like a sideways tree moving in the wind. Next he went to Hosteen Goose and traded for a seashell, and he filled that shell with water. Then he traded with Hosteen Seagull for a beautiful shell necklace that made oceanic noise when shaken. Finally Coyote went to the salt lick and filled both of his cheeks with salt, and then practiced keeping it in place while talking at the same time.

Laden down with all of these items, Hosteen Coyote climbed Fire Mountain. He was so slow and noisy that the monsters heard him coming long before they could see him. They were ready to roast him when he called out, "Yo, monsters, how y'inz doin'? I brought you some presents." This confused the monsters, since no one had brought them gifts before, not even Fire Man, who needed them to guard his mountain. "Oh, yes," said Coyote. "I know no one has been looking after you properly and taking care of you. Probably your skin has even dried out from being up here in the heat without moisture. That would sure make you itch."

The monsters nodded, since they sure did itch. "Move over," said Coyote, "and let me come in and distribute these presents. First, I have a special shell for you that contains the ocean. Put it next to your ear and you will hear." The monsters did hear the roar of the ocean. They were impressed with Coyote's magic—that he could get an entire ocean into such a small shell. Then Coyote said, "I have some beautiful beads for you. When you shake them, water will come to moisturize your skin." As they shook the shell bead necklace, Coyote blew water on them from inside the shell. They felt the cool, moist wind. They were so grateful they didn't see Coyote turning his back toward the center of the mountain and inching closer and closer to the pit of fire. When Coyote heard and smelled his cedar bough catch on fire, he quickly claimed that salt from his cheeks and threw it into the monsters' lidless eyes. They were in agony, with no way to see and no way to stop the pain. Meanwhile Coyote was running lickety-split down the mountain, the burning cedar branch strapped to his tail. Unfortunately, on his way Coyote set all the grass and the bushes on fire, leaving them burning out of control.

How should we interpret this Dene stealing fire story? For our purposes, we might say that the fire Coyote got was like liquid copper dripping down upon that mountain, destroying all the people's favorite stories, maps, and theories about how to get knowledge. But there are other possible interpretations too. The elders teach us that the story exists independently from its tellers and telling. It works on us to change us in its own ways, regardless of our interpretations. Every story is also its own prayer.

What remains when the fires burn out is something simultaneously old and new. It can be represented by either indigenous knowledge or contemporary physics, which has advanced so far as to be unbelievable to the ordinary, uninformed person. Quantum physics suggests that connected people or events change together in ways that are closely correlated. We are all entangled, perpetually embedded in a field of culture, biology, geology, and geography. We can go forward to physics or backward to the wisdom of our ancestors.

In the same way, today's indigenous people are forever interacting with other cultures. They cannot return to an untainted indigenous experience. We will never be able to experience what ancient healing practices were really like. We are all stuck in our modernity with our prejudices, our romanticism about the past, our preferences about what we would like to believe, and our skepticism and doubt that we have learned from Western society. If we can't go backward, we must go forward. However, within quantum physics and the science of complexity, we see ancient insights resurfacing. We see the awareness of connectivity—the idea that everything is related, that what happens to one affects the others.

Biomedicine diverges from narrative medicine with its belief in one, unchanging physiological truth, with disease having natural histories independent of the people who have the disease. Narrative medicine suggests that biology itself is plastic, responding to our stories about ourselves and our lives, faithfully producing those stories upon the raw material of the body. Culture and biology are inseparably intertwined. They forge each other.

Once the structural lesions we can fix surgically are excluded from our diagnoses, physicians enter a land of low correlations and high uncertainty, which is where 80 percent of our practice occurs. Evidence to guide us is sparse. We have to construct a plan, make a map. If the patient improves (whether or not we can prove this was related to what we suggested or did), we proclaim that the map was good. Here we are on the same footing as the world's varied types of health practitioners. Knowing that we have ruled out structural problems, we might have to admit that our traditional Chinese medicine colleagues could construct a map that we couldn't understand but might perform as well or better than any map we could construct.

Indeed, a survey of the world's indigenous cultures might show us that each has a different map that could work as well as our own. On September 25, 2005, *Honolulu Advertiser* reported a story from the *Fiji Times* about the herb kava kava. According to the story, people in Fiji were aghast that University of Hawai'i researchers had just figured out that the occasional liver toxicity caused by the herb was related to the inclusion of stems and leaves in some commercial kava kava preparations. The article from Fiji was quoted as saying, "Why didn't they just ask us? We've known for centuries not to use the stems and the leaves, that these are waste parts of the plant. Everyone here knows that you should only use the root or you could get sick." The *Fiji Times* writer went on to conclude that American pharmaceutical and herb companies probably were using the whole plant because they could make more money that way. The Fijian story about kava kava was better than the manufacturers' story. However, in the modern, scientific story of botanical medicine and profit making, the local indigenous knowledge of the people who live with the plant was dismissed as unimportant—with disastrous consequences.

We largely ignore maps and stories that differ from the ones with which we are most familiar. Medical doctors' preferred stories involve pharmaceuticals because that is how we are trained. However, we actually do not have evidence to support the universal superiority of pharmaceuticals over all other forms of therapy. For example, until 2006, the newer sleeping medications like Ambien (zolpiden) had never been compared in a study to nondrug approaches. Researchers at Beth Israel Deaconess Medical Center and Harvard Medical School finally did such a study and found that a nondrug approach—cognitive-behavioral therapy—was better than drugs.[3] Pharmaceutical advertisements and many modern people habitually tell stories about getting a good night's sleep that involve taking pills. Any indigenous healer could point out our hidden assumptions to us. None of their stories would insist, as we do, that diseases are purely biological, coming from genetic interactions with a physical or infectious environment, and independent of psychology, sociology, culture, or story.

I liken the many belief systems about healing to the many species that live upon Earth. Tom Lovejoy of the Smithsonian Institute points out that there is not a single species we can claim to understand.[4] Our knowledge is embarrassingly rudimentary. This is also true about our understanding of cultures and their healing practices. We academics have not taken the time or cared to respectfully explore with our indigenous neighbors their stories for health and disease and to find out what happens when these stories are applied in the cultures where they originated. We don't even often ask if these other cultures define illness in the same way we do. Lovejoy says that a species that has no apparent use today may, as our knowledge increases, yield astonishing benefits, as did the *Penicillium* mold that served as the basis for the discovery of penicillin. So it may be for the stories about health and healing from other cultures.

A traditional healer may be most effective with members of her own tradition, in the same geographical region where that tradition arose, with people who are most fluent in the cultural practices of that region and who actually live its lifestyle and practice its spirituality. For example, a traditional Cree healer in Saskatchewan might speculate that modern Anglo-Europeans, who live a European lifestyle, take lots of medication, and eat a diet of processed foods and chemicals, might do better with pharmaceutical therapies than a traditional healing approach foreign to their beliefs. The sacred cow of Western medicine—the randomized, controlled trial—is really limited to use within one cultural group within a uniform set of beliefs and practices. It fails, for example, among traditional healers, who are informed by spirits and other entities about herb selection, other treatments, and ceremonies. We need to hear these other stories for their evolutionary possibilities as they interact with our stories. Illness has no natural history, but only emerges as an entity or concept within the stories we tell about it. We can't actually study illness when we exclude or ignore the people who have it.

French philosopher Jean-François Lyotard describes conventional medicine's emphasis on being correct as a "politics of terror," which is the politics of forcing others out of the conversation.[5] Narrative medicine is about arranging the conversation so that everyone can have a voice, and nobody is forced outside the conversation. He believed that the availability of information would make the suppression of other and minority voices less tempting.

The value of diversity is apparent when we realize that we cannot see our hidden assumptions about the world from within our own beliefs (metaphors, maps, paradigms, theories, stories). Only someone from outside of our belief system can comment objectively on our hidden assumptions, since they don't share these assumptions. They can question us in ways we cannot question ourselves. Austrian mathematician Kurt Gödel pointed this out for mathematics when he showed that no system of mathematics can be proven from within.[6] It must be viewed from an outside perspective to see its assumptions. Another way of saying this is to say that some maps are so out-of-date they no longer reflect the territory. Unlike the map of the Spanish mountains, these maps will not lead us out of danger. We are surrounded by mountains that do not appear on the old maps. Here is where our attachment to our maps interferes with the process of living well. We must have the courage to discard old maps and find new ones. Observers from different cultures help us by pointing out when our maps are ridiculously out of date, even when we cannot see it.

American philosopher Stephen Pepper of the University of California at Berkeley believed that each of us functions from what he called a root metaphor or world hypothesis.[7] This is our map that informs us what to expect from the world. Cognitive–behavioral therapy models speak of this as our beliefs, some of which may appear to the therapist as somewhat irrational (which assumes the therapist's view of the world is more correct than the patient's). We can't take any action without a world hypothesis. This is why the map was so necessary for the soldiers. It grounded them. A grounding metaphor like that—a root metaphor—is similar to a tree that must put its roots deep within the earth to survive storms and to gather water and nutrients. Important here is the realization that the root metaphor does not need to be accurate to work. World hypothesis has been defined as "an integrated exploratory or interpretive account of the order and meaning of the full range of things, events, or happenings and their values or significance."[8] In other words, it is our preferred map.

Discovering our hidden assumptions is important because they may prevent our optimal success. Some of our maps have left out the roads to more desirable places than those we have imagined. These places we'd actually rather be are hidden. We need others who do not share our usual assumptions to point out what we have been trained not to see. This is what we do when we compare conventional medicine's story to those of its indigenous counterparts.

No map can include everything. We need maps of mysterious, spiritual, super-ordinary realities that we can't even begin to describe. Like the stories told by aboriginal elders, the stories of quantum physics—like those told by pioneering physicist and philosopher David Bohm[9]—contain maps to indescribable places that can guide and inspire us.

Bohm began his career by studying the interactions of electrons in metals. He showed that their individual, haphazard movement concealed a highly organized and cooperative behavior called plasma oscillation.

This intimated an order beneath apparent chaos. In 1959, working with Yakir Aharonov,[10] he showed that the presence of a magnetic field could alter the behavior of electrons without actually interacting with them. If two electron beams were passed on either side of a space containing a magnetic field, the field would retard the waves of one beam even though it did not penetrate the space and even though no physical possibility existed for the field to interact with the electrons. This was the first instance in which nonlocal action was demonstrated—that is, action that cannot be explained by physical events or properties, or that seems to happen outside of ordinary space and time. This phenomenon, often called "action at a distance," suggested a fundamentally different ordering of the world—one that was more similar to the views of shamans and indigenous healers than that of conventional scientists.

Bohm's universe is a mystical place where past, present, and future coexist. The objects in his universe, even the subatomic particles, are secondary; it is a process of movement, continuous unfolding and enfolding from a seamless whole that is fundamental. In an interview for *Omni* magazine in January 1987 Bohm said,

> When I was a boy, a certain prayer we said every day in Hebrew contained the words to love God with all your heart, all your soul, and all your mind. My understanding of these words—that is, this notion of wholeness, not necessarily directed toward God, but as a way of living—had a tremendous impact on me. I also felt a sense of nature being whole very early. I felt internally related to trees, mountains, and stars in a way I wasn't to all the chaos of the cities.[11]

Bohm's story is that the electron is a particle surrounded by an energy field that is never separate from it and can affect it even from a great distance, as it did in his experiment. The Hungarian philosopher Ervin Laszlo later called this the quantum scalar field, which is a field of information. Albert Einstein didn't like this interpretation because he was opposed in principle to the idea of action at a distance, that things far apart can influence each other profoundly through no recognizable physical means.

Bohm's vision was of enfoldment. He compared the universe to a piece of paper that's been folded into a small packet on which cuts have been made. When the packet is unfolded, the parts that were close are now far away, similar to what happens in a hologram. He believed that the universe is always enfolding, or turning things into smaller packets. The light in a room comes into the room in such a way that the waves of light are all connected and any one of them contains all the information available to any other. When your eye looks at the room, your eye and brain unfold the light to produce a discrete image. When you look through a telescope or a camera, the entire universe is enfolded into each part. When you look, you unfold it to see something discrete like the moon or the sun. Bohm also likened unfolding to what is done when you adjust an old-fashioned television set that is out of focus.

Bohm's science is holistic in that each part contains the whole. Each part refers back to the entire universe that contains it. He is similar to a narrative philosopher who argues that each part is inseparable from its context. This is so different from contemporary reductionist science which is defined as "the idea that everything that exists can be explained as the interactions of a small number of simple things obeying physical laws."[12] Reductionism often works for certain kinds of problems. For example, the kinetic theory of gases can predict most of the important properties of a gas as a whole, given a good understanding of the components of the system. In other cases, emergent properties of the system cannot be predicted from knowledge of the parts of the system. The patterns seen in a traffic jam cannot be predicted simply from a knowledge of the streets and the cars involved. Most certainly the activities of human beings cannot be predicted from a knowledge of their genetic code.

Telling a story is the best way to capture Bohm's notion of enfoldment. Reductionist thinking captures the results of unfolding the piece of paper, sometimes missing the whole or the context from which the observation or event came. The reductionist sees the holes in a cut piece of paper, but fails to grasp the whole. We grasp the larger whole in which we are embedded and connected through stories, because it is too large to be understood in any other way. "Shamans do this when they interpret a complex body of belief, read the power in leaves and the meaning in stones, and skillfully balance the forces of the universe and guide the play of the winds."[13]

Bohm asked us to imagine an infinite sea of energy filling space, with waves moving around and occasionally coming together to produce an intense pulse, similar to the ten- to thirteen-meter waves that sometimes occur on Hawai'i's North Shore. He asked us to imagine that one particular pulse came together and expanded to create our universe of space-time and matter. To us, that pulse seems like a big bang. In a larger context, our big bang is just a little ripple. Even the largest waves crashing upon the shore are small compared to the ocean—the context in which they emerge. Physical matter emerges by unfoldment but is also enfolding back into the implicate or greater order of the larger universe. Bohm called the enfolding process "implicating" and the unfolding process "explicating." Together, the implicate and the explicate are a flowing, undivided whole. Every part of the universe is related to every other part but in different degrees.

> In classical mechanics, movement or velocity is defined as the relation between the position now and the position a short time ago. What was a short time ago is gone, so you relate what is to what is not. This isn't a logical concept. In the implicate order you are relating frames of experience that are copresent in consciousness. You're relating what is to what is. A moment contains flow or movement. The moment may be long or short, as measured in time. In consciousness a moment is around a tenth of a second. Electronic moments are much shorter, but a moment of history might be a century.[14]

Without knowing it, Bohm took a narrative position on memory. He believed that recent events were enfolded more strongly than more remote events. At any given moment, he said, we are surrounded by and feel the presence of all the past and also all possible futures. Both the future and the past influence us in the present. All the events are all present together. Their succession in momentary memory gives us our experience of the flow of time. This succession of moments becomes our story, the story that we live.

Bohm believed that each individual consciousness unfolds the universe for itself. He believed that any high level of consciousness is a social process. He admitted that there could be some level of sensorimotor perception that was isolated to the individual, but that once we reach any abstract level, we depend on language, which is social. The word, which is outside of the individual, evokes the meaning that is inside each person.

Bohm saw meaning as the bridge between consciousness and matter, in the same way that I am arguing that story is the bridge between culture and biology. Story is where we store meaning (as shown by our constantly asking "What is the meaning of that story?"). Any given array of matter (an object like a tree, a fish, a hotel) has for any particular mind a significance or meaning. Similarly, Bohm saw meaning as immediately acting upon matter. He used the example of a shadow on a dark night. If it is interpreted as meaning "assailant," adrenaline pours out, the heart beats faster, blood pressure rises, and muscles tense. "The body and all your thoughts are affected. Everything about you has changed. If you see that it's only a shadow, there's an abrupt change again."[15]

In Bohm's implicate order, meaning or interpretation enfolds the whole world into the individual and vice versa. He believed that this enfolded meaning is unfolded as action, through the bodies of individual people acting on the world (what philosopher Jean-Paul Sartre called praxis). Even the word *hormone* means "messenger," that is, a substance carrying meaning or information. Neurotransmitters carry informative meaning, and that meaning profoundly affects the entire body. Bohm believed that meaning was being. In his view, any transformation of society must result in a profound change of meaning. Any change of meaning for the individual would change the whole because all individuals are interconnected.[16]

To further this discussion of parts and wholes, of unfolding and enfolding, of implicate and explicate, we need a story. Bethany was a thirty-six-year-old woman who had successfully completed treatment for thyroid cancer ten years previously and been pronounced cured. I met her on referral from her internist for help with stress-related symptoms. Those symptoms sounded suspiciously like seizures. An EEG confirmed this, and an MRI showed a temporal lobe tumor. Within one week, she underwent surgery and a tumor called a glioblastoma multiforme was removed. Almost all patients with this diagnosis die within eleven months of diagnosis. Bethany is still alive nine years later. How do we explain this?

Bethany took the standard chemotherapy and radiation therapy. The best estimate at the time was that these treatments would prolong her life by 4 percent—not a dramatic increase. Some of her friends suggested she would be better off skipping these difficult therapies. Bethany disagreed, believing they would have extraordinary benefit for her. To his credit, her neuro-oncologist never disagreed with her optimism. In addition, she joined our weekly healing circle. She requested extra visualization and energy healing sessions. Bethany attended the sweatlodges and healing ceremonies of the local Native American community, along with several others of us.

In Bethany's version of her story, she reinvented her life as she surrounded herself with people who believed that she would be well. She left a stressful job that she hated. She left a relationship that was going nowhere. She created a new, sustainable life and a reason to live. Bethany continues to avoid pessimists. She surrounds herself with loving friends and family, believing that she needs that level of positive culture.

How do we explain Bethany's story? How unusual is it? Skeptics might avoid discussing her, since the pathology reports and laboratory findings cannot be challenged. Nor can her continued existence be questioned. The medical model limits itself with its insistence that the cure of all states of discomfort must be linked to a precise identified pathological mechanism.[17] Treatment must have a mechanism of action in direct correspondence to this pathological mechanism. But Bethany's "cure" cannot be directly linked to any specific treatment. It defies explanation on that level, as do most stories of miraculous healing. Can the concepts of physics, perhaps Bohm's notions, help us explain her healing? Is she connected to the entire universe in such a way that miracles can unfold and manifest in her life?

Bethany's outcome is so far from the mean for the population of all patients with glioblastoma that it would be an act of faith to claim that the chemotherapy and radiation therapy somehow worked amazingly better for her than it did for almost all others, though this explanation is certainly possible. On the other hand, psychological or even New Age explanations for healing appear to be constructed post hoc, as an interpretive effort to explain something that has already happened. Nor have these explanations shown predictive power. For example, people who measure high on the "fighting spirit" construct do not necessarily live longer than people who measure "low" on this construct. Bethany's story is unique to her. What baffles conventional medicine in its attempt to explain healing is the possibility that *no one thing or combination of things healed her.* This new story says that Bethany was part of a transformative effort that involved her and others in ways that were a priori unpredictable. In Bohm's terms, she contained the entire universe and it unfolded within her to transform her in ways that could not be anticipated, replicated, predicted, or controlled.

Bethany's own explanation is completely different from that of another man I know who is a ten-year survivor of glioblastoma. Their stories are so different that an argument would ensue if these two individuals were to meet—at least as long as we keep to the conventional paradigm of stable causes with fixed and measurable effects. Loren's story is about the removal of mercury fillings and other toxic metals, coupled with his passion to share the idea with other people with cancer that they too can heal the way he did. How do we scientifically study such disparate explanations? For Bohm, this would be no problem, since the entire universe is contained within each individual, and it is merely a matter of them unfolding what they need.

What if we move away from medicine as a natural science and toward medicine as a systems science—one that integrates multiple perspectives and levels and draws its inspiration more from quantum physics than from classical mechanics? This perspective moves us away from the search for "powerful healers" or "powerful techniques," to the search for how systems make dramatic changes of state.

This new medicine can embrace the self-healing and emergent properties of systems that physical chemists G. Nicolis and I. Prigogine (recipient of the Nobel Prize) have called "far from equilibrium."[18] Systems maintain equilibrium. They keep things the same. Systems transform only when they are in a state far from equilibrium. Equilibrium states are represented as valleys, while far-from-equilibrium states are represented as mountain passes. Considerable effort is needed to cross the pass into another valley. Once the system is far from equilibrium (near the top of the pass), even minimal effort is enough to complete the journey. This concept offers a potential explanation for the success of so-called "wacky therapies" that only work for some people, sometimes, and cannot be replicated.

Conventional medicine prefers to deal in the linear regions of ordinary life, in the village nestled comfortably in the valley. It's fun to look up at the mountain peaks, but not to climb them or cross arduous passes. That's dangerous and tiring. Narrative medicine, however, must address life on the passes—the transitions between stable states. Conventional medicine seeks biological agents that work the same way for everyone. It seeks reliability and reproducibility of results. Healing, however, is an individual phenomenon. Everyone does it differently. Every person finds his or her own way across the mountain pass, because everyone is situated in different psycho-socio-cultural space. This means that we need to study how people transform, instead of seeking what cured them.

Perhaps our quest for "powerful healers" is just another version of the quest for powerful drugs. The source for healing lies within the internal reorganization of the person as system (including the larger systems within which the person is embedded). The wizardry and power comes from changes in organization, from within rather than without. Perhaps this is more important for even conventional pharmacological therapies and surgeries than we have imagined. Like shamans, we need to address what determines the organism's response to an intervention instead of the intervention itself.

Coherence and Connectivity

Healing is difficult to understand, because it lies outside the cause-and-effect paradigm of classical mechanics. Spiritual healing cannot be traced to a linear series of events. It appears to arise almost out of nowhere from within the entity (person, family, community) being healed. Quantum physics points us toward ideas of coherence and connectivity. We are forced to consider anew exactly how we are all linked. How do we affect each other? A potentially radical shift occurs if we ask these questions not just about psychology or sociology, but also about biology. From this point of view, the separation of disciplines and specialties cultivated by universities, journals, and medical centers is illusory. Separations are acts of perception and not facts of nature. We exist in an indivisible whole.

The concept of coherence, key to the study of quantum physics, furnishes a nonbiological, nonlocal explanatory metaphor involving shared information, rather than a mechanical process of cause and effect. The concept offers some glimmers of awareness into how systems can reorganize themselves in "interventional fields." It provides foundations for an understanding of how the intent of a community can produce biological effects and how embeddedness in a healing environment can be associated with sudden, dramatic shifts in physiology. First, we must understand the phenomenon as it is emerging in physics, remembering that our explanations are simplified stories about something beyond our capacity for understanding.

The ideas about connectivity, coherence, embeddedness, and entanglement emerging from quantum physics represent a dramatic departure from the classical sciences. Classical physics and astronomy studied independent, discrete objects. Classical psychology studied independent, discrete individuals whose behavior could be understood entirely from within them. Classical economics posed a kind of market fundamentalism—that all problems could be solved by the unrestricted actions of the marketplace and that these actions were independent of the other forces at work in society. When particles or people behave in a correlated fashion (and we don't think they should), we proclaim the mysterious existence of coherence, which implies connectivity through nonphysical means.

Coherence represents a correlation between apparently unrelated events, processes, objects, or measurements. Coherence occurs when soldiers march in synchronized step across a bridge. The resonant frequencies augment each other because of the coherence of their steps and can produce such power as to cause the bridge to collapse. This is why soldiers have, historically, broken formation and run across a bridge in a random fashion, only to assemble and resume marching on the other side. Coherence occurs in relation to connections that are not immediately, physically apparent.

Coherence is a powerful explanatory concept in human behavior. Anthropologist Gregory Bateson and his colleagues at the Mental Research Institute of Palo Alto championed the idea of coherence within families—that the actions of individuals are correlated.[19] They asserted that the behaviors, thoughts, and feelings of one member are connected to the behaviors, thoughts, and feelings of other members. Philosopher Michel Foucault presented the idea that the behaviors, thoughts, feelings, and actions of members of a society were related to society-wide conversations regarding knowledge and power—what we think and do is correlated or connected to what those in power think and do.[20] He proposed that these transactions are mediated through knowledge—the flow of information and the relations constructed to regulate the flow of information.

Experiments demonstrating coherence in physics show us that objects are connected. I discussed many of these experiments in *Coyote Wisdom,* all of which demonstrated that changes occur in material objects in physics experiments for reasons that are outside of our usual understanding or grasp of electromagnetic energy. They involve merely the transfer of information and even at instantaneous speeds (much faster than the speed of light). What this implies is a radical connectedness among particles in physics, and perhaps, by extension, everything in the universe. Furthermore, some of these physics experiments showed that the intent of the scientist (to make a measurement or to discover something) radically changed the outcome of the experiment. If it does so in physics, how could it not do so in medicine?

Once connected, what happens to one particle simultaneously influences the other so as to preserve that connection. The particles begin to influence each other through nonphysical means. I think people do the same. The human implication of the scientific idea of coherence is that change in any one of us affects all of those to whom we are related, and vice versa. We cannot escape being affected by those with whom we are coherent, whether we are conscious of this or not. Connection is the rule, rather than the exception. We begin to see that interactions with others modulate and modify our internal states, even create them. Relationships that engender healing do so because coherence has developed among the participants. Conversation and interaction guide mood, and humans may not be able to regulate mood in isolation. Perhaps so-called mood disorders are becoming more prevalent because of our increasing isolation. When we depend on a brain in isolation, mood fluctuates wildly. It has no modulators. "Rather than seeing attitudes and emotions as mentally held, internally generated, and slow to change, perhaps they are a consequence of talk, partial and flexible techniques for communication that emerge in a constantly shifting interaction."[21]

The ideas that link the concepts of narrative medicine to quantum physics include the following:

- Human illness, and its progression or disappearance, is context dependent—related to the network of relationships in which the particular individual is embedded, and depending on cultural and social factors yet to be determined. Disease is not purely biological or genetic. It does not have a natural history, but rather a biopsychosocial, historical, cultural, and geophysical history.
- Systems (meaning wholes that are greater than the sum of their parts) are self-healing (self-correcting), demonstrate emergent properties (meaning that new things emerge that cannot be anticipated or predicted), and are capable of developing unique, novel outcomes that are not relevant or applicable to any other system. Even biological treatments, with their powerful mechanisms of action, also have informational components in which they stimulate self-healing and system reorganization.
- Dramatic biological change (healing) is associated with an internal reorganization of the system of the person and of systems surrounding the person. Information transfer that facilitates this reorganization may be more important that the provision of external agents.

The hierarchy of systems principle says that behavior is similar at all levels.[22] Systems theory postulates that the operating principles of any level of discourse or explanation (*hierarchy* in systems terminology) are similar to those at any other level. Demonstrating the existence of a phenomenon at the smallest possible and the largest possible levels suggests that it might operate at levels in-between. If coherence exists on the level of photons, could it also exist on the level of social relationships? Are we humans inextricably interconnected? To borrow quantum physics terminology, are we hopelessly entangled in each other? Does the entanglement (of people who are embedded in a natural (social and geographic) landscape) form a society and a culture?

Family coherence suggests that I instantaneously sense shifts in the thoughts, feelings, or behavior of my brother, and then compensate to preserve symmetry or relatedness to him (without necessarily being conscious of this). Coherence provides an explanation for the mysterious changes family members make during family therapy—for example, Gregory Bateson's description of family members passing around the identified patient role.[23] Family coherence means that I must change if my brother changes in order to preserve symmetry in my relationship with him. It means that I am not independent from my brother. We are correlated or entangled. What he does affects me—*even at great distances*.

Family therapists Jay Haley and Paul Watzlawick implicitly described coherence when they wrote about the mysterious ways that family members changed individuals to keep patterns of interaction the same (maintain homeostasis) within the family.[24] Philadelphia psychiatrist Salvador Minuchin proposed this idea, especially in his studies of families with anorexic or psychotic members.[25] Gregory Bateson explained this phenomenon using information theory or cybernetics, specifically with the thermostat metaphor.[26] Families try to regulate the affective climate to keep anger levels the same, even though the anger passes through different family members, appearing first in one, then in another. Similarly, he wrote about depression being constant within a family with different members expressing it at different times. The concept of coherence from quantum physics becomes a more elegant metaphor than a thermostat for familial interaction patterns. It provides more explanatory power, suggesting the power of relatedness across all levels of nature and the need to preserve symmetry. We behave like others who originate from the same source as we do (family members). We sometimes radically change directions to maintain symmetry when others from the same source as us change.

One of my favorite examples of self-regulation and the need to preserve symmetry comes from the Gaia hypothesis.[27] This hypothesis arises from evidence such as the narrow temperature range maintained on the surface of the earth since life began, compared with the temperature range experienced in the universe. Even the great ice ages were small blips in an otherwise even life of constant temperature. Lovelock calculates the probability of this occurring by chance to be a ridiculously infinitesimal number, concluding that Earth is self-regulating. Astrophysicist Robert Nadeau discovered a similar phenomenon operating at the macroscopic level of the whole universe and concluded that homeostasis in the universe can be maintained only through cooperation and coherence among its parts, not random chance.[28] This lends support to what philosopher Ervin Laszlo calls the God hypothesis, which states that the universe is self-regulating and therefore worthy of the ascription of consciousness.[29] (Bateson argued that all self-regulating systems are entitled to be called conscious, though the subjective experience of consciousness within self-regulating systems might vary dramatically.[30])

Why should we care about coherence from the standpoint of the social world? Descartes is credited with the idea that the social interactions of two minds are independent from their embeddedness in the physical world of bodies. French philosopher Maurice Merleau-Ponty championed the opposite idea—that all of our perceptions (whether of direct sensation or the reading of complex physical instruments) are embedded in a world constructed through our bodies.[31]

We are connected through social interaction (which is simultaneously nonlocal or energetic as well as based in verbal conversations) so that we know at faster-than-light speeds what is happening with another person and respond to that information sometimes without even consciously registering that we are doing so. We may dream the same dream as another, we may choose our clothing in the morning in relation to what the other person chooses; our attitudes and beliefs vary in relationship to this ongoing dialogue of connectivity that occurs on multiple levels (some wordless). These nonverbal, possibly even energetic exchanges modulate our internal states. I suspect we have as little awareness about these as we do about how conversation changes us. Most of us believe that we are guiding the conversation, while conversation may be the milieu in which we are embedded—we are inseparable from the conversation and from the others within it.

All of these concepts shatter our ideas about independence and objectivity. We are far less autonomous than we might have imagined. If everything is connected, how can anything be independent? If healing emerges through this relatedness, this coherence, how can there be an objective place from which to study it? The existence of coherence forces the destruction of our conventional concepts of the individual—especially the autonomous, freely choosing, rational man of the Enlightenment or the romantic ideal of the rugged individualist of North America. Such people only pretend to themselves and others that they operate in isolation from the rest of us.

The demonstration of coherence in physics (and its slowly evolving demonstration in social life, as reflected in studies of distance healing, the power of prayer, psychic phenomena, spiritual healing, and the like) inspires us to deconstruct our concept of the individual and the self. If I am hopelessly entangled with other people, then who am I? I am certainly not an autonomous being who rationally chooses what I do, especially when family–systems studies demonstrate that I will change without even realizing it in order to maintain symmetry within the family, as Bateson suggested, to regulate the affective climate.[32]

Coherence inspires me to realize that my concepts are largely products of my fear of uncertainty, my wish to know, and to recognize that I know for sure what's going on, when I don't. It means we can never be certain where we stop and others begin, which is exactly the situation in physics today where matter is seen as a wave of energy with varying densities and structures spreading outward in a probability distribution. I'm hopelessly unable to decide what is self and what is non-self, and I'm relatively unable to know with certainty why I do anything, though my creative mind can generate any number of fantastic post hoc explanations for my actions (past lives, penis envy, fear of castration, sibling rivalry, hormonal imperatives, and on and on). My concepts are only a story I create to satisfy my need for certainty.

Evidence for Coherence and Connectivity in the Biological Realm

Entanglement is central to the science of connectivity. Entanglement refers to the interaction of distant states that are not capable of interacting within the rules of classical physics and biology. Their interaction cannot be predicted by knowledge of their individual attributes, but arises from relationships rather than from intrinsic, internal properties. Quantum biology, the newly emerging science resulting from the application of the ideas of quantum physics to biology, describes a state in which individual molecular reactions occurring at specific space-time points carry out their individual functions, with an overall coordination that cannot be explained except by coherence. What I am suggesting is that stories are the means through which we can grasp that coherence. Stories are shorthand means of keeping track of what is happening, even on a molecular level. It is not that the story causes anything. These processes run deep. It is just that the story contains the overview we seek, the sense of the bigger picture, to which all these smaller processes are subservient.

In these biological systems the uncertainty principle holds and we cannot know everything about the system all at once. R. P. Bajpai writes about the remarkable capabilities that these processes bestow on living systems, including perfectly secure communication, virtually perfect information transfer, and signal detection below noise thresholds.[33] The emerging picture places control outside of the individual and his or her consciousness, and within a broader self-regulating system or pattern to which we belong. Properties emerge without individual design. The self-made man of the Enlightenment or the winner of the Darwinist competition disappears.

Evidence is accumulating to overthrow molecular determinism (the view that all life processes can be adequately explained by referring to underlying molecular interactions). Biological psychiatry as it is currently practiced is the sine qua non of molecular determinism, operating as if all psychological phenomena have molecular explanations and can be modified by pharmacological means. Quantum biology is also challenging the beliefs of genetic determinism—the claim that the set of genes in the genome contains a complete set of instructions for building and operating the organism. Quantum biologists are beginning to suspect that some basic developmental processes are outside of genetic control or only indirectly affected by genes. Biologist Lev Beloussov suggests that genes themselves may merely be obedient servants fulfilling powerful commands from the rest of the organism or even larger entities—an opposite view to those held by the genetic-control hypothesis advocates.[34]

Laszlo points out two impressive paradoxes that weaken the genetic-control hypothesis. First, a simple amoeba has two hundred times more DNA per cell than a human cell. The number of genes of closely related rodents can vary by a factor of two, and the housefly has five times more genes than the fruit fly.[35] This is called the C-value paradox. The genetic-control hypothesis predicts that more complex organisms should have more genes, which is not the case. The complexity of the organism in its phenome (the actual physical expression; what it appears to be) is not reflected in the complexity of the genome; in fact, the opposite is found. The second paradox is the gene-number hypothesis: in the organisms, more genes are always found without functions than genes with functions. The set of functional genes is far smaller than the set of all genes—another embarrassing finding for the genetic determinism hypothesis.

What should we study, if not molecular and genetically determined events? What about the relations between organs in a biological system, or the flow of information from external sources into and outside of the organism? These studies are proceeding in the biological realm as they are in the human realm.

Evidence for Coherence and Connectivity in the Human Realm

The first controlled experiments on connectivity between humans separated in space and in time date to J. B. Rhine's card- and dice-guessing work at Duke University in the 1930s.[36] These experiments showed that some individuals could guess much better than could be attributed to chance alone. Since then, experiments have become progressively more sophisticated, and no evidence has emerged to suggest a role for hidden sensory cues, machine bias, cheating by subjects, experimenter error, or incompetence in explaining the often positive results.

In 1976, Russell Targ and Harold Puthoff conducted experiments to explore the possibility of telepathic transmission between individuals, one acting as "sender" and the other as "receiver."[37] The receiver was placed in a sealed, opaque, electrically shielded chamber and the sender in another room where he or she was subjected to bright flashes of light at regular intervals. Electroencephalographs (EEG) recorded the brain-wave patterns of both. The sender exhibited the EEG pattern that usually accompanies exposure to bright flashes of light. After a brief interval, the receiver began to produce the same patterns, even though this person was not exposed to the flashes or receiving sense-perceivable signals from the sender.

Targ and Puthoff conducted further experiments on remote viewing.[38] In these tests, sender and receiver were separated by distances that precluded any form of sensory communication. At a randomly chosen site, the sender acted as a "beacon" and the receiver attempted to see what the sender saw. To document his or her impressions, the receiver gave verbal descriptions, at times accompanied by sketches. Independent judges found that roughly 66 percent of the time, the descriptions of the sketches matched the characteristics of the site that was actually seen by the sender. (Remote-viewing experiments reported from other laboratories, involving distances from half a mile to several thousand miles, generally reported success rates of around 50 percent, considerably above random probability. The most successful viewers appeared to be those who were relaxed, attentive, and meditative. They reported receiving a preliminary impression as a gentle and fleeting form that gradually evolved into an integrated image. They experienced the image as a surprise, both because it was clear to their perception and because it was clearly elsewhere in space and time than the physical location of the experiment.)

Between 1964 and 1969, Stanley Krippner and associates carried out what they called "dream ESP experiments" at Maimondes Hospital in New York City.[39] A volunteer spent the night at the laboratory. He or she would meet the sender and the experimenters on arrival, when the laboratory procedure was explained. Electrodes were attached to the volunteer's head to monitor EEG and eye movements. No further sensory contact occurred with the sender until the next morning. One of the experimenters threw dice that, in combination with a random-number table, gave a number that corresponded to a sealed envelope containing an art print. The envelope was opened when the sender reached his or her private room in a distant part of the hospital. The sender then spent the night concentrating on the print. The experimenters woke the volunteers by intercom when the monitor showed the end of a period of rapid eye movement (REM) sleep. The subject was then asked to describe any dream he or she might have had before awakening. The comments were recorded, together with the contents of an interview the next morning when the subject was asked to associate with the remembered dreams. The interview was conducted in a double-blind fashion—neither the subject nor the experimenters knew which art print had been selected the night before.

Using data taken from the first night that each volunteer spent at the dream laboratory, the series of experiments produced sixty-two nights of data for analysis. The data showed a significant correlation between the art print selected for a given night and the recipient's dreams on that night. The score was considerably higher on nights when there were few or no electrical storms in the area and sunspot activity was low—that is, when Earth's geomagnetic field was relatively undisturbed.

Psychologist Jacobo Grinberg-Zylberbaum, at the National University of Mexico, also demonstrated these concepts using EEGs.[40] He put pairs of people inside soundproof and electromagnetic radiation-proof Faraday cages (devices that prevent any known energy from entering or leaving) and asked them to meditate together for twenty minutes. Then he separated the pair into two different cages and stimulated one member of the pair at random intervals with a series of 100 events—things like flashes of light, sounds, or short, intense (but not painful) electricity to the index and ring finger of the right hand. The other member of the pair remained relaxed with eyes closed and was instructed to feel the presence of the partner. There was no known way (in terms of energy that we know) that the "unstimulated" partner could know what was happening to the "stimulated" partner. The EEGs of both subjects were then compared. Among subjects who had prior relationships before meeting at the laboratory, the EEG changes that were seen in the stimulated people were also seen in the unstimulated partner in 25 percent of the cases. A young couple, deeply in love, provided a particularly poignant example. Their EEG patterns remained closely synchronized throughout the experiment, during which they reported feeling a deep oneness. In a limited way, Grinberg-Zylberbaum was able to replicate the results of these experiments. When an unstimulated subject showed EEG changes in one experiment, he tended to show them again in other experiments. A variety of control conditions also demonstrated no effects.

A related experiment investigated the degree of synchrony between the left and right hemispheres of a person's cerebral cortex.[41] In ordinary waking consciousness, the two hemispheres of the brain exhibit uncoordinated wave patterns in the EEG. This study showed that when people enter a meditative state of consciousness, these patterns become synchronized. In deep meditation, the two hemispheres fall into a nearly identical pattern. Experiments with up to twelve subjects showed an astonishing synchronization of the brain waves of the entire group when people meditated together. These experiments provide some experimental justification for the belief that we are all connected.[42]

Psychotherapists have reported memories, feelings, attitudes, and associations experienced during sessions that were outside the usual scope of their experience and personality.[43] At the time these strange experiences occurred, they were indistinguishable from the memories, feelings, and related sentiments of the therapists themselves. Only later, upon reflection, did they come to realize that the anomalous events stemmed not from their own life and experiences, but from those of their patients. In the course of the therapeutic relationship, some aspect of the patient's psyche was projected into the mind of the therapist. In that location, at least for a limited time, it integrated with the therapist's own psyche and produced an awareness of some of the patient's memories, feeling, and associations.

William Braud and Marilyn Schlitz carried out trials regarding the impact of the mental imagery of senders on the physiology of receivers who were at a distance and unaware that such imagery was being directed to them.[44] They reported that the mental images of the sender caused changes in the physiology of the distant receiver—effects comparable to those that one's own mental processes produce in one's own body. People who attempted to influence their own bodily functions were only slightly more effective than those who attempted to influence the physiology of others. The difference between remote influence and self-influence was almost insignificant: "Telesomatic" influence by a distant person proved to be nearly as effective as "psychosomatic" influence by the same person.

Embeddedness of Consciousness and Experience Determines Meaning-Making

Individuals are not meaning-makers apart from the social milieus or systems in which they operate. Sociologist Erving Goffman asserted that we bring our interpretations to any social circumstance, and, with them, our sense of what our part should be in that circumstance. Goffman wrote, "A teammate is someone whose dramaturgical co-operation one is dependent upon in fostering a given definition of the situation. . . ."[45] Our interpretation of a social circumstance is forged by our participation or embeddedness in that social system. The system itself emerges through the coherence of individuals who belong to that system. The system maintains itself through the connectivity of individuals who are embedded within it.

Healing is difficult to understand because of this embeddedness. If we are all interlaced with each other and each has something to say about the others' conditions (including health and disease), then we are all responsible for sudden shifts in health and disease, though in what way is often a guess. The nice linear cause-and-effect relationships so desired by modern medicine and biology rapidly break down in the bog of healing. We have to abandon our quest for simple explanations and certainty when we embrace embeddedness.

Another way of thinking about context and embeddedness comes from Goffman's concept of the frame—the boundary between action within and action without.[46] The frame is the context in which action occurs and those participating in that action are firmly embedded in that frame. For Goffman, the frame marked off local events from the ongoing flow of surrounding events through a special set of boundary markers or brackets occurring before and after the activity in time or surrounding it in space. His standard example was "the set of devices that has come to be employed in Western dramaturgy: at the beginning, the lights dim, the bell rings, and the curtain rises; at the other end, the curtain falls and the lights go on."[47] A story is framed when we introduce it by saying, "Once upon a time . . ." A school day is framed by the opening bell, the closing bell, and the physical boundaries of the school.

Goffman's frame represents a kind of fluid boundary between the system contained and the containing system. One frame for an individual is the family. A frame for a family is the extended kinship system in traditional societies, or a looser network of friendship circles in modern, Western societies. But unlike earlier versions of systems theory applied to the human condition, quantum physics has destroyed the neat metaphor of boxes within boxes, each larger box nicely containing the smaller box. Quantum physics reveals an absence of clear boundaries between boxes or frames, with multiple intersections and a breakdown of the classical notion of hierarchy. We are all contaminants in each other's frames. We are embedded within each other's systems in ways we cannot even guess. The human drama exists within the bio-geographical frame, referring to nature and the specific geographical region in which our particular human drama of interest unfolds.

The term embeddedness arises from physics, while framing comes from theater and art. Hence, we can create an equivalency between the metaphor of the theater and the metaphor of physics—the essence of systemic understanding—that common processes underlie operations everywhere. Goffman saw framing as a constitutive act that people accomplish through their interaction. He saw attunement in understanding and purpose as coordinating social interaction. When we ground this attunement in the concepts of coherence and embeddedness, we show how attunement is a characteristic of all systems, and not just human ones. Goffman viewed attunement as coming from participants meeting "system requirements" (demonstrating that they were capable of participating within the frame). The system imposes its requirements or constraints upon its members who naturally adjust to comply. Attunement and coherence both result from and create shared membership.

Systemic evolution occurs when systems find themselves far from their usual equilibrium and then transform. This is what we commonly call healing. Goffman says, "In these circumstances, the whole framework of . . . constraints—both system and ritual—can become something to honor, to invert, or to disregard, depending on the mood that strikes. On these occasions, it's not merely that the lid can't be closed, but that there is no box."[48] The system reaches such a far-from-equilibrium condition that it reorganizes itself. It transforms and reinvents itself. It reconstitutes itself. It *heals*.

New properties emerge from this transformation. Evolutionary leaps happen suddenly—not through Darwin's progressive process of natural selection, but abruptly, dramatically, and in a hurry.

Making Maps for Healing— Which Selves, Which Worlds?

We are stuck within the frame of our culture and must work within it. Stepping outside of this frame is impossible, though some individuals can become truly bicultural (and rarely, tricultural). Our own frame changes as it interfaces with other frames. While we cannot escape having a culture, the forms and structures taken by the cultures of the world do vary widely. The abundance and diversity of different cultures suggests that their forms are somewhat arbitrary and created by us.

What makes indigenous methods of healing unusual to Western culture is that they potentially work through what physicist and Nobel laureate Erwin Schrödinger called the dynamic order, instead of by making mechanical changes—what is within biomedicine's comfort zone. Dynamic order exists because of system-wide correlations that involve all parts, even those distantly related. Dynamic order refers to the organization of system components and system-wide correlations between parts that permit smooth functioning.[49]

People of antiquity saw (and today's indigenous people see) human health and disease within the context of the world in which the person is embedded, including their cosmic context.[50] The indigenous view is like the systems view which reacts to the classical scientific method by putting people back into the world in which they live, and seeing them as embedded and emerging in this world. By emerging, I mean new properties appearing that could not be predicted prior to their appearance. Regarding the classical scientific method, Laszlo wrote that it "led to the fragmentation of our understanding of human beings. In the midst of all the complex special theories, we have gained little real insight into human nature itself."[51]

The study of healing must expand beyond the worldview created by classical methods. A larger view is needed that can consider the multiple, interacting and interrelated frames within which people live. Classical medicine stops at the frame of the body, ignoring the social world and the importance of human relationships with multiple frames, including the natural world. The realization that all levels affect all other levels renders meaningless the concept of independent variables and the separation of disciplines, which is the current frame of conventional medicine.

Having looked at the world in which healing occurs, we must also consider who or what is being healed. All systems show evidence of reactivity to elements from the external world, and respond in an effort to increase or decrease exposure to those elements. This assertion is a definition of subjectivity, suggesting that humans are not unique in having this property. Laszlo wrote, "We must end by acknowledging that subjectivity is possessed by all natural systems, although the grade of subjectivity differs from level to level and species to species. There is no unique correlation between the nervous system and the capacity for subjective sensation."[52]

In this view, the subjects (including humans) are interconnected with each other and the world. We abandon the notion of discrete human beings entirely enclosed by their skin.

Studies of non-ordinary reality must also inform our understanding of the self.[53] The work of Stanislav Grof with altered states of consciousness (ASC) induced by psychoactive drugs or breathing techniques showed that ASC embraced a large part of the human psyche; the states of normal waking consciousness being but the tip of the iceberg.[54] Studies of non-ordinary reality are important in understanding the person who heals and the healing process. More than one hundred years ago, William James noted:

> Our normal waking consciousness . . . is but one special type of consciousness, whilst all about it, parted from it by the flimsiest of screens, there lie potential forms of consciousness that were entirely different. We may go through life without suspecting their existence; but apply the requisite stimulus, and at a touch they are all there in all their completeness.[55]

Because people are connected, embedded, and entangled, their physiological processes are influenced by systems outside of the conventional limits posed by modern biology. Healing is actually internal systems reorganization occurring at far-from-equilibrium conditions, and it is dependent upon the historical, sociocultural, and geological matrix or frame into which the person is embedded. The frame provides the conditions under which internal reorganization can occur. The common observation that healing requires a community recognizes that the thoughts and beliefs of those to whom we are connected cohere with our own to produce a sustained output that influences everyone's physiology. Our cells are informed of our common intent by those to whom we are connected.

We can summarize these observations in the following points:

- Human disease and its progression or disappearance is context-dependent—it depends on the network of relationships in which the particular individual is embedded and on cultural and social factors yet to be determined. Disease is not purely biological or genetic.
- Systems are self-correcting and self-healing, demonstrate emergent properties, and are capable of developing unique, novel outcomes that are not relevant or applicable to any other system. Emergent properties are novel events or transformations appearing without explanation from interacting systems, except to point to the role of internal reorganization of elements of the system in producing novel behavior or properties that could not have been anticipated.

- Healing can result from the internal reorganization of a system. Information transfer that facilitates this reorganization may be more important than the provision of external agents.

Systems, including human systems, undergo remarkable internal reorganizations when their contexts shift and they find themselves far from equilibrium. Healing is our ordinary-language way of talking about these dramatic shifts. Because of the idiosyncrasy of these internal shifts, related to preexisting organization (also called history) and to the new contexts that are being formed, formulaic attempts to predict healing are doomed to fail. Each system must be considered by its own merits.

Instead of ignoring the natural sciences, we can contextualize them. In doing this, we find a basis for the scientific study of healing. Through our progressive broadening of context or frame, we may encounter other provocative hypotheses, including the idea that the geological region in which we are embedded conditions and influences the shapes and forms that our thoughts (art, writing, science) take, helping to explain differences in the music, shapes, and rituals of the earth's geographic regions. How far embeddedness will go as a hypothesis remains to be determined.

Once we have come to appreciate this, we can understand why healing is not rational, why we need new science to study healing, and why one size does not fit all to explain healing. We can look at systems of healing and how they provide information for component parts of systems to reorganize themselves, and can understand the pivotal role of dialogue (in all of its definitions) in this process. I think then, we will stop arguing about the efficacy of individual techniques and will abandon our obsession with the randomized, controlled trial or even the idea that we can control anything at all. We will adopt methods of current physics and systems engineering to study systems that are moving toward transformation so that we can learn how to influence those processes to move in the directions we prefer (health and wellness) rather than toward the directions we do not prefer (illness and disease).

We can develop a different kind of science—a descriptive, hermeneutic methodology. A science with which we learn how to study the process of transformation, how to recognize when conditions are ripe for transformation, and how to predict when transformation will occur, even if we cannot know what the result of that transformation will look like. We can learn how to ask the right questions to discover how specific systems transform. Perhaps a science of necessary and sufficient conditions will emerge. Perhaps we can learn to recognize systems that are too close to equilibrium for sudden, dramatic reorganization to form. Perhaps we can learn how to assist systems in questioning prevailing assumptions and allegiances so that transformation becomes more likely.

When we shift our focus from the action of external agents to the flow and organization of all kinds of information, we arrive at a radical new science that is more quantum than mechanical. We can come to understand how small interventions for far-from-equilibrium systems provoke reorganization, while large interventions for systems close to equilibrium have no effect. We can gain that understanding only through hearing the stories of systems that change and systems that don't change, perhaps bringing them together to consider similarities and differences, to compare each other's contexts. I propose that this work will further the conventional natural systems by bringing a context to biology, allowing us to better understand why some people respond to treatment and others do not.

4
Master Narratives

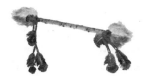

The truth is the thing I invented so I could live.

NICOLE KRAUSS[1]

We were biologically destined to become cultural creatures, but biology did not determine what kind of culture we would have. The values of a group (or the morals of their stories) determine its growth, persistence, or decay. Cultures are value-guided systems, just as stories have plot. Cultures satisfy value needs. Values guide our concepts of rationality, meaningfulness in emotional experience, richness of imagination, and depth of faith. The form in which cultures satisfy our needs is dependent upon the specific kinds of values people hold.[2]

The concept of values can be used to tie the behavior of cultural systems to other systems. The narrative perspective emphasizes the role of values in determining the plots of stories. While stories are created as products of human brains trying to make sense of the world for a variety of purposes, these stories are often about larger systems in which we find ourselves or with which we are interacting. Our stories try to explain the values we perceive these systems—including other people—to be operating from. We have an implicit understanding that events make sense if we capture the underlying values that lead others to perform specific acts. Even a simple thermostat pursues the value of keeping the temperature constant. The universe pursues the value of maintaining the cosmological parameters in a narrow, constant range, preventing excessive expansion or immediate contraction, and allowing things to be as they are—meaning stable. The earth pursues the value of temperature regulation and climate control.[3]

To the extent that we absorb the stories of a culture, we absorb the values or morals of those stories. The ways we get caught in pursuing those values mirrors Michel Foucault's description of how people become unwitting constituents of power-knowledge systems or Erving Goffman's description of the experience of membership in a frame. We do what we're supposed to. We do what we are expected to do. We perform in the ways that our roles demand from us. How else can we explain ordinary people committing the atrocities of the Native American genocide in North America, the massive and tortuous executions of the French and Spanish Inquisitions, the killing fields of the Khmer Rouge, and current suicide bombings? What the narrative perspective adds is the realization that we have a story to explain what we do and that this story emerged through dialogue with others. This story is cocreated through our social relationships, some of which take the form of power relationships, in which others demand actions from us based upon their power over us.

The world's traditional cultural stories have historically held a society together. They orient the people about what to think, feel, and believe. They teach the values of the group. They inform the people how to behave. They come from distant ancestors. They may contain or inform rituals or important events. Storytellers alter or edit, combine, and adapt tales for changing times and conditions. Stories change as culture changes, and the two may be synonymous. Traditional stories are passed from generation to generation and from the old to the young by word of mouth. This is the oral tradition. It helps people organize their experiences into meaningful patterns. While cultures do not share the same emotions or values or beliefs, a striking similarity is found among folktales from different parts of the world.

As best as we can understand, precontact aboriginal culture revolved around stories. Today, many aboriginal writers say that we are our stories. Storytelling in this past was not mundane. People narrated their lives to their community as a means of teaching and as a form of entertainment. This was how they came to be understood and to understand each other. This is how shared or group identity was constructed. It was how values became consistent among group members. This narration was the original documentary. The presentation of one's life story before an audience revealed not only what happened but also gave a somewhat authentic sense of the person telling the story. With the exception of the most venerated elders, surely this narration involved certain challenging and confrontational interactions with the audience in which some versions of stories shared were contested, modified, and revised.

Psychologist Theodore Sarbin said, "We live in a story-shaped world."[4] He believed that every aspect of our mental and social lives, from our dreams and nightmares through the rituals of work, family, and worship, to the experience of life as a daily tumble of events, is fashioned by story. This occurs through both *plot* and *action*. We use plot to link seemingly disconnected events together into an understandable story with a beginning, middle, and an end. The actual behaviors of individuals must make sense within the intentional, goal-directed context of a story. Our stories also have moral dimensions that permit listeners to weigh the motives of the characters as well as give meaning to the action(s) detailed within the story.

The larger stories in which we often unconsciously dwell have been called "master narratives" and provide the meanings and values within which people position their identities.[5] While master narratives establish sequences of actions and events as routines thereby normalizing them, they also give guidance and direction to everyday actions. Without this guidance and sense of direction, we would be lost. Master narratives become habitual, and, to the extent that their enactment becomes our routine, the more we become subjected to them; they constrain and delineate our freedom to choose to do otherwise, effectively reducing our range of potential action. They are not automatically bad or reflective of one up–one down power relationships. Complicity with them does not automatically result in our supporting those at the top of power-knowledge hierarchies.[6]

Participation in the master narratives of cultures does us a favor. It allows us to function automatically. We need to be able to concentrate on a task and block out distractions. To illustrate this, New York University psychologist John Bargh gave participants in an experiment ten sentences containing at least six scrambled words, and asked them to make a correct sentence with at least four of the words.[7] Subjects did this quickly and accurately, but then walked out of the room much more slowly and with a different gait than they had used to enter the room. Within each sentence was a word related to old age. Bargh explained this by positing an adaptive unconscious that attends to all that we do not so that we can concentrate on a task. This adaptive unconscious attended to those aspects of the tasks that were not related to the test subjects' immediate purpose and intention.

Our brains do many things that lie outside of our conscious awareness. These things influence our behavior and beliefs. While the intentional searchlight of consciousness directs itself to a goal, our nervous systems and "non-intentioned" or free-floating consciousness watches our backs.

This principle is illustrated nicely in the experiments of psychologists Claude Steele and Joshua Aronson, which involved black and white students answering questions from the Graduate Record Examination, the standardized test used for entrance into graduate school.[8] When the black students were asked about their race before answering questions, the number of questions they answered correctly was cut in half. This is an example of a master narrative of American culture that says that blacks are not as smart as whites and don't deserve to succeed. When the psychologists asked the black students if it bugged them to be asked about their race before the test, they answered, "No," and added that they just didn't think they were smart enough to be at the university.

These examples show the subtle power of master narratives, but also show how we do need to be able to do some things automatically, without having to think about them, for, as neuropsychological experiments have demonstrated, our conscious mind cannot actually "multitask," and trying to do so simply reduces our efficiency. The master narratives that we must oppose are those that support values that we actually don't want to enact—like the belief that whites are smarter than blacks, or that Indians are stupid. In describing an aboriginal family, a nurse told me just this morning, "You can never find those people. They're not like the rest of us. They're always running around and not locatable." She was speaking to me on the phone and was incorrectly assuming, because I was the psychiatrist for this patient, that I was not aboriginal.

In my context, one of the subtle master narratives that I am actively recruiting people to oppose is the idea that "you can't get well. A doctor has to fix you." Or, "You have to take or do something specific (and mechanical or objective) to be fixed." My counter-narratives run like this: "You do have the capability to influence your health and disease through your own actions and the supporting actions of others in your community. You can do something on your own to move toward greater wellness without waiting for the doctor to do it for you. You don't have to understand how to do it. It will emerge through talking with your friends and family and through engaging in those actions that make sense to all of you. Healing sometimes just emerges."

I am grateful to journalist Malcolm Gladwell for some other metaphors related to this concept.[9] He wrote about how tennis professional Andre Agassi never hit a forehand shot on videotape the way he said he did. Baseball great Ted Williams never hit a baseball on videotape the way he said he did. People rarely use the formulas they say they use to pick their dates. We don't actually do things the way we think we do them. The stories we tell to explain what we do are just stories, albeit stories that work for us on important levels. What seems to matter is intent—the intent to hit the ball, to make a date, to get well. Intent seems to initiate an unseen process that produces results. That's the counter-narrative I'm advocating for healing.

How much awareness of this do we actually have? I suspect very little. We sometimes achieve some modicum of awareness when we are confronted with contradictory stories, both of which we have espoused. In those contexts, we often feel like both stories cannot be right and we must pick one. I think we fall into contexts and conversations in the sense that the existentialists write about being thrown into a world that was not of our design. I suspect that the negotiation of partially contradictory positions is forced upon us through our membership in multiple contexts with different participants. Another way of speaking would be to say that we play multiple roles for many audiences. Some of these audiences overlap. Sometimes we get caught in situations where the audience is so overlapping that half of them expect one role from us and half another, and we can essentially play only one role at a time. Then we are interactively forced into the collaborative design of a new role (or voice or story).

Australian psychologist Michael White and New Zealand psychiatrist David Epston have created a therapeutic technique from just this—showing people stories that contradict the usual master narrative that the person lives.[10] White and Epston call these contradictory (and sometimes isolated) stories "unique outcomes" because they are incompatible with the story the person (and his community) is telling himself. These occur at times when a different value is operating than what is customary. These events can be used to cast doubt and to help the person gain some awareness that other stories and values are possible. Reflection and the awareness of differences, including contradictions, helps us to see that our stories and values can be changed.

White and Epston have achieved some fame for extending this concept into what they call externalization, which says that people need to separate themselves from problems. Of interest is the common occurrence of this approach in indigenous cultures. When problems and conditions become master narratives they actually provide people with a sense of identity. For example, in medicine, we have lupus patients, cancer patients, and arthritis patients, and all of these labels carry prescriptive power for identity. According to White and Epston's concept, change is easier if the person does not view the problem as her identity.

Each context or frame has a different conversation in which we are embedded and which generates different stances or positions that may contradict the stances and positions made in other conversations from other contexts. This is why membership in multiple frames can promote awareness, but membership in only one frame is sometimes stultifying. If we actually have relatively little agency (as I am suggesting), then assuming any degree of agency is a radical act of empowerment. We empower ourselves when we become critically aware of the master narratives that we live and that live us. I believe that most of our conversations are rather automatic within a set of shifting, internalized values and loose allegiances to several particular plots (not getting fired, getting the girl of our dreams, making more money). We have little understanding of the nature of the resources that enable people to take positions that contribute and ultimately lead to change. The master narratives operating in any given culture or context are usually powerful and stand over and above any locally situated alternative stories.

My goal is to foster liberation and emancipation from the devaluing and disempowering master narratives of conventional medicine, though in moments of weakness—like the time I was accused of being in a cult for sweating alongside patients as part of the spiritual life of our First Nations community in Pittsburgh—I have felt quite discouraged. We have to work to avoid being swallowed and absorbed by these master narratives. We can only succeed by enacting our alternate counter-narratives on a daily basis through our interactions with the world. These are the daily practices that I emphasize with people. To change, we must carry out at least 101 consecutive days of a new practice—something we have never done before, or at least not consistently.

Most of the master narratives that we enact are inaccessible to conscious recognition and change. We have to learn *how* to perceive before we can perceive. These master narratives even include what we should perceive. These master narratives structure our perception and interpretation of the world as intelligible and therefore permeate our everyday language. We generally lack all awareness of our enactment of these narratives and only rarely challenge what they teach us to take for granted. The more people heal, the more able people are to question and challenge the master narrative that makes healing external and mechanical.[11]

You cannot challenge too many plot lines or master narratives at the same time. I think this is why the healers I know don't pray for cure of cancer, but rather, keep moving forward the length of time in which the person will remain well and alive. The idea of cure from cancer is too radical (opposes too many master narratives). Lengthening of life is still a big stretch, but it is only one master narrative, the idea that we can do something (pray, for instance) to improve our health or lengthen our lives. In other contexts, the master narrative that is being challenged is the idea that spiritual beings can intervene to help us. I think this is why seemingly excessively ambitious projects for personal growth, change, healing, and curing often fail. They challenge too many habitual ideas.

Psychologist Michael Bamberg writes about one story that repositions characters to transform a stereotypical dominant narrative in which the heroic male prince battles the dragon to save the beautiful princess so that he can possess her. In *The Paper Bag Princess*, author Robert Munsch first introduces Elizabeth as "a beautiful princess." Through the plot of the story, she undergoes a transformation into a dirty, "normal" girl (the girl dressed in a paper bag), who outsmarts a dragon in order to save her prince.[12] At the end she decides not to marry her prince, because he insists on maintaining his male, hegemonic gaze of her as "*his* beautiful princess." The sequence of events of the usual "prince slays the dragon and gets the girl" story is kept intact with only minor changes necessary to keep the character in line with other master narratives (for example, girls are generally expected to be nonviolent, though recent movies show that this perception is changing) and maintain intelligibility. Because of the nonviolent constraint that intelligibility with the master narrative requires, the dragon in this tale must not be defeated by physical force. Therefore, Munsch has his heroine defeat the dragon by the force of "artful smartness." Bamberg tells us that the *The Paper Bag Princess* is a good example of how master plot lines (only boys can be heroes and slay dragons) can be appropriated and transformed by inserting "counter-characters" (a girl in a paper bag who overcomes a dragon through her smartness and saves the prince only to refuse to marry him in the end). Bamberg tells us that these counter-characters must not be too different from what people expect.[13] A radically different character would lead to an immediate dismissal by the audience. To tell a believable story that challenges people's perceptions of what is supposed to be (the master narrative)—as in changing a story that expects progressive disease and death to one of healing and curing—we must proceed in this same manner and with the same level of subtlety and grace.

So many of the characters in the stories I tell are engaged in the same struggle—to leave some of their culture's dominant stories intact while at the same time reshaping and reconfiguring their own role within that culture. We always remain somewhat complicit with our culture and its master narrative and must work to change components of it from within. In addition, we need to remain sensitive to possible counters from the audience about our stories. They are also the voices of our culture. For example, in almost every audience I address, someone doesn't believe the stories I tell. They must reject these stories on first principles. As one woman said, "People do not get well from cancer. It must have been misdiagnosed." We always operate on the edge of disputability and must maintain an interactional subtlety and rhetorical finesse in order to be even partially believable. This is what we mean when we say we are being politically correct. Our stories don't always make the stars shift in the sky.

We are always juggling several story lines simultaneously. We must use stories to juggle our claims so as to make them acceptable to those around us. Claims that are too far-fetched will be rejected. A claim that noni juice cures all cancers if drunk in sufficient quantities is unlikely to be believed by many people. To claim that noni juice was part of a person's overall program of immune stimulation is more believable. The challenge is first to introduce in an acceptable way the idea that what we do does influence our health, that cancer is not a fate determined and dealt by a genetic blow which cannot be countered. We must position ourselves so as to be seen as *both* complicit with and as countering a dominant narrative (paradigm, story, voice, etc.).

Psychologists Neill Korobov and Michael Bamberg of Clark University are doing exciting research on how adolescent boys develop a sexual identity through the subtleties of their dialogue with each other.[14] The instantiation of maturity occurs in starts and stops and each person evaluates the other and negotiates an acceptable position, which could change in another group that generates a different dialogue. We are shaped by the conversations in which we participate and our values shift as those of our larger groups do. Our stories about who we are and what our purpose is continue to evolve as changes occur around us. Our values and our feelings are not isolated inside us, but, rather, are generated through our involvement with others. They are the ingredients of a social life or drama.[15] Korobov and Bamberg emphasize the developing sophistication of adolescents' abilities to play up motives against facts, the strategic use of concessions to reduce the seriousness of a denial, and the inventive ability to style the other through caricature. They believe that these "finely tuned positioning skills" are necessary to forge identity and manage relationships in a social milieu. "Creating a . . . self involves reconciling the disparate or potentially incompatible features of social categories . . . *in the moment* into an ongoing synthesis that is dynamic and ever changing. Rather it may come into existence in the way talk is accomplished; that is, as highly flexible and fragile projections of identity that involve a continuous refinement of 'finely tuned positioning skills.'"[16] So it is through dialogue that we evolve to become how we see ourselves today, and it is through the negotiation of dialogue that we will become we who will be tomorrow.

Bamberg further shows how people position themselves in conversations as "misunderstood," "aware," or "knowing," and thus *not* as naive, childish, desperate, or shallow (or other qualities).[17] They do this by orienting to each other with subtly crafted, hedged responses and delayed or weak disagreements that preface strategically organized accounts or evaluations. He describes how these strategies are appropriated to avoid conversational trouble. In other words, these strategies reflect the interactive development of "finely tuned positioning skills," which refers to the dexterity of speakers in being able to constantly interpret and negotiate conversational possibilities. He argues that the development of conversational skills does not necessarily reflect the progressive acquisition of *internal* states, cultural principles, or cognitive scripts, but rather, just skills through which each person explores what others expect from him and experiment with what to do about that. We try different approaches as "conversational experiments" with quick retractions if we don't like where a particular approach takes us. We end up where we feel most comfortable in that dialogical space. It's an important argument for the social maintenance of so-called internal states like depression, anxiety, suicidal behavior, or bipolarity. Bamberg refutes the claim that conversation merely reflects internal processes within the speakers, arguing instead that conversation involves culturally relevant ways in which speakers *move to* the edge of the disputability that is inherent in talk about potentially charged topics, such as sexuality. The art of conversation involves appearing desirable or "cool," but not extreme or weird. What constitutes cool or weird changes as different speakers enter and leave the conversation, thereby requiring a constant repositioning and renegotiation depending upon who is present. He describes this as an evasive, inscrutable, and insinuatingly strategic project. In this approach, we are more interested in what people say in response to each other, and especially to their contradictory and inconsistent descriptions of people, motives, states of mind, or events.

The study of narratives is remarkably different from the more conventional use of attitude scales and inventories. Bamberg writes that answering a forced-choice question is entirely different "than expressing an attitude in daily social interaction."[18] Questionnaire items tend to reify issues by reducing them to relatively stereotypical and simple descriptions that may be easily rejected. Second, the forced-choice format systematically strips off the interactive subtleties and rhetorical finessing that are part of the daily expression of attitudes, evaluations, and assessments. On a questionnaire, the boys may predominantly disagree with the attitudes that are purportedly associated with the items, especially if those items are measuring something like overt sexism. But in their daily interactions, they may actually put such attitudes to use in myriad ways, constructing them as caricatures, displacing them onto other boys, orienting to them in ironic or tongue-in-cheek ways, or at times even claiming them in order to resist being positioned as effeminate, soft, or weak.

People actively position themselves in conversations to accomplish something. They enter dialogue with the intent to produce a result. Our actions and statements are part of a plot. If we pay close attention to the ways in which what the talk is "about" is presented and described, we can begin to make sense of the dialogue and the evolving intents of its participants. We gain further understanding when we look for descriptions and evaluations of characters in the conversation as well as descriptions of time and space in the way that these relate to other people and to potential future actions. People choose their descriptions and evaluations for interactive purposes, using them to signal each other about how they want to be understood.

We work from two levels of observation—the content of what is being said and the sequence of the speakers—to understand the underlying intent and values driving how the speakers position themselves and present who they want to be seen as. Each person in the dialogue evolves through simultaneously acting and being acted upon by others.

Becoming aware of our roles and the values that we assist larger entities in pursuing can facilitate change and transformation. Awareness of our roles as roles and of potential alternate roles, gives us potential resources to rebel and change the way we participate in larger systems or groups. Change simultaneously involves different dialogues with others outside of ourselves and different internal conversations within ourselves. These different dialogues lead to different physiologies and different biology. Here is where healing can happen. When our awareness increases, we gain some sense of agency, some sense of authorship in the play in which we appear to be acting. We discover that we have some ability to change scripts in process, that we can make little changes as we go that sometimes have big reverberations. Suffering, illness, and problems diminish our sense of agency and personal power.[19] As we become more and more defined by a problem or an illness, we become less able to see competent action for ourselves. Through collaboration with other humans (sometimes healers), we begin to see a possibility for personal power that didn't exist before.

A story about Leopold, a man with AIDS, will illustrate this. He was very sick. He didn't have much personal power or sense of agency. He felt trapped, isolated, and alone. I wanted to give him a different sense for his life. Consistent with my approach, I knew better than to disagree with him or argue with him that there were small things he could do to improve his health, so I told him the Dene story of the journey from the Fourth World to the current Fifth (or Glittering) World.[20]

What resembled Leo's situation was that the story begins with people's lives being threatened by something completely beyond their control—in this case by something Coyote did.

Conditions in the Fourth World had been pretty ideal, with a relatively constant and comfortable climate and temperature. Food was plentiful and no one suffered. But all of that changed suddenly because of something Coyote did. Unknown to the people, Coyote had stolen Water Monster's beautiful fur coat, not knowing that Water Monster's two babies were each in a pocket of that coat. When those babies went missing, Water Monster flew into a rage. Convinced that the newcomers (the people who had come up from the Third World) had stolen her babies, Water Monster dived down to the bottom of the sea to dig a hole, causing water from the Third World to come up into the Fourth World and flood those people out. Turkey and First Woman's son were the first to see the water rising. They were out walking when they heard an unusual sound. They looked in each of the four directions for that sound until finally, they saw huge waves in the west and realized that the ocean had already leaped its boundaries and was rising toward their homes. They ran back to the village to tell First Woman. No one knew until later why all this had happened, that Coyote had inadvertently stolen Water Monster's babies and was too afraid to return them, fearing that Water Monster would eat him on the spot. Coyote preferred to let everyone suffer for his misdeeds than bear the consequences himself.

The story matched Leo's own sense of victimization in contracting HIV and then AIDS. He had been in a relationship with another man who was HIV positive and hadn't bothered to tell him. He might have avoided that relationship had he known, which was probably why the other man didn't tell him. He would at least have taken precautions. His life was now threatened because of the acts of another. I could tell that I had his attention with this story. I didn't have to make a direct link. People are smart; they figure these things out for themselves. I also thought the parallels between the Christian and Dene flood stories would interest Leo, who had been raised Christian in Finland. He liked North American stories very much, the way many Europeans do. He identified with the characters quickly.

First Woman mobilized the people swiftly in the face of the rising water, urging them to collect their belongings and climb to the highest point on the land. Maybe the flood would stop and they could return home. Secretly, Coyote knew this wouldn't happen, since Water Monster would not stop the flood until her babies were returned, and Coyote was not about to do that. Coyote knew the flood would continue and was worried about how to get out of the Fourth World and into the Fifth.

Similarly, I wanted to mobilize Leo. I wanted the spirit of the story to enter into him, to stir him up in the same way that First Woman mobilized the people. I sensed an urgent need for him to act, to either live or die well, with meaning and purpose intact. I also had a sense that others (like Coyote) knew what was happening in his body from lab tests and other clinical determinants, and actually knew things that he didn't know. There were secrets (like Coyote's knowledge of the prognosis for the flood) that made this story parallel his situation. I wanted Leo to survive—physically, emotionally, and spiritually—in the same way First Woman was concerned with her people's survival. Later I would tell him stories I had heard about northern peoples living through winters in which the winds blew so hard the caribou froze, dogs died, and people were reduced to eating spruce bark.

> *The people gathered their things and started climbing. Most remembered the journey from the Third World and didn't want to repeat that terror. The Fourth World had been kind, with ideal growing conditions. Weather was temperate, without storms or other hardships. Food was so plentiful that only minimal effort was required to live well. The people feared that the next world would not be so kind. Reluctantly they abandoned what they could not carry and followed First Woman to the heights of their land. Some stayed behind, saying they were too tired.*

I wanted Leo to gather his things and start climbing. I wanted him to rise out of his passivity and become more active. I wanted him to respond in time to the challenges facing him. I didn't know where he was going. I didn't know what his Fifth World would be like. I didn't know whether his Fifth World would be a spirit world or a material world, but I knew he needed to go somewhere with urgency, just like the people in the story. I knew he could just say he was too tired and give up the way some in the story did, and the story mentioned that possibility as well, naming it for him.

> *The train of people snaked their way toward the top of the highest peak, even as the floodwaters filled the landscape of the valley. When they reached the top, they realized that the waters would soon cover them. First Woman urged them inside a hollow tree that stood at the top of that peak. One by one, they climbed through the inside of that tree to the top of the tree. By the time they reached the top, all the land was covered and water*

was rising up the tree. First Woman needed someone to open a hole in the sky. Woodpecker volunteered to go first. With effort that took him beyond the point of exhaustion, he finally made a small hole in that ceiling. When he pulled his beak out of the hole, he almost fell into the water, but First Woman caught him.

With this story, I anchored these characters in Leo's mind so I could use them again later. I wanted the spirit of Woodpecker, who makes the first hole, to impress Leo. Woodpecker almost sacrifices himself for that first effort, which doesn't seem so large but is really quite momentous. First Woman saves Woodpecker. I later used Woodpecker as a reminder of how great change begins with small events, and that we need others to catch us when we spend energy to start the change process and then collapse. I also wanted to build a sense of teamwork between Leo and me.

"Who can widen this hole?" First Woman asked. Duck came forward. "I have a strong bill," she said. "I can widen the hole." Duck flew up to the hole Woodpecker had started and proceeded to pound away with her bill. Just as she reached her point of exhaustion, Duck managed to make a crack that stretched from North to South. Then Hawk volunteered to resume where Duck had stopped. He managed to make a crack from East to West. Now there was a small hole and two intersecting cracks. Something would have to be done fast to widen that hole, for the people could hear the wild water rising and didn't believe they could get out in time.

I used this story repetitively as an example of how a whole community was required to break through into the Fifth World. One person or animal could not do it alone. Leo needed help from others. He couldn't do this alone.

When First Woman asked for volunteers to widen the hole, the Beetle People stepped forward. "We can do it," they said, "if someone will carry us there." A temporary truce was made so that the Bird People could bring the beetles to the hole in their beaks. The various beetles worked upside down to widen the hole. The dung beetles widened the hole from Center to East. The striped beetles widened it from Center to South. Then the yellow beetles widened the hole from Center to West, while the staghorn beetles made a bigger hole from Center to North. The hole was much bigger and the cracks were wider, but the beetles were spent, so Grasshopper stepped in to give her best effort to make it even bigger.

Thus, even the smallest, seemingly insignificant creatures were crucial to the community process and to the creative effort. I used the contributions of the insects in the story to remind Leo that the small can have tremendous power, no matter how unimportant, small, and cast aside he felt at present. He had Beetle and Grasshopper power, and could still get things done. The insects also teach us how the repetitive application of small steps eventually led to big change, another point I wanted Leo to get.

Locust went next and broke through into the Fifth World. Birds from the Fifth World met her and tested her. Crane tossed a black cloud at her, and she turned it into rain and hail. Next blue mist was thrown at her, and she turned it into lightning and summer rain. Then a yellow cloud was thrown at her, and she turned it into sheet lightning and thunder. When she turned a white cloud into ice and snow, she won the right for the people to live in the Fifth World. Locust returned in triumph. Dragonfly agreed to carry Spider to the hole in the sky where she began to spin a heavy rope, so strong that even Bear could climb through.

"Leo," I said. "Something similar to what happened to Locust will happen to you too. Once you break through your own personal ceiling of wellness and your health improves, people will challenge you. They will test you in the same way as the birds throwing winds at Locust. I don't know why people are like this, but apparently animals do it too and it has been going on since the beginning of time. They will tell you that your improvement is only temporary and will demand that you abandon any hope as false. But you know that no hope is false. Like the animals that helped First Woman, you will not give up. Some new part of you will come forward when an old part of you is exhausted. You will succeed in breaking through your ceiling like the animals did in breaking through theirs."

The Termite People volunteered to widen the hole still further. Small birds carried them to where they could apply their chewing power. By the time they were exhausted, the hole could pass very small animals like Mouse and Shrew, but not large animals like Bear. The Ant People responded next to First Woman's call for more help. "We can widen that hole," they said. They made a living ladder to reach the hole. With their rapid industriousness, they soon had a hole large enough for Beaver and Otter.

"Who can help next?" asked First Woman.

Badger stepped forward. "I am a digger," she said. "I can make that hole big enough even for Bear."

"Leo," I said. "Like what happened for First Woman, your small efforts will grow bigger and bigger, like a tiny seed growing into a giant redwood. As smaller parts of you succeed, eventually bigger parts of you, like your inner Badger who's a real champion digger, can step forward and complete the task. You can 'badger' your way to empowerment. Like the progression from insects to badger, every part of you can make a helpful contribution, breaking open a hole into a new world of wellness. Parts of you as seemingly insignificant as ants and locusts and beetles can help. You will learn of the healing power of the small, about how little efforts can really pay off."

"I will help," said Coyote. "I can dig just as well as Badger." First Woman had her suspicions about Coyote's motives, but she couldn't fault his enthusiasm. Maybe next life he would come back as a less lazy animal, she thought.

"Alright," First Woman said. "Get to work." (Coyote had gotten distracted admiring his reflection in the ceiling of the sky. He was even plucking out some extra nose hairs, priding himself on his good grooming and overall appearance, which others saw as little better than scruffy.) "Make us a hole big enough for Bear." Coyote painfully suppressed his desire to demand food first before any work. So they got to work, or rather, Badger did, for Coyote only pretended to work. Badger led the way with ferocious digging. Coyote stayed behind Badger, pretending to dig furiously, but mostly just pushing Badger's dirt around. He still had a big

sack on his back filled with Water Monster's fur coat, one of her babies in each side pocket. He wasn't about to let that fall. But he did drop some of the precious stones he had won gambling. He was acting so hard at digging, that he lost some of his things. With all this furious digging, little pieces of blue sky got mixed in with the dirt. Today these chunks of Fourth World sky are called turquoise. Many of Coyote's other precious stones also got buried in the dirt, and people are still finding them today as gold, silver, and gems. Badger and Coyote's fur never got clean after all that digging. To this day, their paws are black from the dirt, and black streaks run the length of their bodies.

Eventually Badger broke through, and the animals made a chain, standing on each other's shoulders, to climb through that hole. Bear was the last animal to go, followed by First Woman and First Man. Strong magicians used their medicines to make Bear lighter and pull him through the hole. Once he had gotten through, it was easy for the people to follow. First came the Hopi, then the Zuni, then the other Pueblo people, then the Apache, the Plains people, and finally the thirty-two clans of the Dene. When all the people and animals had crossed through the hole in the sky, Wolverine replaced the dirt and packed it down so that the water from the flood could not come after them. Bear helped, and this is how everyone got to the Fifth World, which was still looking bleak and needing a lot of work, but that's another story.

Every champion deserves a Coyote, and Badger certainly had one. For this story, for Leo, I used Coyote to represent the idea that even when a disaster is caused by a reprehensible act, something positive can emerge and arise from it. The flood that destroyed the Fourth World started because Coyote stole Water Monster's babies; Leo had gotten AIDS through the negligence of another. Nonetheless, Leo's efforts could still make a difference in his life. I continued to reinforce this point throughout our work together. By telling him a traditional story, anchoring the characters, and embedding him in the story through visualization and guided imagery processes, the story became his story. His story became one of triumph emerging from tragedy.

At the time of this writing, six years have passed, and Leo is still alive with AIDS. He is living triumphantly in each moment, weaving stories like spider ropes to carry bears—other people with AIDS—up to his level of meaning and purpose, peacefulness and contentment. This and the other stories I told him stayed with him to encourage his efforts.

The Relationship of Healing and Truth

We must accept the lack of a certain, ultimate truth. We cannot know truth, only the stories we create about truth. Humility lies in the recognition that our stories will require constant modifications to keep up with our own evolution. Maturity consists of the ability to manage multiple, competing ideological tensions while negotiating an identity that works for the various, sometimes conflicting communities to which we belong.

Knowledge about healing is diverse and context dependent. It differs by locality. We are limited to observations from particular measurement systems that generate explanatory hypotheses (stories) that we must refute or confirm with further observations or tests of hypotheses. Philosophers of science Karl Popper and Kurt Gödel both argued persuasively that nothing can ever be proven.[21] Michel Foucault showed how ideas come to achieve truth status through political and not scientific means. Various bodies of experts (representatives of the ruling class) set the rules and decide what they will support as true. They set the standards for what is considered normal and how people should live.

Through a narrative perspective, we try to reject totalizing, essentialist, or foundational concepts. A totalizing concept puts all phenomena under one explanatory principle—for example, genetics or molecular determinism. An example of an essentialist idea is that the concept called "anxiety disorder" is a real entity that can be uniformly applied to explain a certain kind of mood or behavior in any given person, independent of culture, biology, and other human constraints. Foundational thinking suggests that there are stable systems of meaning that can be discovered and proven through rational thought and scientific inquiry.

Contemporary medicine's belief in totalizing, essentialist, and foundational concepts prevents an adequate study of the phenomenon of healing. The totalizing concept of medicine states that all of health and disease can ultimately be explained by genetics. Its essentialism is biological—that a basic, underlying biology exists independent of culture, the circumstances of our lives, and all other constraints. Conventional medicine's foundationalism is expressed in its belief that there is one best way to heal, which can be discovered through randomized, controlled trials.

Quantum physics describes a reality so vast as to contain everything and to be beyond description except in mathematical terms. Quantum physics is anti-foundational. Stability is a joke. With his uncertainty principle, physicist Werner Heisenberg taught us that we can only be certain about one thing at a time and never about the whole picture.[22] Einstein's theory of relativity taught us the impossibility of finding an absolute reference point from which to make measurements. These are considerations relevant to the study of healing.

Haverford University philosopher Ashok Gangadean wrote that the experience of independence is an illusion of predicating thought, the artificial division of perceiver and perceived.[23] If we are inextricably embedded and entangled in nature, any thought of separating us from nature is absurd. Our very lives and consciousnesses may have arisen as an emergent property of nature's internal dialogue.

Independence is an illusion. Only interdependence exists. Essentialism posits independent or transcendent concepts. Even the equations posited by quantum physics are just descriptions or stories of a universe in which we are hopelessly embedded. Mathematics qualifies as a language in that regard—it has grammar and syntax. It tells a story to those who can speak the language. Quantum biologists consider these phenomena responsible for our capacity to even think. We cannot escape. Erving Goffman emphasized the impossibility of considering human behavior and actions apart from the stage or frame upon which, or in which, they occur. Healing cannot be studied in isolation from the frame or stage in which it occurs. I suspect this is true for all biological treatments, but we don't study pharmaceuticals and the responses to them from this perspective.

A similar theory of emergent processes is taking hold in psychology under the term "microgenesis."[24] It assumes that developmental changes (such as learning or better understanding) emerge as individuals create and accomplish interactive tasks in everyday conversations. In this view, through what Bamberg dubbed "talk-in-interaction," people establish a sense of self. The interactive space between the participants, whether situated in interviews or other social locations, is the arena in which identities are performed and consolidated and where they can be accessed. It is also the arena in which healing evolves.

The explanations people give about healing are suspect. Goffman said, "What is presented by the individual concerning himself and his world is so much an abstraction, a self-defensive argument, a careful selection from a multitude of acts, that the best that can be done with this sort of thing is to say that it is a lay dramatist's scenario employing himself as a character and a somewhat supportable reading of the past."[25] People's descriptions or explanations of their own healings are similar. Fundamentally, healing or internal reorganization and transformation operate through means that are invisible to us and whose understanding is poorly attainable at best.

The pathway to healing for the individual is contingent upon the larger systems to which he or she belongs. Individuals are completely interconnected and nonlocal. People's identities are created through relationship interactions and occupy various culturally based sites of meaning—family, work, social class, geographic region, gender, sexual orientation, club membership, psychotherapy client, president of the Parent Teacher Organization—every site evoking a different identity, different language uses, different foci of value and energy, different social practices, and so forth. Each person will have a different pathway to healing, depending upon the facts of each site with which they are associated.

People are embodied in a physical world, entrenched in the material practices and structures of their society—working, playing, procreating, and living as part of the material systems of society. People are social in origin, taking meaning, value, and self-image from their identity in groups, their activities in society, their intimate relations, and from the multiple pools of common meanings, symbols, and practices they share with other members of their sub-cultural groups and with their society as a larger unit.

A narrative approach sees "reality" as more fragmented, diverse, tenuous, and culture-specific than would contemporary medicine, with the following consequences:

- Greater emphasis on the body; the actual insertion of the human into the texture of time and history,
- Greater attention to the specifics of culture, and its arenas of discourse and practice, a greater attention to the role of language and context in our construction of reality and identity, and
- Greater attention to the specific stories or histories of individuals, groups, or families.

These emphases are essential for the study of healing. We must attend to each specific story of healing as if there were no other. We must consider how biological change is contextual and dependent upon the actual multidimensional placement (time, location, culture) of a human body into a particular time and history. We must pay greater attention to the role of culture and its practices as relevant to our discussion about healing, and we must look at how people's identities are formed—those who are well and those who are sick. We must ask the question, how do these differences (sickness and wellness) come about? When we do, we are drawn to the many big stories (master narratives) of our lives as well as the smaller stories and vignettes circulating around us.

5
The Power of Large Groups in Shaping Identity

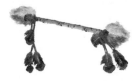

A few people have a bed for the night
For a night the wind is kept from them
The snow meant for them falls on the roadway
But it won't change the world
It won't improve relations among men
It will not shorten the age of exploitation.

BERTOLT BRECHT[1]

Imagine a ceremony in a rural area near Duncan, British Columbia, on Vancouver Island. In the longhouse, a youth is being initiated. Two hundred people are singing. The rhythm of multiple drums and rattles sets the pace. The youth is lying flat. He is lifted up and carried on the shoulders of eight men. He remains this way for four days after which time he is returned to the vertical. The collected energy is awe-inspiring. Even the trees outside are vibrating in the thick fog.

Western culture has forgotten the power of large groups. Modern culture's closest version is the sports spectacle, which has a very different intent from ceremony and ritual. Religious services provide us with some sense of group power, but modern religion has vitiated the power of its ceremonies so greatly that it is hard to feel.* While we can still go to ceremony in areas rich in aboriginal culture, it has vanished for much of the urban world.

In my teachings about ceremony and ritual, I like to show people how easy it is for a group of strangers to come together, create shared ceremony that is inclusive of elements of all their cultures, and then enact it. Whenever people gather with the same intent, coherence occurs. Coherence implies connectivity. In essence, we hook up. Hearing stories is healing. It requires a group setting to produce those stories and to hear other people's stories. Within the group, we can hear the story and consider its source. Others are present to corroborate the story, thereby demystifying it. We have a diversity of sources supporting a common story. As people become more and more isolated, however, such group experiences have become progressively less common in modern life. Lost along with the sense of community group experiences engender, is the opportunity to take a storied approach to health care through a process of group re-authoring. Groups that can provide this do still exist, and include Alcoholics Anonymous, the Native American church, and others in which people give testimony and the group reshapes the story, in a sense "re-authoring" a new story in a collaborative framework.

Life is storied and narrative is the mode in which meaning and values are stored. This allows for multiple techniques for transformation. We are not limited to one set of local practices and values, regardless of how successful they are in that locale. They may not generalize. As one elder told me, "When you think you know what you're doing, you don't. When you think you know what's going on, you're wrong." That's an important perspective to keep. We can talk about what we think we're doing and what we think is going on as we work collaboratively with others, but in the spirit of remembering that we're probably wrong and we're only making gross approximations anyway. Transformative practices and results spontaneously emerge in large groups when people gather with the same intention, defying rational explanation.

In medicine, we doctors are faced with the difficulty that most of us

---

*Notable exceptions to this generalization exist, including in some Roman Catholic masses, evangelical revival meetings, and Gospel churches.

don't know that we have a story. We think everything we do is the factual truth. We forget that history really means "his story" or "her story." When we talk to someone about her illness, we are actually helping her tell her story, how she came to be where she is. Having other family members and friends present results in a much richer story than would emerge with just the individual there. Health care is supposed to build on the story with each contact, but if we don't know the story, each contact becomes a closed episode of its own, disconnected from every other episode. Fragmentation results as the outcome of a nonstoried approach to health care.

Whenever we consider the group, we need to think about the various groups to which we belong. Some indigenous elders believe that we are nothing more than all the stories that have been or will ever be told about us. We cannot consider individuals apart from groups, because people do not exist apart from groups. Galveston-based family therapists Harry Goolishian and Harlene Anderson wrote that problems gain their meaning when they diminish our sense of agency and personal liberation.[2] Another way to look at this is to consider that individuals are constrained by the groups to which they belong. Opportunities for solutions arise when people feel capable of new action and when they feel more freedom to act. Our goal is to find more ways to achieve this freedom. The stories that we tell ourselves about ourselves and our lives, the ways in which we interpret the events of our lives, are intertwined with those of other members of the groups to which we belong, and become integrated and coherent through dialogue with other group members. These stories change through our and others' personal efforts. If our story is one of hopelessness, then we don't even begin to consider the possibility of changing our stories, regardless of who is willing to help.

Our culture, as the largest group to which we belong, contains a repository of stories and roles that we could play. Our birth places us into ongoing stories. Our community further constrains the stories we are allowed to play.[3] The group is the holder of the stories about us until we can learn and absorb language. As we grow and develop, the group becomes the audience for the stories we start to tell about ourselves and others. They provide the feedback for what works and what doesn't. By the time we reach adulthood, we have learned a broad range of socially validated roles and have mastered the linguistic and behavioral aspects of those roles.

Some experience is unstoried. It hasn't been interpreted yet. Perhaps it doesn't fit into our usual perceptual frameworks, so we ignore it. An important aspect of narrative therapy is to story experience that is previously unstoried. That means to give uninterpreted experience an interpretation, a meaning. We do that in collaboration with other people, through participation in the groups to which we belong. Philosopher Paul Ricoeur said that the story of a new life grows out of the events that have not yet been storied.[4] These are the stories that have not yet been told. Life becomes human and meaningful through the assignment of meaning to its events. That meaning is communicated and reinforced through the key events being put together into a story.

The groups to which we belong serve to shape our identities through the stories they tell about us. We hear and internalize these stories and tell them to ourselves. Identity is the story we tell ourselves about ourselves. Identity differs from awareness, which is primary and pre-narrative. Meditation techniques aim at awareness without interpretation, which is pre-narrative. Achieving a pre-narrative awareness is an important tool for deconstruction, for removing our usual assumptions about the world, so that we can reflect upon what is essential and what is not; what we prefer and what do we not prefer; and more.

As we remember conversations, engage in them, anticipate what the other will say, and rehearse future conversations, we develop the ability to converse internally, to imagine that we are talking to people. I suspect this has some disadvantages. I've suspected that a pre-narrative awareness of spirits exists within children. I don't think it's just synesthesia or sensory mix-up when infants focus on a point that contains nothing so far as I can see, and smile, and then laugh and laugh. I believe they are engaged in some pre-verbal spirit communication or recognition. Perhaps it is even telepathic, an instant communication of ideas and emotions. We seem to lose this ability as spoken, interpersonal language becomes primary. Schizophrenics can regain the ability, as do other psychotic people, but at great personal cost. In some indigenous communities, this ability is never lost. Mainstream culture labels these people as primitive. Indigenous healers retain the ability to speak to spirits. Others of us have had to work for years to recover this ability (through meditation, prayer, ceremony, fasting) and believe that we do have dialogue with animals, plants, rocks, and spirits. The experience is largely unnarrated, though sometimes stories are told and instructions are given.

A primary insight of family theory and therapy of the twentieth century was to show that psychotic utterances are communication and do make sense when considered in the context of the larger group. Nonpsychotic lives have plots that are readily understood in some relatively linear fashion. We can make sense of how the person plans to get from A to B, or we can understand a life as a refusal to make linear plots, but psychotic plots are harder to understand. We look to the plot to understand what might happen next, to get a sense of what is permanent and what might change. A killer is expected to kill again. A policeman is expected to apprehend criminals recurrently. A teacher will teach again. We are taken aback when we encounter stories that appear to contain no plot. These are stories of minimal agency and high levels of subjugation, meaning that others appear to control the plot and the individual appears as a minor character, stage prop, or supporting actor with a very fixed role in stories seemingly created by others (members of the larger group). These individuals lack a sense of agency. They feel powerless to influence the plot. They feel hopeless that things will change. They feel stuck in a role. Their lives lack flexibility and playfulness. This absence of joy is one of the most striking elements of what is called schizophrenia, in which suffering and despair can be immense.

Juha Holma and Jukka Aaltonen, members of the Finnish Integrated Approach to the Treatment of Acute Psychosis, have written about the pre-narrative quality of psychosis.[5] They use the power of groups to shape narratives as a way to improve psychosis. Psychotic individuals lack well-constructed narratives, they believe. They often lack reflectivity because the stories that do dominate them fix them in roles that lack the capacity for choice and change. They cannot see a way out. They cannot perceive other possibilities. Their lives are limited. They are subjugated by other stories from larger groups in which they are contained (society, subculture, family). Their identity appears to be copied or borrowed. They seem to contribute little to its construction and absorb the stories heard around them in a somewhat haphazard fashion. They are minor characters in other people's stories. In twenty-first century psychiatry, they are usually caught in the mainstream psychiatric story of having defective brains and being hopeless cases. These stories deprive them of agency and fix their role as being chronically mentally ill people whose utterances are meaningless, by definition, since they are psychotic. They have disorders of thinking, so their thoughts are, by definition, invalid and irrelevant.

One of the principles stressed by Holma and Aaltonen, with which all elders appear to agree, is that we must empower people to feel more of a sense of agency in their lives, which is why it is essential to include the larger group in our work. Regardless of what we do, when we collaborate with people who are suffering, that suffering diminishes when they feel a greater sense of influence over conditions around them. When they perceive that they can make a change and get feedback from their environment that they have been perceived as having agency, things improve, whatever the basis for the suffering. Empowerment is good. It can lead to change, though some people are so stuck in roles that we must empower those around them to see them different and demand different responses, which is where the larger group comes in. The group expects its members to perform certain roles. Resistance to change occurs when members start modifying those roles. This resistance is diminished when dialogue occurs about everyone's roles, thereby allowing everyone to change. When everyone changes, change can be permanent.

Holma and Aaltonen discuss the importance of narrating a new story that captures the pre-narrative quality of experience. This concept is basic to all that we do for people who suffer. However, Holma and Aaltonen worked with the larger family group to create new narratives about individual family members. One patient they describe was a twenty-two-year-old man who presented with "peculiar thoughts." Morgan felt depressed and attributed his depression to brain cancer. He had been a student, but moved back home to live with his parents. The family story about his changes went like this: "Morgan feels depressed and peculiar because he has brain cancer, and/or an extra flow of testosterone during exercise, and/or because policemen gave him LSD when he was arrested."[6] Consistent with the family's embeddedness in mainstream culture, their initial stories attributed agency entirely to others (someone did something to Morgan) and to biological mechanisms. Their story was entirely compatible with the underlying principles of contemporary psychiatry, with the exception of their resistance to the concept of no others being involved, that Morgan merely had a defective brain. No one initially likes this aspect of the psychiatric story. Most of us want someone else or something else to be at fault, as in their story about excessive surges of testosterone.

Through a series of family group meetings, Morgan's family's story changed. The family therapists situated Morgan's metaphoric language into a narrative that they could understand and told it back to him. They said things like, "This is what I feel and think when you tell me what you just said." When Morgan talked about being an "architect of the end," they constructed a narrative of potential suicidality, which Morgan denied. When discussion of Morgan's anger and aggressiveness emerged, the team members talked about how they handled such feelings and impulses themselves. They told stories about themselves. They also constructed hypothetical stories that might explain Morgan's anger and aggressiveness and wondered if these stories might be true. Their actions represented the first time anyone in the family had ever attempted to construct a story to explain inner psychological experiences. These had never before been discussed openly in the family. These experiences were not storied. Unstoried experiences are not amenable to discussion. Father and mother began to reflect upon their roles in the family and to wonder if these roles should change.

Over time, the identified patient developed a new story about himself. He saw himself as more self-sufficient. He had better impulse control and more ability to discuss his emotions. He eventually rented an apartment and lived reasonably well on his own, with some occasional resurgence of mild psychotic symptoms. His father was creating a new self-story in which he was less irritated by things left undone. His mother was creating a new self-story in which she was able to discuss feelings and inner psychological events. The larger group (the family) had changed, allowing all its members to change and to maintain those changes. Their narratives about each other and themselves now allowed for different role enactments that produced different physiological responses from the brain. The brain is inseparable from the story. Brains respond to what we perceive. Perception is created by the stories we live. We see what we expect to see and the brain responds accordingly. The brain cannot be expected to be responsible for brain-environment mismatch. This is the responsibility of the larger group to correct misperceptions through changing the story that everyone lives.

We could speculate that Morgan's psychotic symptoms emerged when his role became too rigid to contain him. I believe the mind-body-spirit has an innate drive to self-correct, to restore balance and harmony. This is my story and has indigenous origins. I would explain the psychotic symptoms here as a necessary flow of energy that could not be released in any other way. New stories allowed that energy to flow in different ways and the psychotic symptoms diminished. There are other stories, however, that could just as readily be constructed, and, our explanatory stories are less important than the stories about what changed and how we think we influenced the change process.

Here's a story about a group with which I collaborated in a similar way. The presenting complaint was paranoia. Isaac was a twenty-eight-year-old man who was convinced that his ex-girlfriend had organized a plot to torture and drive him mad. He was very convincing on many levels, but when we persuaded him to take part in a meeting of everyone who knew him, we were able to ascertain that the likelihood of a plot against him was slim. Isaac's ex-girlfriend was very angry with him and upset that he was not financially supporting the child they had together, but she didn't strike us as capable of or interested in hiring hit men or a goon squad to beat up Isaac.

Isaac's confirmation of his story was that he kept getting assaulted. Things kept disappearing from his trailer, which was constantly being sabotaged. Isaac drove a taxi and told a story about a fellow driver who had been beaten almost to death by a man who kept asking where Isaac was. We were able to confirm that the driver had been dangerously mugged, but the perpetrator had never asked about Isaac. Isaac was hearing secret messages over the dispatch when he was driving the cab. He would go to the locations discussed and find no one there. His behavior became sufficiently erratic that he was asked to stop driving and to work instead in the dispatch office. He actually performed very well there, because he was so attentive to the secret messages that he never missed an actual message. His employer came to one of our meetings and told us how much he valued Isaac's work, though he knew that Isaac was not entirely grounded in reality. "But everyone's entitled to a conspiracy theory or two," he said.

We tried to confront Isaac with the apparent absence of a plot, but this backfired. He hid from us for two months. That was good feedback for an incorrect move. When Isaac came back we apologized for not believing him. We began to wonder how we could help him to protect himself. We wondered about karate as a thought. He had already begun to take tae kwon do. We wondered at the wisdom of him confronting certain people known in the community as outlaws. (When Isaac confronted them, they inevitably beat him up for pleasure, not, apparently, because they had been paid to do so. However, he took their response as proof that they had been paid to beat him.)

Over time we were able to help Isaac develop a strategy of protection. We tried Risperdal briefly, but he rejected the drug, saying it "took off his edge." He felt he needed that edge to be on constant guard to protect himself. We were going to have to do this without medication.

We also presented Isaac with a series of experiments to see how much influence he had over the process. We wondered what would happen if he started paying child support. We speculated that his ex-girlfriend might be so surprised and pleased that she would stop hiring the guys to beat him up or asking family members to hurt him, as Isaac believed they were doing. Isaac argued about this for a couple of months, but agreed to "try an experiment" with us. It worked, and he began to spend time with his son. This reduced some of his anxiety. Then we wondered what would happen if he slowly started fixing up his trailer. We suggested he leave something in plain sight for sabotage. When it usually remained safe, Isaac began to relax even further. During this time, we had convinced him to cut way back on marijuana, suggesting smoking decreased his ability to protect himself. It was when he was stoned that he usually got beaten up. Isaac eventually tried this and found that he was being bruised less often.

Over two years and with the help of large group meetings with others from his community, to which he agreed on the condition that he would get to listen to tape recordings of the meetings, Isaac slowly lost his paranoia and became happier and more relaxed. He developed a sense that he had some agency in affecting what happened to him, and began to apply that belief to produce more agency. He did this without any medication. The addition of his larger group was important to keep the community involved in collaborating with Isaac to help him to be more relaxed and to avoid irrational acts that could get him in trouble.

Another example from my practice is about a lonely man who had been arrested for threatening a social worker with an ax. There were limits to how much he could change by himself, so we needed the community to shift the way that it thought about him. No charges were pressed and we were called to evaluate him. We saw him in his home. He insisted on talking to us for two hours about his spiritual visions.

Alfred recounted amazing visions in between paroxysms of a raspy and repetitive smoker's cough. He primarily trapped and fished out in the bush and described beavers standing up on top of their houses in the middle of ponds to tell him about the second coming of Christ. He pointed out stains on the walls of his cabin that he interpreted as signs of the Virgin Mary's visitation. We wanted to give him the benefit of the doubt for his visions. What we wanted to stop was his threatening the social workers.

An immediate intervention was to call together everyone who knew Alfred. It turned out that he had a large family and many contacts in the community. Twenty-five people came to that first meeting. Everyone liked him on some level, but not everyone trusted him. He was known to use drugs on occasion and to manipulate others into buying him plane tickets to where he wanted to go, ostensibly for mental health treatment. When he got there, he would check out after one day and do what he wanted. Alfred, of course, disagreed with all of this.

We developed a story with which everyone could agree. Alfred's brain had been frozen from sleeping out on the snow for too long. He needed help thawing his brain. Medication could help with that. On the other hand, his experience in the bush had caused a spiritual awakening that could be inspirational for everyone. We found some young men who would volunteer to spend time with Alfred, to write down his visions, and to return to read them back to him so that he could confirm the accuracy or make changes. In fact, we suggested maybe the community needed to start an archive of visions that happened in the bush. The young people were enthusiastic about this, especially since we had negotiated with the tribe to pay them for this effort.

Alfred was lonely and isolated. His psychotic symptoms brought him attention and notoriety in the community, which was preferable to being alone. Probably all stories told about him had an element of truth. He could be manipulative. He did take drugs sometimes. He did occasionally drink to excess. But he could also be kind. After a successful hunt, he brought the poorest people in the village meat to eat for a month. He shared everything that he had, sometimes to excess. We praised his efforts to live like a saint.

Over time, we worked with the community to shape Alfred's life into a more saintlike form and to give him more attention. It cost less to provide him with attention than to ship him to the psychiatric hospital. His relatives helped care for him. Alfred settled down and stopped causing trouble for social workers. He usually had a smile on his face. He still disappeared at times into the bush, but always came back with new visions and fish and meat for everyone. We reduced Alfred's psychotic symptoms by helping his community make his actual life more interesting than his psychotic life. Also, the community created a narrative for him as a visionary hunter. He liked this story. It gave him meaning and purpose. He began to see himself as someone who could help everyone and upon whom others could rely for food in times of need. He preferred these new stories about him. They brought him into closer integration with the community.

Involving the larger community to change the stories about a person and create opportunities that didn't previously exist can be much more effective than private, one-on-one treatment confined to a small room. Since communities hold the stories about us, it is more efficient to change those stories all at once than to change the affected person's story in secret and then to expect those changes to generalize.

We need the group to re-author our stories. Rarely can re-authoring be done in isolation. Some stories are compatible with some types of problems; others are not. How we change or re-author stories remains a mystery. Some of the process relates to our increasing realization that we have some freedom to act to change our lives. When we begin to "de-identify" with the life we have been living, we can ask ourselves (and others), was this really the life I wanted to live? Could it be different? If so, how would I want it to be different?

Of course, every member of the group has his or her own thoughts about how things could change. The important thing is that we have an audience. The groups and communities to which we belong hold us accountable. All communities have criteria for how to be a good member. If we belong to the community, we are expected to conform. This becomes an internalized audience. How this happens is mysterious, but we do imagine others hearing and reacting to us. These others are commonly the important members of our various communities.

And we can change our audience—and thus change our world. When we act in the world, we get feedback. When our performance changes, our feedback changes. When we collaborate with others and realize that we get different feedback when we act differently, we start to conceive that we have some agency, some sense of personal power. Achieving new results by acting in a new way teaches us that we can influence our world.

6
Narrative Medicine in Action

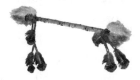

*If there is anything that human history demonstrates, it is
the extreme slowness with which the academic and critical
mind acknowledges facts to exist [that] present themselves
as wild facts, with no staff or pigeon-hole, or as facts [that]
threaten to break up the accepted system.*

WILLIAM JAMES[1]

I learned the hard way why we need more than one story for approaching the world. I was planning my 2006 trip to Santa Fe for the annual summer Creativity and Madness Conference. I had carefully saved my money in a Canadian savings account that I could access with my ATM card. I was planning to take out cash when I got to the States to avoid the high fees associated with currency exchange.

To my chagrin, my ATM card demagnetized on the trip to Santa Fe, leaving me without access to my cash. Luckily some true friends responded to my plight and loaned me money until I could resolve the crisis. Fortunately, I was able to quickly pay them back with income from private sessions with clients during the conference. Suddenly I realized why people carried traveler's checks and a credit card or two in addition to an ATM card. I used this story to introduce the talk I gave in Santa Fe that year, telling the audience that my story had direct parallels to medicine and psychology. Having only one explanatory story for how healing occurs is like putting all the money in one account with only one means of access. If something happens that doesn't apply to this story (like the ATM card being demagnetized), there is no backup plan, no alternative.

The central idea of this book is that illness makes sense within the overall stories and contexts of a person's life. This is not a new idea. Indigenous cultures have believed this since long before recorded history. Narrative medicine tells us that people have many stories and that they enact these stories. We can create a master story or an anthology of particularly important stories in collaboration with people and their families and community. These are the "bigger stories" that reveal how an illness makes sense within a life. From these stories we can see the meaning of the illness to the person, family, and community.

A narrative approach to medicine helps us understand there are many ways to interpret what patients tell us. We can create many, equally valid stories that represent how we interpret our own world and that of our patients. We pick one of many possible stories, often not even conscious of the stories we have ignored or discarded. When our preferred story doesn't work, we tend to blame the client, saying that they are treatment resistant, noncompliant, or just don't want to get better. Instead, we need to recognize that our story may just not sufficiently match our patient's story, and that we need to look for other stories than the one that has become our default mode. The more we can do this consciously, the easier it will be for us to be helpful to many different people.

Some of our explanations (stories) in medicine have evolved because they work really well—for example, placing a chest tube to relieve a pneumothorax saves lives. However, some medical stories are forced onto people because we are committed on principle to prefer a certain way of seeing the world (biological, genetic) over other ways (energetic, spiritual). Some of these stories don't always work very well. Conventional medical treatments for chronic allergies, schizophrenia, and heart disease, for example, are woefully limited.

The stories that we all internalize and tell ourselves over and over again inform us as to what our values are, tell us what we should find meaningful, and sustain the stage upon which suffering and illnesses unfold. I am suggesting that the stage actually plays a big role in determining what forms our suffering will take and what diseases we will develop. This means that physicians need to know the stories their patients are living or enacting. Knowing the story and the stage upon which it is being performed will help us understand the patient's implicit values and anticipate the next events to occur in that person's life (the plot). We will be much more effective in reducing suffering and illness when our treatment stories make sense in the context of the illness stories told by the patient, the patient's family, and the patient's culture.

We might even wonder if the brain's neural networks actually develop their connections and structure in response to stories we internalize at an early age, stories that tell us who we are. The neural connections change as we acquire new knowledge. Stories and conversations become patterns of information within the brain.[2] I am suggesting that the brain (which controls an amazing amount of physiology) is structured through our social interactions. Culture actually directs brain development even selecting for the emergence of some potential brain functions and not others.

A man recently presented to me with a sense of emptiness. He was an artist who had undergone twenty years of psychotherapy. He had also been to multiple shamans, but no one had helped him with his emptiness. As I sometimes do to save time, I asked him to tell me about any characters from movies, books, plays, or stories with whom he strongly identified. Immediately he enthusiastically mentioned Batman. He loved the Batman movies. "What appeals to you most?" I asked.

"Righting wrongs," he said. "Making things right."

"And how are you doing that?" I asked.

"I'm not," he said.

"Maybe that's what you need to do," I said. This led to a discussion of how he could right wrongs as an artist, and he began a series of creative, sculptural pieces on the theme of George Bush's administration and what he as Batman would perceive to be wrong with that group, including wrongs that needed to be righted. He had a sudden awareness of how he could incorporate political criticism into his sculptures, which the Republicans from Texas would buy anyway for their homes, building lobbies, and corporate boardrooms. He was enlivened to realize that he could probably be as outrageous as he wished, and it would only increase sales. He could really be Batman—righting wrongs invisibly and anonymously. I kidded him, telling him that I expected him to sculpt from now on wearing his Halloween Batman costume. His sense of emptiness disappeared as he became more like the character he admired and began living the story he wished to live.

Becoming a more authentic character to his own preferred story served as a kind of tipping point to allow all the previous psychotherapy and traditional healing to coalesce into a different, more desirable outcome. This was not an artificial health that would soon fall apart, leading the person to collapse back into sickness. Two years later, he was productive and still fulfilled, producing more art than ever, but now with his hidden political agenda.

Even risky behavior makes sense within the values contained in the stories of the people involved. Structured interviews or questionnaires cannot capture these stories. What we lack in medicine is a context from which to make sense of human suffering, of people getting sick, getting well, staying sick, being born, and dying. Literature does much better than we do; hence, the proliferation of Literature and Medicine courses. But beyond this understanding of the contexts of patients, we physicians need to realize that our treatments are also contained in stories and are presented in story fashion. If we really want to change suffering and illness, we must renegotiate the stories within which we all work and live. Change the story and the illness may change.

It is human nature to make story and talk story. When we do, we create meaning that did not exist before. Our stories evolve and change in dialogue with others. The medical dialogue is one of these conversations. Patients and doctors interact to shape the story of an incipient condition into a narrative that the doctor can understand and to which she can then respond. People have to be taught to be patients, and the learning occurs through the dialogue surrounding medical contacts and visits. People achieve medical identities through these stories (for example, cancer patient or arthritis patient). These storied identities can then maintain them as members of communities of sufferers. The way we respond to one another is a primary factor in shaping who we think we are.[3]

It is through our connectedness with others that we create our social networks, concepts, and culture. Creation involves dialogue, the medium of connectedness. By dialogue, we mean information exchange, the essence of what connects the universe, a flow of data that creates reality, maintains feedback loops, keeps Earth's temperature within a narrow range, and melts iron at 98.6°F (37°C) within the human body.

Local environments provide the stage upon which the human story is performed. Aboriginal cultures have taught us that the local environment is simultaneously geological, social, biological, and spiritual. We invent the separations, not nature. Nature is a seamless whole. Information exchange (dialogue) among all levels maintains the integrity of the local environment and provides the stage for the unfolding of human concerns. The stories, stages, and characters that populate our lives create the biology of our lives, and vice versa. Aboriginal culture and neurophysiology both confirm the same basic fact—that the brain cannot be separated from the environment it evaluates and acts upon. Language is one tool for evaluation and action, and includes gestures, acts of expressing emotion, and the results of prior learning. Our bodies allow us to interact because our bodies are embedded in nature; they are nature.

This means that, acting together, people cocreate the concepts by which we live. We do this in conversation with each other.[4] Through conversation, we set a stage upon which our biology either falters or thrives. Because we are embodied, everything we create must be "bodied forth." Biology is inseparable from sociology. Without bodies, we could not interact and our interactions would not affect our physiology. Theodore Sarbin said, "People live and understand their living through socially constructed narrative realities that give meaning and organization to their experience. It is a world of human language and discourse."[5] A narrative reality is the world created within a story.

In the Hawai'ian creation story, the narrative reality is the world of the gods and goddesses, the sacred beings, one that plays itself out in the heavens, on land, and under the sea. The world within these stories can feel very real when we live the stories as if they are true—a crucial point of narrative philosophy. We must at least acknowledge that we can't ever know for certain which stories about the world are true, so we must pick and choose in accordance with our desires and interests.

Once we settle upon a story, however, we must live it *as if* it were true. We must perform it by living it. By enacting the story, by living as if it were true, we make it so. We make it true. Pieces of our stories took place long before we were born and are contained in the traditional stories passed down to us from our ancestors. They are contained in the stories our parents tell us. We modify them as we live the stories and find that some pieces no longer apply in our changing world culture. This means that our realities, our worlds, are cocreated through the stories that arise from our conversations with each other. These stories then give meaning to our experience. The meaning that comes to be attached to experience has profound impact upon our biology, giving rise to illnesses, risky behaviors practiced both as solace and communication, and response tendencies. Smoking cigarettes, for example, can be understood only in the context of the person who smokes, as a means of responding to a situation.

Let's look at the Native Hawai'ian narrative reality as example. We begin with the Kumulipo poem, translated by Queen Lili'uokalani in 1895:

> Time begins with darkness. Her name is Po.
> *O ke au I kahuli wela ka honua.*
> At that time that turned the heat of the Earth,
> *O ke au I kahuli lole ka lani,*
> At that time when the heavens turned and changed,
> *O ke au i kuka'iaka ka la,*
> At the time when the light of the sun was subdued,
> *E he'emalamalama I ka malama,*
> To cause light to break forth,
> *O ke au o Makali'I ka po,*
> At the time of the night of winter,
> *O ka walewale ho'okumu henna ia,*

Then began the slime which established the Earth,
O ke kumu o ka lipo, i lipo ai,
The source of deepest darkness,
O ke kumu o ka Po, I po ai,
The source of deepest night,
O ka lilolipo, o ka lipolipo,
Of the depth of darkness, of the depth of darkness,
O ka lipo o ka la, o ka lipo e ka pa,
Of the darkness of the sun, in the depth of night,
Po wale ho'i.
It is night.[6]

Our creation stories situate us within a view of the world that colors our perception and our reaction to ongoing events. In the Hawai'ian story, Po is the night. Po is the darkness. She is the first to come forth. Everything begins with her.[7] Beginning here, darkness is my Creator. Life emerges from darkness. Unlike the Judeo-Christian story, here the struggle between light and dark does not mirror good and evil; rather, light is born from the darkness. Differences like this, the color metaphors used by the peoples of different cultures, can contribute to subtle misunderstandings. We must understand that differences in points of view arise from the traditional stories of the respective cultures and can be anticipated when we study these stories. In the same manner, illnesses of different people can be understood and anticipated when we contemplate the stories of the families in which the illnesses develop.

When I work with indigenous people, I use their traditional stories to situate them within a context of ancestral power and cultural pride. Creation stories have power because they tell us how it all began. A Hawai'ian family came to see me because their son, Kimo, was causing trouble. He was beating up his younger brother without warning for minor annoyances. He was sneaking out at night. He was cursing his mother and ignoring her rules, refusing to do his chores, and letting his schoolwork slide. The teachers were sending him home with angry notes. The school referred the family to me. They suggested that perhaps Kimo should be on a medication that "would fix him up." Essentially, they hoped medication could help make Kimo into "a better person."

As we began, the family was saturated in a biomedical story that says "people are defective and need to be treated with medication to make their brain chemistry right again. If everyone is on the right medications, the family will be happy and problems will be solved." This would be a good story if it worked, but it rarely does. To begin, I had to fulfill my psychiatric role in the conventional biomedical story. I had to ask the questions defined to determine if Kimo could be assigned to any of the conventional diagnostic labels. If I were to ignore the reality of the family presented to me, they would simply exclude me. Then I would have no opportunity to influence their story and no opportunity to coauthor a revision with the family, an approach that might be more friendly and kind.

From my role within the conventional narrative, I had to consider depression, anxiety, attention disorders, schizophrenia and other psychoses, mood disorders including bipolar disorder, oppositional defiant disorder, conduct disorder, and other potential diagnoses for Kimo. The boy was lucid and attentive for the entire first hour-and-a-half-long interview. He did not fidget or seem distracted. Attention deficit hyperactivity disorder seemed unlikely. He did not appear depressed or particularly anxious. He was in control of his rebellion. He was not psychotic. Within the DSM-IV categories, possible diagnoses included conduct disorder, oppositional defiant disorder, or adjustment reaction of adolescence with disturbance of conduct. DSM-IV is frustrating in that the stories generated through its diagnoses have no magic or power to change people. They embed them in a label of disease to the exclusion of healing.

Obviously, I am not a conventional psychiatrist who would insist on giving Kimo a drug, no matter what. When nothing else makes sense, our profession usually tries selective serotonin reuptake inhibitors (SSRIs, such as Prozac, Paxil, and Zoloft), since they are the "safest" psychiatric medications and usually work for everything, somehow. I didn't see an urgent need to start Kimo on the road to the defective brain story. Our first session ended with the idea that maybe Kimo did not have a disease that needed a medication and that we could have another session with the whole family present to explore other options. I asked each person to keep notes about how the various family members influenced one another.

Kimo's father and mother were divorced. In the next session, I learned that Dad lived with his mother, who drank heavily every day. Dad had a history of heavy drinking while married, but currently had his drinking more under control. He worked itinerant jobs when he needed money. His ex-wife, Kimo's mom, worked for the local school board and saw her former husband as a derelict and a failure. "He's a bum," she said. "He's a worthless bum alcoholic who'll never work a real job for the rest of his life."

"Why do you call him to come over?" I asked, more than a little puzzled.

"I call him when I'm at my wit's end with Kimo. I tell him, 'Get your butt over here or I'm going to prison for killing the kid.'"

"And then he comes?"

"Then he comes."

"And then what happens?"

"He calms Kimo down. He stays a few days. He eats all my food. Then I kick him out and he goes back to his mom's place."

"So if Kimo wants a visit from his dad, all he has to do is act bad?" I asked. Mom looked at me quizzically.

"It's not like that," she said. "He can see his dad anytime. He even lived with him for a short time, but I had to take him back. There was too much drinking at that house."

"I'm sure he'd prefer to see his dad at his own house," I said. "After all, kids prefer their own rooms and stuff to other people's houses and other people's stuff." We talked more about the concept that Kimo was actually smart and organizing his world to get what he wanted, instead of defective and needing medication. This was a new perspective for his mother.

"Let me read you a poem," I said. "Perhaps you will recognize it?" I read her the Kumulipo poem. The tone changed. The energy shifted. Things seemed more serious, but in a good way.

"What's that got to do with me?" she asked.

"It's the creation story of the Hawai'ian people," I said. "I'm not Hawai'ian, but you guys are. It's your story and I wanted to honor it. I wanted to invite us all to imagine that we are starting in darkness just like Po did, that we don't have a clue what's going on with Kimo, or anyone else for that matter, and we are going to spend some time together and let something emerge, the way light broke forth *(mala-malama I ka malama)*, the way Earth formed out of deepest darkness. You're feeling as if you're in deepest darkness about Kimo and the stress of your family. I thought we could honor your heritage's knowledge that wisdom comes from darkness."

"That's nice," she said. "I never thought like that before."

"Always a first time," I said. "Guess it could be now. So let's practice ignorance. Let's drop all our theories about Kimo and what's going on. Let's stop calling him lazy. Let's stop thinking he's just stubborn. Let's sit and talk without any set ideas about what's going on and see what emerges."

"I know what's going on," announced Kumu, the younger son.

"What do you know?" I asked.

"Mom's always saying Kimo is just like his dad." Now it was time to focus on the wisdom of the youngest child.

"In what ways are Dad and Kimo alike?" I asked.

Kumu was quick to respond. "They're both lazy," he said. "That's what Mom always says. She always says Kimo is just like his father when she's mad."

"Is he your father, too?" I asked.

"Sure he is," Kumu said. "But I'm not like him. I'm just like my mother. That's why Kimo and I fight so much."

"So what should we do about this?" I asked.

"Everyone should have to work for their smokes and money," said Kumu. "Mom's always complaining she buys all the smokes and makes all the money and Dad never helps her and Kimo never does his chores, so they should all have to work for what they get."

"Even Mom?" I asked.

"Yeah, well, she works, but she should lose points for being grumpy and crabby and yelling at us," he said in a challenging tone. Kumu had shared new stories, especially the story that the two children were like the two different parents. Now we had something to work with.

"Alright," I said. "Let's run with Kumu's version. We've got two teams here—Dad's team and Mom's team. Mom's team gets work done—money work and homework. Dad's team has more fun. Let's see if we can come up with some ideas for how both teams can benefit. Let's see if we can be different from Pele and her sister. Do you guys know that story?" They didn't.

"Let me tell you this story," I said. "It's a bit like what's going on with you guys. Maybe it will give you some ideas."

Namakaokaha'i and Pelehonuamea were both daughters of Haumea, the great goddess who gave birth to so many of your sacred people. Nama is the powerful goddess of the ocean and Pele is the great goddess of volcanoes. When you see hot lava flowing down the mountainside, you know her temper has flared. The two began fighting almost at birth, just like Kimo and Kumu. Nama always won, however, because ocean water cools hot lava and turns it to stone. I'm not sure which of you guys always wins. I suspect Kimo does, because he is older and stronger, but, on the other hand, Kumu is sneakier, and maybe he can win on that basis.

The boys nodded enthusiastically, seemingly proud of their attributes.

Nama won so often their mother feared she would quench Pele's flames forever. Haumea got so scared she gave Pele a canoe and asked her to get as far away from Nama as she could.

"That would be like sending Kumu to live with your relatives in Hilo, which I know you have considered, because Kimo is strong and gives Kumu bruises," I interjected. Both parents nodded.

Pele asked her brother, a shark god, to guide her canoe, which he did, but Nama followed in close pursuit, chasing her across the ocean and putting out her sacred fires wherever they burned.

From the northwest atolls to Ni'ihau, from island to island they battled. The mountainous remnants of those battles can still be seen. Finally, on Maui, Pele thought she had climbed higher than Nama could reach, but Nama's last wave reached the top of what we now call Hale'akala. That wave smashed Pele's body onto the ground, breaking every bone. Pele entered spirit form and continued to flee from Nama all the way to the

Big Island, to the top of what we now call Kilauea, which was so high that
Nama could not reach her. Pele found a home at last.

"So is that like your fighting?" I asked Kimo and Kumu.

"Just like it!" both of them exclaimed proudly, almost simultaneously. I had their attention. They liked comparing themselves and their fights to the epic battles of sacred beings. It was almost as good as identifying with superheroes.

"Any clues about how to solve this fighting?" I asked.

"Separate rooms," said Kumu quickly. "He needs his mountain. I need my ocean. We need our own rooms."

"Then we need a new house," Mom said. "I've got no space for them to have their own rooms."

"Alright, then," I said. "We have a goal to work on—separate rooms! What other goals could we work toward?" I looked at Mom. "Could you come up with a reward system? Could everyone, including Dad, have to work for their smokes, or something like smokes? At least I hope Kumu isn't smoking yet." Kumu nodded his agreement. "How could everyone work for privileges and benefits, like money?"

"There's no money to work for," Mom said.

"I'll bet there is," I said. "I bet you buy them things for school. You buy them food. You buy them shoes, and you buy them other stuff they want. Maybe they should work for their stuff. Maybe they should get rewards for good behavior and lose money for bad behavior. Would that work?"

Mom thought it over. "We've tried such things before," she said, "and they never worked longer than a few weeks."

"Maybe you didn't try them longer than a few weeks," I wondered. "And maybe you and Dad weren't part of the game, and because you're the team leaders, it matters what the two of you do. You have to be part of it, too. You have to work for your luxury items, including smokes. Make Dad work for his smokes and beer. Everybody has to do it, or Kumu will say it's no fair."

After some thought and discussion, Mom declared, "Well, we've never tried that before. I guess we could do it." Her tone was now thoughtful, as if she thought they might be able to succeed, not skeptical, as she had sounded before. I credited the sacred story for helping to guide the tone and mood toward potential acceptance of new ideas.

"Do you want to sit here and figure this out?" I asked. "I have another appointment coming, but I could put you into an empty room to work it out, and then we could go over it after my next appointment."

"No," Mom said. "We can do it ourselves, tonight, at home. We can work this out on our own."

"Great," I said. "Write it down and mail me a copy of what you come up with. We can see how it works next time we meet. And one more thing. I wondered if you'd all be willing to look into the ancient gods and goddesses and each of you come next time with your favorite and tell me a little story about why you like that one the best." To my surprise, they all agreed to bring that information next time. Mom had an auntie in Hilo who knew kahunas and kapunas who could be asked about such things. Kimo and Kumu said there were books at their school library to look at.

In the next session, three weeks later, we reviewed their scheme for rewards and fines. We fine-tuned some difficulties and closed some loopholes. I was impressed at their sophistication. They had created a system better than I could have imagined for them. Smokes played a predominant role, but there were other rewards. They also brought their favorite gods.

Kimo's favorite was Nanaue, the son of Kamohoali'i, the supreme shark god, and Kalei, a human woman who lived at the mouth of the Waipi'o River on the Big Island. Kimo told a story about how this guy had a big shark's mouth all across his back.

His mom hid the big shark's mouth from other people all through his childhood. He had to wear a cape over it so no one could see it. And he couldn't eat meat of any kind, or he would go crazy. The problems began when he got old enough to eat alone with the men. His grandfather fed him pork by accident, not knowing it would drive him crazy. That gave him a taste for meat, and all sharks know the best meat is human meat.

Soon he started going down to the water to hide, waiting for people to go swimming so he could eat them. For years he ate anyone who went swimming alone. He'd even ask people if they were going swimming so he could run down to the water and wait for them.

Nanaue's mother began to suspect that he was the man-eating shark who lived in the shallow waters outside the village, but her love for her son prevented her from saying anything to the other people. But one hot day the men were working in the taro patch. Wondering why Nanaue would wear his red cloak on such a hot day, his friend yanked it off, and suddenly everyone saw the big shark's mouth. Seeing that mouth, the men grabbed their spears and chased Nanaue, but he was too fast for them and jumped into the sea, turning into a shark as he went under water.

Nanaue went to Hana on the island of Maui, and everything was fine for a while. He married a woman and they had a son. Life was good, but he could not overcome his desire to eat human flesh. Soon he was back to his old tricks. But the people found out again and chased him away.

He went from island to island and village to village, until everybody had heard the legend of the man-eating shark. When he came to the island of Moloka'i, the people were expecting him. They captured him and killed him. If only he had listened to his mother. If only all had obeyed his father's advice about never feeding him meat, this tragedy would have been spared.

Kimo wished to be Nanaue, the man-eating shark, despite this tragic ending (which is quite telling as an aspect of his story). I wondered at his identification with a "bad boy" character, one whose tragic flaw only emerges when he begins to eat with the adult men, no longer under his mother's protection. In a sense Kimo was experimenting with being an adult. He wanted his own smokes. He wanted to go out when he wanted to and stay out as long as he wished. Kimo was at the same stage of life as Nanaue when he first tasted human flesh. Maybe Kimo was identifying with this character who tasted forbidden fruit and couldn't get enough of it, even though it led to his demise. This is a story that could lead to addiction or excess. It warranted further dialogue and potential transformation.

Kumu proudly announced that he was Kimo's dad, the great shark god. Kumu had a way of one-upping Kimo, which frustrated Kimo greatly. Kumu was attached to the idea of being the younger child who comes out on top. He seemed to pride himself on being smarter and more devious than his older brother—the attributes possessed by the great shark god.

Mom announced that she was most certainly Haumea, the goddess who gave birth to so many wonderful children. We all laughed at her tongue-in-cheek playfulness. Mom told us about how Haumea's spirit occupied the trees from which came the power objects men used to increase their chances of success in war or politics. She also provided the wood for carvings of the goddess Makali, who attracts fish. Most importantly, her spirit gave beauty to the young people of each generation in order to make them desirable, so they could create powerful offspring to increase the *mana* of every family line. "Just like my Kimo and Kumu are going to do," she said.

Dad chose Kahi'uka, one of the guardian shark gods of Pu'uloa in 'Ewa, O'ahu. These shark gods defended the fishermen from man-eating sharks. The fisherman showed their appreciation by giving them the first of their catch, bringing them food and *'awa*,* and scraping barnacles off their bodies. Here was Dad, picking a character that has little real work to do and has his livelihood handed to him, just as was currently happening within his own family.

Now we could talk about each family member in terms of his or her ritualistic roles and names. We could explore Kimo in the role of the tragic man-eating shark. I joked with them, "If only Kimo had never gotten a taste for cigarettes. Think of what he might have accomplished." We saw that Kumu was perpetually off the hook, since he played the great and powerful dad who disappeared. We talked about Dad's role as Kahi-uka, coming home for a while to rescue Mom from the kids, bumming cigarettes, and eating the food in the refrigerator (the first of the catch). Mom's role reminded me of the Hopi dolls of mothers with many children. She carried all the burdens on her shoulders. She was seen as the creator of the children and the family and all revolved around her.

Through the use of characters in the stories, we could explore the roles of each family member and hook these roles into their origins

---

*Kava

within the traditional culture. We could also slowly transform the characters, because Kimo really didn't really want to be killed by the people of Moloka'i. Dad wanted to become equal in stature to Mom. Mom didn't want all the burdens she shouldered. And Kumu wanted to be more vulnerable and connected, less aloof and above it all. The use of traditional characters and stories allowed us to talk about family members and issues in an "as if" manner. We could discuss the stories and the characters as if we were discussing the family members who identified with these characters, which reduced defensiveness and helped everyone maintain a sense of humor.

Conventional medicine is based upon a certain style of dialogue with nature. For the most part, it rests upon machines and reductionist science. Nature is supposed to behave the same way each time. The conversation is limited to biological responses—the strength of an enzyme reaction, the level of a biochemical compound in the serum, the appearance of red blood cells. Narrative medicine includes those conversations and more, including some that lie outside the realm of what conventional medicine considers acceptable. These include conversations with what might be called the spirit of illness, death, pain, the Universe, ancestors, other humans, plants, animals, and minerals, expressed through movement, perception, and sensation. Indigenous cultures have historically relied upon and valued these kinds of conversations. Western cultures have not.

Narrative medicine presents a dialogue in the broadest possible sense—information exchange—about the concerns that arise when we live in a physical world, in a body, facing the inevitability of death and the possibility of disease, dysfunction, and restrictions on our freedom of thought, mobility, and interaction.

It gets even more interesting when spirits or ancestors give us information. I remember sitting in ceremony with a woman who had endometriosis and very clearly hearing the voice of my grandfather saying, "Her problem is she has stopped painting. She is trapped in her tiny house, in her sadness and fear, and she has no outlet. At least when she painted, the feelings had somewhere to go. Now they go into her pelvis." I told the woman and her husband about this and it opened up an entirely new level of discourse. The original topic had been whether or not to take steroids. I had invited us to consider this topic in ceremony and through prayer, once we had exhausted the medical story about steroids and endometriosis (which is an inconclusive, uncertain story, occasionally fraught with peril, like so many medical stories).

I sat in ceremony with another woman who suffered from migraine headaches. I saw a mental picture of an older woman and described her. My description turned out to fit her immigrant great-grandmother. This matriarch of the family invited the woman to change her life, saying the migraines would go away. Changing her life meant moving out of New York City and finding a more expansive, less stressful life with room for nature, art, children, and dogs. Two years after moving to the country, her migraines were forgotten.

We can't assume that the information we think we are getting from spirit communication is correct. Even when I do things that could be called psychic, I don't assume I am psychic. I just happened to stumble into a conversation with nonphysical entities. I could distort or mishear. I could misinterpret. I could be hearing someone else's conversation. My purpose is to start a dialogue. It is through the dialogue that meaning emerges, not through my actions or knowledge or expertise.

Here is a traditional Dene story about the importance of integrating multiple stories into the final narrative that we live by, the story we call our own. This is a story about how the people learned to build their homes.

During those early years in the Fifth World (our world as we see it today), the land was reshaped to resemble the previous Fourth World. The people made their homes near springs or rivers, or beside the lake that had arisen at the place of emergence, where they had come up through a hole in the ground. The rivers and mountains were still being created. Once rain began to fall, it was no longer necessary to huddle in two or three places. Water was plentiful and the land blossomed. Food was abundant, except in those two or three places that were now almost barren.

The people divided and began to follow the myriad dirt paths to the lakes, mountains, hillsides, and flat tops of the mesas. As they spread apart, silence descended upon their former homes. Looking back, they could see Coyote greeting the sun as he stood alone on what used to be fertile crop fields and grazing land.

First Woman informed the dispersing people that they could build houses however they wished. "Look to the original inhabitants of this land for inspiration," she said. "From the nests of the swallows hanging under the tops of rocky cliffs to the burrows of the badger, all have something to teach you." She reminded them to consult these original inhabitants before using the clay, tall trees, cliff rocks, or other natural materials. The Bird People had reached the Fifth World first and had been building homes the longest. Standing at the foot of the mountains, First Woman asked them for advice on how to make a warm house that would furnish protection at night, but would not be blown away by strong winds nor destroyed by hard rain or hail.

Gray Eagle rose to the task, proudly offering to show his home in the rock crevice roofed by an overhanging ledge, high on the crest of Blue Mountain. He demonstrated how he carried sticks and short poles to build a hollow circle twice his height, which he lined with spruce twigs and his own breast feathers. "Never will my house be reduced to riffraff and piles of dust," he said, "for it is sturdier than the wind and rain and will keep my children safe." The walls to Gray Eagle's house rose more than one thousand feet above the lush valley, impossible to reach by anyone who could not fly.

First Woman thanked Hosteen Eagle for his advice, saying, "We cannot defy the pull of Mother Earth the way you do. We will use your example, however, to go to the mountains in the summer and build cool shelters of pole and brush. We are grateful for your teaching us how to put poles together to form a circle. We would not be warm enough in your house in the winter, even if we could reach it." Gray Eagle rose toward snow-covered peaks, his feathers buffeted by wind currents, announcing that he and his kind just flew elsewhere for the winter, returning in spring when conditions were more favorable. First Woman thanked him for his council and offered him white shell beads to wear on his headdress as he rose up into his blue-sky home of space and light. She thanked him for the inspiration to make their houses round, like the sun.

Another bird rose up to present a different design, one that would be warm even in the winter. Hosteen Oriole led them to a cottonwood tree standing high above willows and marsh grass, beside a rushing creek. She showed the people how to pick a stout branch that would not break in a storm. She wove a snug basket with strips of willow bark and marsh grass leaves with an opening at one side, lining the inside with milkweed pod fuzz and cliff rose. The people admired her ingenuity, but sadly informed her that they could not live in the tops of trees. First Woman thanked Hosteen Oriole, giving her yellow beads to wear around her throat, telling her that she had inspired the people to weave ropes for tying things together and baskets for gathering seeds and nuts.

As they were taking their leave, Hosteen Woodpecker bade them follow him to his house. He showed them how to make a hole in a hollow tree, into which he stuffed grasses and soft moss to make the most desirable kind of house ever. First Woman thanked Hosteen Woodpecker, giving him red beads to wear in his headdress, for he had inspired her quite differently than he had anticipated. He had given her the idea for drums, which would become very important to the people.

Next Cliff Swallow came forth to demonstrate his style of home-building. He led the people through his beautiful valley, past meadows and rocky ledges, to his home beneath the highest overhangs of the towering cliffs. He showed how he brought adobe from the stream and mixed it with bits of grass to build walls underneath the cliff. His home was round, with an opening to the side, well protected from the elements. First Woman thanked Hosteen Cliff Swallow as he proudly sat swaying on the top of a juniper tree, for he had taught them how to make adobe walls. Most people could not live in a place so high. They thought they could not build long enough ladders to reach such homes, nor would they have anywhere to store food for the winter. However, some of the people stayed in this place to emulate the life of the cliff swallows, building similar dwellings from which they climbed down long ladders just to get water. They became known as the Cliff House People. First Woman gave Hosteen Cliff Swallow a gift of black beads to decorate his coat, to thank him for his contribution.

The four-leggeds who lived in caves were not worth visiting, for they constructed nothing. The people continued down the river, looking for Hosteen Muskrat, whose home was a tangle of brush and branches completely surrounded by water, the entrance accessible only through swimming. Although similar to Hosteen Muskrat's, the homes of Hosteen Otter and Hosteen Mink were closer to the shore and more accessible, but were dark and damp and smelled of fish.

The homes of the Beaver People were quite the exception. The people loved the dome-shaped roofs and appreciated the two-story construction. Crossed logs were stacked in beehive fashion with an opening for ventilation at one side. The second story was comfortably dry because it was above water level. Fresh air and sunlight entered through the roof; reeds closed off the underwater opening. Since the people did not want to live in water, First Woman announced that they could copy this design for use on dry land. As they left, she offered the beavers a gift of an abalone shell.

Moving further downstream, the people passed a cottonwood tree with silk netting strewn over several branches. "This is the home of Hosteen Caterpillar," announced First Woman. While quite innovative and protective for caterpillars, the people agreed that this method was of little use to them, since they could not make silk from their bodies nor hibernate in cocoons for the winter. Next they encountered the Spider Family, who played tricks on them, but promised to teach them how to weave once they had thread or yarn. They especially liked the way the Spider People divided the rooms of their homes with woven blankets.

They visited the Ant People last. Their home was covered with earth to make it harder for enemies to find them. The one opening in the roof had a hidden doorway facing the east, where the ants entered through a long passageway. The rooms underneath the floor could store food for the winter. The walls were plastered and floors made of hard clay. They left the ants brightly colored pebbles as gifts to use for decorating the roofs of their homes.

The people had learned enough. Their homes would be round, as were most of the animals' homes, like the sun and the full moon. They would build walls of logs and make these walls higher than their heads, the *way the eagles and beavers did. They would have a dome-shaped roof with an opening to the sky and a doorway to the east so the sun could awaken them in the morning. They would plaster their floors and walls as the swallows and the ants did. When their homes were finished, they would cover them with earth and place a woven blanket over the doorway to keep warm. And that is how homes are built even to this day.*

Just as First Woman taught the people to do, narrative medicine teaches us that we must integrate multiple points of view to arrive at appropriate solutions. Thus, narrative medicine is more a philosophy than a set of practices. We don't reject the biological story or the genetic story. We don't reject the stories surgeons or internists or gastroenterologists tell. We contextualize them. We fit these stories alongside the other stories told by people themselves, their families, and their cultures. We hear the story as the product of dialogue, and we start new dialogues to generate new stories.

Just as conversations involve speakers, some dialogues involve bodies interacting with other bodies. These dialogues are called physical examinations or bodywork or chiropractic adjustments. Even diagnostic imaging is just one type of conversation with the body, one that we cannot understand at times. Sometimes the answers the body provides to radiological queries are unintelligible.

In narrative medicine, we take the medical history very seriously, because the medical history becomes the story of the illness. I like to have multiple histories. I'm especially interested in the one the illness tells about itself. That story emerges through dialogue, often facilitated by helping the person achieve an altered state of consciousness using imagery or hypnosis. The person who carries the illness has a story about what it's been like to live with the illness. All members of the community should contribute to that story or history, because it does not belong to just one individual, but to the whole community of the illness. People in the community have stories about the person who carries the illness—perhaps their experience of being around the sick person, or their stories about what happened to the sick person's relatives because of the illness, or even associated stories about illnesses they have had. Everyone who knows the person has something to contribute to the story that unfolds about the illness.

The levels encompassed by these dialogues (or stories) include:

1. Family
2. Our own inner subjective world
3. Spirits
4. Animals
5. Plants
6. Minerals
7. Our physical body
8. The illness

The essence of these dialogues includes:

1. Reflection
2. Questions of differences between observations (which anthropologist Gregory Bateson said is the beginning of knowledge)
3. The emergence of unexpected properties during the process
4. Reorganization
5. Transcendence
6. Transformation (which often involves moving far away from what could be considered equilibrium)

Psychologist David Smail writes,

The majority of those who find themselves in distress in Western society turn to the clinic because there is nowhere else to go that carries the same promise of relief. They, as well as most of them who treat them, believe that they are hosts of a personal illness or disorder that can be cured by established medical and/or therapeutic techniques. That belief, however, is in my view (and the view of others) false, and it is clinical experience itself that reveals it as false.[8]

Here is an interesting example of a medical story in which reality becomes confused with the story. This story, published in a medical journal, is called "An Ache in the Abdomen: Severe Stomach Pain Cramps a Young Lad's Life."[9] The story is about an eight-year-old boy presenting to the emergency department with severe cramping and abdominal pain lasting one week. The pain occasionally woke the boy from sleep. Narcotics were given for pain relief. No other findings or symptoms existed. His physical examination was completely normal. A full laboratory investigation, including an abdominal ultrasound, came back completely normal. An upper GI series and abdominal CT scan were normal. In between episodes of pain, the child was playful and had a good appetite. He appeared well. At the next episode of pain, he was taken to surgery, and here was what the surgeons found:

The laparotomy revealed that the child had a normal anatomy, no malrotation, and no damaged bowel segments. The surgery did show a moderate amount of small bowel adhesions, specifically one segment that was firmly attached to the anterior abdominal wall, close to the umbilicus. The surgeon surmised that this was probably related to the boy's previous surgery after birth (eight years ago) in which an omphalocele was repaired. Following the procedure, the child made a remarkable recovery.[10]

What I love about this story is its innocence of interpretation, its absolute belief in the curative power of surgery. In fact, adhesions do not necessarily cause pain and the removal of adhesions does not necessarily cure pain. The story avoids all alternate explanations. What about surgery as ritual? A *New York Times* story, based on a study from the Houston V.A. Hospital, tells us about the effectiveness of sham surgery for relieving knee pain.[11] How is this surgery any different? Anyone with any scientific training should see that this story doesn't prove anything. It simply shows how firmly the medical and surgical stories are entrenched in our culture. Sequential events do not establish causal relationships.

Why and how this boy improved is a mystery and should remain a mystery, regardless of our speculations. I am not saying the surgical story is incorrect. I am saying the story is indeterminate. We can't know that what was done during the surgery mattered at all. All we can know is that the child was well after the surgery. Nevertheless, we are emotionally required to construct a story to explain the healing, and the surgeon in this case, naturally, wanted a story that gave him the credit.

This leads us to Sarah's story, a different kind of yarn about healing, but structurally similar to the surgical story described above. In both cases, we actually have no clue why healing occurred. We just know that it did, and we proceed, as humans do, to construct satisfactory explanations to guide us in the future. Whether they will or not do so adequately is another question.

Sarah came for a healing retreat because she intermittently lost the use of her legs and collapsed to the floor. Friends and family feared multiple sclerosis. She refused to be tested. As I prepared for Sarah's intensive, I spent time each day praying and contemplating the work we would do. I projected enhanced well-being for her long before we started working. I think all effective people do this for their clients. Effective business people do this for the bottom line—the financial health of their business.

Sarah and I started with guided imagery so we could develop a shared map for the territory in which we would be working. Sarah saw an Everest-like mountain she needed to climb. Her legs were freezing in the cold and the snow. Her guide had abandoned her. People were dying in the village below and would continue to die unless she reached the peak to find an exotic flower and return it to them for their medicine, but how could she climb Everest with frozen, useless limbs? She saw that she needed a guide, and how she would find that guide and what he would do became the focus for later work.

Next we moved to Cherokee-style bodywork. What was immediately remarkable was that Sarah appeared not to breathe. For traditional healers, the most important expression of the connection between the human and the Creator is the physical coming and going of breath. Cherokee bodywork emphasizes this principle and aims for the person to breathe freely and without restrictions. The goal is to bring breath into every part of the body. Our work became teaching Sarah to breathe, of making slow and deep breathing into a habit, of finding a way for Sarah to release the tension in her body that prohibited her breathing. That led to an awareness that breath is spirit. We focused our efforts on enabling Sarah to breathe spirit into every part of her body.

William Lyon helped me to realize how ubiquitous is the linkage of breath and spirit in North America. After talking with him, I sought out literature about this connection and was able to use these facts with Sarah as truisms to give prescriptive force to what I was advising her to do. I told her the story about the Hopi saying it is possible to access the Creator only "to the extent that [we] align [the] breath with the cosmic breath that is 'very something.'"[12] I told her that a Hopi word for God translates as "giver of the breath of life." I told her that the Creek word for Creator means master of breath,[13] and that the Zuni word for Creator (Awonawilona) translates as "symbol and initiator of life, who is the breath of life and life itself."[14] I told her the Zuni believed that Awonawilona made all of Creation from the breath of his heart.[15] And that the Seminole word for Creator translates as "breath-maker" or "life-maker." Another of their terms for Creator translates as both "breathing" and "living or alive." I told Sarah that the White Mountain Apache believed that breath and life are the same thing, both bestowed by the Creator. I mentioned the Klamath word *hokis,* which simultaneously means "soul, breath, and life."[16] I told her how the Zuni strived to develop deep, slow, long nasal breathing as one aspect of their training in achieving altered states of consciousness.[17]

All of these facts created for us a small story about the importance of breathing for bringing spirit into her body and sending spirit to all parts of her body. This story would ultimately provide her with vital healing imagery. She would start to see herself as participating in a process of opening up her whole body for the entrance of spirit. I finished by telling Sarah about the Lakota word for breath, which is *ni.* I told her how it was used to create words such as *inipi,* meaning breath of life—the term for the sweatlodge ceremony—or *yuni,* meaning the act of making one conscious of something.[18] I told her that even the English word *spirit* comes from the Latin root *spiritus,* meaning breath, among other things. I introduced her to the idea that we obtain our creative wisdom, our in*spir*ation through our breath. After this long parade of facts and stories, she believed. I had inculcated an idea about breathing bringing spirit and healing into her body. This led her to consider a more spiritual approach to her problem, one that involved inviting her own spirit to fully occupy her body and provide her with the energy she needed for healing.

The aim of a spiritually guided approach is to launch people on a quest in which they have a direct, internal experience of the spiritual domain. In short, they have their own conversations with spirits. Faith is unnecessary after these journeys. Perhaps you already know this from your own experience. But we must keep in mind, from the perspective of narrative medicine, that this too is only one story, or one collection of stories. It is my preferred story, but not one that everyone accepts. I use it when I can. A story is only as useful as it is acceptable to those for whom it is intended.

Sarah asked me, "How do you know when you are talking to a spirit?"

I answered, "Because they are different from me. They have different ideas. We have a conversation. I hear things from them. But you have to have an internal, ecstatic (or at least slightly joyful) experience to know what I am talking about. In order to understand this way of working, you must have your own experiences. You must be on your own inner quest or spiritual journey, or none of this will make sense. But maybe that's not so important anyway," I said. "What we are doing can work even if you just think it is a metaphor. And maybe it will be just as powerful."

Psychologist Abraham Maslow has written about transcendental experiences—those in which we feel the presence of the Divine (Great Mystery, or whatever name we choose) and return changed for the better.[19] We are more complete after these experiences. This is what the psychiatric establishment fails to grasp about traditional healers—that their altered states and extraordinary experiences actually make them more stable community members, more solid instead of less. They become progressively more loving and compassionate people as a result of their trance experience, the opposite of what the DSM-IV describes for psychosis or even "magical thinking."

In Sarah's imagery, she saw a cloud leopard breathe life back into her legs. I asked her to keep this image in her mind during her bodywork—seeing her legs come alive and become capable of carrying her up the mountainside. This reawakening of her legs was an image of empowerment, of building personal power.

Shamans and healers everywhere build personal power. This comes with some caveats. They may be very powerful in ceremony and effective in healing, but scoundrels in some other aspect of their lives. Apparently we are not required to excel in every area. We get to pick and choose, or perhaps our character pushes us in specific ways. I have realized that I do cultivate personal power, but I pass it off to the spirits who help me. I imagine it is their power and that my role is to be able to contact them, ask for help, and get out of the way when the help comes. I still believe that, but I have also recognized I can teach skills that apply to accumulating personal power and pass them on to others in an inspirational sense. It just has to be done. Beyond that, it is important simply to connect people with their own vital force, what Aristotle called "entelechy," meaning a vital force that moves one's being toward self-fulfillment.

Ultimately, my goal with Sarah was to assist her in getting in direct touch with her spirit helpers. Together they would be able to contemplate their position as small beings enclosed within the Great Mystery. Perhaps they could help her find healing or curing. Perhaps not, but they would be there for her long after she left me, so her direct connection with them was far more important than whatever connection she had with me. Lyon has told me that all sacred rituals are actually about getting directly in touch with the Great Mystery. Healing rituals are designed to put a human being back into "walking in beauty." When we operate in ceremony as if we are in harmony, we become so.[20] In relation to this, Dene healing, for example, centers around restoring balance with the self and the Creator, which may incidentally relieve physical symptoms.

Sarah's dreams were filled with leopards. Each day we were doing ceremony. A vision came to her of a tribal people living at the base of a great mountain. They were taking her hunting. They were hunting her soul. Each day they caught small creatures for their meal, but not yet her soul. The night before her sweatlodge ceremony, they found it, roaming the side of the great mountain like a snow leopard. They lassoed it and pulled it back into her body.

I like to do one or more sweatlodge ceremonies each week, depending upon the needs and health of the participants. I also wanted to help Sarah deepen her trance ability before she left for home. This entering a trance goes on at the beginning of just about everything we do. The deeper the trance, the better it seems to work. I think this is because our everyday minds need to get out of the way. We carry too many accumulated thoughts and beliefs from modern culture that are counterproductive to healing. We must transcend or step aside from these beliefs. Singing, drumming, and rattling in the dark always help. Spirits seem to arrive more readily in the dark, but that is probably because of what the dark does to our consciousness, not the spirits' preference. The Tlingit believe that the spirits "only permit themselves to be conjured by the sound of a drum or rattle."[21] We need unified consciousness in order for spirits to appear.

Through the bodywork and the ceremony, Sarah was developing her own skill and personal technique in summoning her helper spirits through breathing. Through calling upon her breath and entering into a kind of trance with breathing, she was becoming able to visualize her helpers at will. She could call the leopards and the tribesmen. Whether these were real or not is immaterial. They came and gave her that greater sense of empowerment and strength that said, "you can walk." When she felt their presence, the strength returned in her legs.

Several years later, Sarah is walking. Her weakness is gone. Her strength is back. She has changed her story. Now she sees herself as the mountain climber, like those early explorers of Everest, who can reach the loftiest heights and bring back gifts for the people. She needs the strength in her legs to be able to do so. She has traveled several times to Nepal and Tibet to raise funds for local communities. She has helped bring ecotourism into the area. She has been responsible for bringing medical care to underserved areas. I hadn't realized her fascination with this area when Everest emerged as her image, but I followed it with her to see where it would go.

Sarah's earlier story had a plot line of progressive deterioration and decline. It was a tragedy. She had adjusted to it. Through interaction with the story of aboriginal healing, her own personal story changed. She developed a story of renewal, of being kissed by the breath of a cloud leopard, and being able to rise off her bed of weakness to climb Everest. The aboriginal story competed within her for the conventional story, which is quite boring: You get multiple sclerosis. Through a series of waxing and waning episodes of symptom relief and exacerbation, you gradually get worse and die. The end.

The aboriginal story does not accept the medical pronouncement of prognosis or diagnosis. You are here in this territory of living in multiple sclerosis, it says, like being in Nepal or Tibet. Only Creator knows what is possible. Let's work together to see what we are able to do with the help of the spirits and your mind and all the personal power we can build together. Let's see what emerges. Let's expect everything we can imagine or dream. That's a radically different story from that offered by conventional medicine.

I prefer the underlying assumption of narrative medicine (that we can change) to those of conventional biomedicine (that we are prisoners of our genetics and our biology). We are born into history—political histories, spiritual histories, histories of science—a collection of stories about how things got to be the way they are. Similarly, we are born into a history of ourselves. We become the person that is projected by this history. Some of these characters have diseases. In this chapter we have seen that transformation and change occur when we have an inspirational story to guide us. We aspire to become our hero, or the character of our inspirational story. We may aspire to be like Ghandi, Jesus, Muhammad, Martin Luther King, Mother Teresa, or even fictional characters like Batman. We try to live up to the story that we want to be. The most central point of the practice of narrative medicine is this—change the story, change everyone's stories about the person, and you change the person. Changing the person often changes the illness. This is called healing.

7
Talking with Asthma

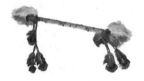

A good scientist has freed himself of concepts and keeps his mind open to what is.

LAO-TZU[1]

Asthma has a well-established conventional story. In this story, genetic factors influence the interaction of the membranes of the respiratory tree with the environment, which leads to excess mucus production, inflammation, constriction, and spasm of the smooth muscles. In this story, how the person lives, influences of family stress and relationships, and personal and cultural beliefs all are irrelevant to asthma, which appears because of genetic mutations that lead the immune system to respond in "asthmatic ways." Pulmonologists rarely care about the story of the person's life. This is unimportant to their conceptualization of the disease.

Conventional medicine gives the doctor the responsibility for respiratory well-being, though the patient is expected to "comply," to follow "doctor's orders." The emphasis is on external treatment and cure. Treatments lie within a body of expert knowledge that the specialist applies to the suffering person. The expert and his knowledge are more important for treatment decisions than is what the person who suffers with asthma knows.

An underlying assumption is that all people with asthma should respond similarly to a particular treatment if it is good (meaning reliable, replicable, predictable). I call this the "one size fits all" assumption. Mind-body medicine can venture a bit further from the mainstream by saying that mind is important, but then falters in its search for essential traits to predict asthma severity, a search that rarely succeeds, because our usual questionnaire-based research misses the richness, individuality, and diversity of human stories and human interaction. The focus remains external—what can I do for you, the patient? Rarely does anybody wonder, what can we do collaboratively, working together?

The assumptions behind aboriginal healing are collaborative and dialogical, a fact that is sometimes obscured by some healers' poor grasp of mainstream languages (English, French, Spanish). Traditional elders can sound illiterate and even stupid when they speak a noun-based language that they know only poorly, or when they are translated by others who do not fully understand their concepts, which can be quite sophisticated and are normally expressed in their own verb-based languages.

The aboriginal healer focuses upon the person with asthma rather than the asthma, and on the dialogues that can ensue with that person. Through conversation, a healing space is constructed that can involve healers, family members, and friends. Change comes from engaging in the dialogue. Conversing changes people through mysterious (non-rational) means. As noted earlier, dialogue implies connectivity. Given sufficient dialogue (synonymous with information flow, which is what happens in dialogue) reorganization can occur. Some possible reorganizations do not include asthma.

Asthma can be conceptualized as one thread that runs through a life, just as multiple themes may run through a novel. Asthma wants to be recognized, for it is not just a theme. It is also a character. It has a life. It has its own story. It has its own spirit. Small miracles can occur when it is recognized. It rejoices when recognized. Asthma is a kind of person who wants to be encountered. This is not the daily fare of physicians, who work with signs and symptoms, much as historians work with documents. In the context both of medicine and history, the voices behind the signs, symptoms, and documents are silent.

In her French book, whose title translates into English as *The Taste of the Archive,* Arlette Farge writes about how historians begin with mute voices and proceed to make them speak.[2] Healers are called upon to be historians of a different sort. We even call the stories we collect "histories." We speak of the history of the illness. We construct an oral testimony. We reassemble a living voice. We create a triangular relationship among the doctor, the patient, and the illness. We give asthma the opportunity to testify before us. Once asthma can tell its story, then the patient can tell her story, family members can tell their stories, doctors can tell their stories, and we end up with a rich archive of stories from various perspectives about this character called asthma. Narrative medicine begins at the confrontation with and between testimonies and, in particular, gives voice to testimonies that have been reduced to silence.

Here is an example. Karen had long suffered from asthma (as well as Crohn's disease, hypothyroidism, and arthritis). She was only in her mid-thirties and felt her body was betraying her, as all the men in her life had done. She said she had "tried everything" for her asthma, and all had failed.

We began with a dialogue with the spirit of her asthma. These dialogues emerge as part of a guided imagery process in which we enter a relaxed state of mind and then slowly allow a scene to appear in which the spirit of the illness wishes to present itself. For Karen, it appeared as a huge spider that was eating her bronchial tubes. The spider said it had been there since her birth and that it fed on shame. It thrived on humiliation, which had been a major issue for her parents and their parents as well. We learn from the aboriginal healers not to try to generalize this into any principles about asthma. This is Karen's story and only Karen's story. Nothing more. Her story tells us nothing about what the next person will tell us. Next we looked for a helper spirit. It happened to be Gauguin. Was it really the historical person? Does it matter? Gauguin told Karen the story of his frustrated life as a banker in Paris and how he overthrew it and ran off to Tahiti to become a painter. He told her to do the same.

Now we could shift the focus of the dialogue to wonder what form her escape might take. We began to plan a "jail break." I suggested we contact several "future selves" to inquire how each of them had handled the transition to wellness. We found beings with whom to talk. One had moved to San Francisco and opened up a gallery. Another version of her future self moved her social work practice to a low-key job with an agency. All involved her starting to paint again, with a dramatic increase in her exposure to light and space. I playfully invoked Max Tegmark's parallel universe story as a rationale for our journeys.[3] Within this new story, even dietary changes and micronutrients could take on new meaning and new effectiveness. As Karen made these changes, she began to improve. The biomedical story cannot explain Karen's changes, except to say that they were random, which dismisses the personality of her asthma and the richness of her narrative about what happened.

Ceremony was pivotal in Karen's healing journey. Healing ceremonies like Karen's require focused, concentrated effort—more human consciousness than can be attained in ordinary life. In Karen's context, this was accomplished through guided imagery, visualization, and other dialogue.

Here is another teaching tale that will help us understand this process of dialogical healing. It is a story about Crystal, a twenty-eight-year-old woman who had tried every medication and combination of medications known but was still wheezing. She had even gone to Columbia University and the Mayo Clinic, to no avail. Her example illustrates how useless a diagnosis of asthma or really any diagnosis is in an aboriginal context. We simply have to start the dialogue to learn about this particular woman's asthma. We need to converse with the spirit of her story, or, if that is not possible, to simply talk.

We start with an altered state of consciousness. We need trance. Why? To stop the internal chatter. We can't hear anyone else when we're doing all the talking inside our heads. Trance helps us suspend any unusual beliefs or ideas about the world so we can see it afresh. Historically speaking, the world's aboriginal cultures have been adept at trance states because the information obtained was so crucial for their survival. In altered states of consciousness, instructions came for how to find water, how to store milk, how to avoid getting caught in storms, where to find game, and other vital information. Within these cultures, people learn to be discerning about the quality of story they want to accept and use.

By externalizing conversations with the spirit of illness—talking to illness—we are able to re-create or "rewrite" the illness as an "other." This allows for more ready healing. I told Crystal the story of Red Swan to stimulate her to look for the spirit of her illness. This is a traditional Ojibway story from Manitoba.

Our story begins with three orphaned sisters who lived isolated in the woods. They were old enough and had learned enough from their parents to survive. The oldest taught the younger sisters what she learned, and they took care of each other. As time passed, the youngest sister began to wonder where the other people were. She wanted to go looking for other people. Her older sister reasoned that their parents would have lived among other people if other people were worth the trouble, so probably they were better off staying where they are. The younger sister acquiesced, but still secretly wished to seek out others.

One day, the oldest sister proposed a game: The winner will bring home the most exotic food for the evening meal. All the sisters were excited. This promised to be an interesting hunting game. Each went off in a separate direction.

After walking some distance, the youngest sister, the heroine of our story, began to notice the strangest phenomena. A red glow filled the sky. It seemed brightest in the west, which is where she went. Heading toward the source of the glow led her to a lake. In the middle of that lake was Red Swan, emanating the light. Thinking this must be the most exotic dinner anyone could capture, she aimed an arrow and fired, but the arrow bounced off the swan, causing no damage whatsoever. She fired again and again with the same result. Frustrated, she realized this must be a magical swan, and only magical arrows would affect it.

She remembered her father's medicine bundle, which had not been opened since his passing. Ignoring all taboos, she ran home, threw open the door to their dwelling, and tore open her father's bundle, removing his four prayer arrows without even taking the time to fold up the bundle after herself. She was running now, trying to get back to the swan before it flew away. Inexplicably, she found herself drawn to the swan, unable to resist its pull. She had to have it. She ran and ran, and, almost exhausted, broke into the clearing before the lake. Luckily the swan was still there, next to the island in the center of the lake.

She fired her arrow and missed by a hair. The second arrow passed through the swan's outstretched wing. The third arrow lodged in its neck—certainly a killing blow, but one the swan seemed not to notice at all. Unfolding its wings, it rose above the surface of the lake, arrow and all, and began to fly toward the west.

Our heroine found herself running after the swan. Faster and faster she ran. Soon she was running so fast that she could shoot an arrow into the sky and catch it on its way down. She was running with no thoughts of her sisters or any other consequences. She simply had to have the red swan.

After running all day, she came upon a ridge where she saw the sun passing down below the horizon. Below her was a village. She was amazed to see so many people. Before she could collect her thoughts, the sentry challenged her, and she responded with the simple request to grant her food and shelter for the night, for she had traveled far. She was taken to the dwelling of the chief, who welcomed her warmly. He had clearly heard the story of Red Swan before. He bade her sit and eat. When she had finished, he asked her about the swan and why she was so dedicated to following it. "Many have come this way," he said, "but none have returned. I fear this is a fool's errand. Why don't you stay here with us and marry my son?" He pointed toward a young man in the corner of the dwelling, laughing with others. "He is handsome enough," said the chief, "and certainly better than the sure death that will come from following the swan."

Our heroine contemplated the chief's son, who indeed was handsome. Clearly the family was wealthy, with many more opportunities than she had ever imagined. But the swan still lured her. She realized that the promise of the swan was more important than the certainty of the chief's son. "No," she said, "but thank you. I must follow the swan. I have no choice in this matter. It is my destiny."

"Alright," said the chief. "You have spoken. I am sorry, for surely we will never see you again, as we have never again seen any of the others who followed the swan."

"So be it," she said, thanking the chief for his hospitality and promising to be gone before the first edge of the sun had crossed the horizon.

That day she ran and ran and ran, traveling faster than the arrows she shot into the sky. By sundown, she was again exhausted and came upon a ridge overlooking another village. Again she greeted the sentry and was taken to the lodge of the chief. The same offers were made. This time the chief's son was even more handsome, but she had already entertained the question and knew immediately that she could not stay. "No," she told the chief. "I am in search of Red Swan." Again, the chief was disappointed, but gave in gracefully. The next morning she was running again.

Another day of running passed, and the young woman found herself at the edge of a meadow, overlooking a single dwelling in its center. She heard the sounds of one lone man. She silently walked toward the entrance, waiting for him to turn and notice her. The old man stood still by the entrance, his back facing her. Eventually he turned his face to her. "Why are you just standing there?" he asked her. "Why do you not come inside?"

"You have not invited me," she responded.

"You are expected," he said. "Come," he said, motioning her inside. She entered and sat in the place of honor. Eventually he completed his task and turned to face her. "I know why you are here," he said. "Our brother has called you through the Red Swan. He needs your help. You will learn more about this tomorrow night at the home of my other brother. Tonight, you must rest and eat and relax."

"Kettle," the old man said suddenly. "Come here and cook for us." To her surprise, an ancient kettle at the edge of the dwelling waddled over to the fire and set itself down.

"What do you want, old man?" the kettle asked.

"Food for this fine young woman," the man said gruffly.

"Then feed me so I can feed you," said the kettle. The man filled it with water and threw in a single kernel of corn and a blueberry. This will be a terrible dinner, thought the woman, who settled back to rest, adjusting to the idea of having no food that night. Within minutes, however, the

most delicious aromas filled the room. To her surprise, a thick stew was bubbling in the pot.

"Eat your fill," said the old man. The more she ate, the more food there seemed to be, until she was so full she drifted off to sleep. The next morning, she awoke early, refreshed. After a quick meal of berries and dried fruit, and with the old man's blessing, she was off and running again.

The same things happened to her the following evening. This time, the old man was older. The kettle was bigger. Everything was the same, until the kettle refused to cook. "I will not cook," said the kettle, "until we ask her some questions. We need to know if she's the one."

"Oh, alright," said the older man. "Ask her what you will." The kettle demanded that the young woman tell him her dreams. She tentatively began, but none of them satisfied the kettle, until she told him her oldest and longest dreams of reuniting with her parents. To her surprise, that satisfied the kettle. "You may just be the one," it said. "I like those dreams. Now I will cook." And cook it did. Using the same minimal ingredients, the kettle made a stew, the likes of which the young woman had never tasted before. When she had eaten her fill, the older man told her about their brother. "He has been sending that swan for a long time. He has been cursed. He wronged some people, and they took his scalp. He cannot get it back until someone unrelated to him comes to do him an act of kindness, and, believe me, he is not someone upon which many would bestow kindness. He has sent that swan as his only recourse. He will give you the swan if you succeed, for that is what all who come are seeking. If you do not succeed, the people who cursed him will kill you. So turn back if you are not sure of yourself."

"I will not turn back," said the young woman, "but how will I do what is necessary?"

"He will give you three powers," said the old man. "Use them wisely and you will succeed."

"Alright," she said. She left with the rising of the sun.

That night she came to another meadow with a single dwelling in its center. No one could mistake the hideous cries of pain that came from within. It sounded as if someone was being beaten. She gingerly crept to the house and saw a man crying out as if he were being struck. She waited until this fit ended. "Come in," he said, weakly. "You must be looking for Red Swan."

"I am," she said.

"He is here and you may have him, but first you must recover my scalp. Evil people have cut it off and cursed me. You must sneak into their village and steal it back for me. Succeed, and the swan is yours."

"I am told you have powers for me."

"I do," he said. "I will give you the power to shape-shift three times. But be careful," he said, "for there is no fourth chance." He performed a ceremony and through the smoke of unknown herbs and prayers and songs, painted her forehead with dye and oil. "When you awaken in the morning, the powers will be yours," he said. That night, they ate sparsely, not at all like the meals of the previous evenings. She wondered where Red Swan was, but did not ask.

By mid-morning the next day she had reached the village. In the center of the village was a pole on which the man's scalp rested. The villagers were beating it with a stick. She could imagine the man crying out every time the stick hit his scalp. He must have really done something terrible to them, she thought, wanting to get the scalp and the swan and escape before he did something terrible to her, too. She sat and prayed for guidance until it came to her. Quickly, before she could change her mind, she used her first power to turn herself into a hummingbird, a creature these people had never before seen. She readily flew past them to the scalp as they watched in awe and wonder. When she reached the scalp, she used her second power to transform herself into the north wind, blowing the scalp all the way to the edge of the clearing. There she used her final power and turned herself into a hawk, carrying the scalp high into the sky, gripped by her talons. The villagers quickly recovered and shot at the hawk, almost hitting her with their spears and arrows.

However, she got away, and from high in the sky, she could look down and see the top of the man's head, where the scalp was supposed to go. She positioned it in her talons and then dived, shoving it as hard as she could back onto the man's head. She knocked him out in the process, quite by accident. When he awakened, she was apologetic. "No matter," he said, rubbing his head. "I am so grateful to have it back. You did well to put it back on my head so quickly and neatly." They shared supper and she waited to hear about Red Swan.

When she had heard nothing by morning and was already preparing to leave, she worried that this man was going to cheat her. Finally he mentioned Red Swan, just as she was going out the door. "Don't forget your swan," he said. "Come," he shouted to the back of the dwelling. "Come here, nephew." A handsome man emerged, more handsome than either of the two chiefs' sons. "This is Red Swan, my nephew," the man said. "You may take him and do what you will with him. He doesn't want to stay here and I've grown quite tired of him and his never-ending appetite. He can be your problem now."

I suppose it was love at first sight, and love it most certainly was. The young woman led Red Swan along the trail home, stopping the first night at the older man's dwelling. He was glad to hear that Red Swan had been liberated from their somewhat evil brother. "Take good care of him," the old man said, "and take the kettle with you. Trade it to the first village for something really valuable. They need the kettle far more than I do, but make them give you a really good price." She thanked him for the kettle and left in the morning. The following night, events repeated themselves with the other old man. Now she had acquired two kettles and one man.

The following night she struck a hard bargain for the first kettle. She was thinking of her sisters and of preserving peace and harmony in their home. She held out until the chief traded his son for the kettle. The next night she repeated her bargaining, and now she had no kettles and three men.

Weren't her sisters surprised when she came home? They had given her up for dead. Little did they know that she was bringing home a man for each of them, though she kept Red Swan for herself. They lived a good long life and had many more stories to tell, none of which we have time to describe here, but they are the stories that come after the honeymoon and keep everything interesting.

The links that we created for Crystal included investing the swan with meaning toward a desire for health and wellness. Obstacles were the challenges met along the way. The chiefs offered seduction just as pharmacology does, as do drugs, alcohol, and relationships. We must perform the tasks that allow us to overcome our challenges and capture the swan.

I believe we humans are capable of internally, creatively solving all our health problems, though I can't say I know how, and certainly can't be called upon to make this happen on command. Nevertheless, this is a guiding principle that I prefer. It is practical in that it allows me to collaborate with people to learn what to do. Even when we don't "solve the problem," other elements change, so the whole process is constructive, sometimes even fun.

Crystal went on her own imagery journey to find her Red Swan. We loosely followed the template of the story. The swan revealed that asthma was an "evil spirit" that had tormented Crystal's family for generations, getting stronger and more malevolent over time. It fed on a need for status and prestige, a need for appraisal based upon money and power, and individual competitive strategies. It would starve in the face of internal peace, internal approval, and a cooperative, community strategy, which could include exorcism of the spirit of the illness. Crystal took to the possession metaphor. Sometimes we do feel as if illnesses possess us. She could relate to the idea that her family's issues had affected her health. She began to strategize with her community of friends about how to bring more peace and internal approval into her life. Eventually we did do a ceremony to relieve her of the asthma spirit. We waited until we had built up enough power in the form of a story that everyone believed so that the ceremony would work. Crystal progressively stopped using medication after the ceremony, and her asthma has not come back.

In narrative medicine, one of our goals is to avoid insights and interpretations until entities and illnesses literally shout their meanings to us. The narrative approach demands that we find a person's own story and see how it is supported by the stories of his or her community. Through those stories, we find the locations of disharmony. Amber's story shows how this works. She was undergoing continual hospitalizations for asthma exacerbations with more and more prescribed medications. The standard medical approach was not working for Amber.

Amber had been to a naturopath and had been treated unsuccessfully for allergies and parasites. She believed she was allergic to soy and milk and had toxoplasmosis, and a special diet had helped. She thought her chi was deficient. She had taken micronutrients in phases. She would alternate between eating only organic food and eating only at McDonald's. Spirulina made her sick. She tended to go to extremes.

What could a narrative approach add to her treatment?

Amber and I decided to initiate a dialogue with her asthma. After relaxation and trance induction, I invited Amber to allow a scene to appear in which her symptoms could be understood. She saw a peaceful river with trees. The trees were healthy; the branches swayed in the breeze and light played on the colored leaves. The grass around the trees was plentiful and healthy. However, the water was murky, with trash floating on the surface. The banks of the river were muddy. A mountain stood in the background, covered with snow. It reminded her of an ice cream sundae with a cherry on top, covered with whipped cream.

I asked her to look around to see if any clues could be found for the river's pollution. She couldn't see any source. "Let's go upstream," I said, "and find where the pollution comes from." We traveled upstream until we found a factory dumping its waste into the river. We went inside to learn why. Inside, the walls were gray, and the place had a desolate feel. The factory was full of sadness. "Who is there," I asked Amber, "that can tell us what's going on?"

"'Cynic' is there," she said. "He protects me from bad feelings. He's standing there with his arms crossed, disapproving. He's standing there wearing a white Dutch Boy painting hat. The workers in the factory remind me of my grandmother's ceramic dolls. Cynic is short and looks Danish. The workers are dancing as if they are in a ballet, perhaps the Cinderella ballet."

"What do they make in this factory?" I asked.

"Clogs," she said. She added that she felt helpless in the factory.

"Why is the factory being allowed to pollute like this?" I asked.

"The environmental police are corrupt," she said. "They chase me all the time in my dreams. They're after me. They're trying to kill me. They're trying to hurt me. I'm always running down the streets of the town that surrounds the factory."

"Who's in charge of the police?" I asked.

"My father," she said.

"We've got to get in to talk to him," I said. "How can we do that?"

"We have to tie up his secretary who protects him from appointments and walk-ins," she said. "Tying her up is the only way we can get in to see my father."

"Who is his secretary?" I ask. "Do we know her?"

"My mother," she said. "My mother is his secretary."

"Why are the police corrupt?" I asked. "Why do they allow the environment to get polluted?"

"So my father can make more money," she said. "He doesn't care what happens around him as long as he makes a profit."

"Is there anyone who can clean up the river?" I ask.

"My Grandpa Bernie," she said. "He's come to clean up the river. He's brought a good fairy to clean up the river. It will take her some time, though."

"Alright," I said. "Let's allow them to get to work, and let's visit another place in your body that needs our attention. Where do we need to go?"

"My knee," she said. "The cartilage is red and messed up."

"What do the cartilage cells look like?" I asked.

"They're red and bloated," she said. "They're eating french fries. They're hanging upside down like bats. They're not moving. They look like statues. There are single molecules there that look like white M&M's. They're thin and long. They're upside-down hanging statues. It's like they're covered with plaster of paris. That's a good thing. All the bats are encased in this white plaster of paris stuff."

"What can we do here?" I asked her.

"We can't do anything here," she said. "We have to go somewhere else."

"Where do you want to go?" I asked her.

"To the heart," she said.

"OK," I said. "What does it look like inside your heart?"

"It's white and bulging," she said. "I go inside and open it up and there are more bats in there. They're covered with black gunk. We need to wash them away with blood. They have faces like lions and tigers.

"I have a bat problem," she said. She described the faces of the bats, screaming and in pain, almost insane. Bats were everywhere, covering the inside of her heart. They were eating her heart. Bats, including baby bats, were everywhere inside her.

"What are we going to do about this?" I asked her.

"We're going to have to feed them," she said. "Maybe mosquitoes or something. We're going to need a guru or a teacher to do this."

"Where else do we need to go?" I asked her.

"To the lungs," she said. "They look like the bat cave inside," she said. "It looks just like the inside of the knee. There's a windstorm coming," she said. "It's going to be like a sand blaster. It's going to blast out these layers of bats. The bats want our attention. Their faces are like paintings," she said. "I see their eyes, snouts, and other parts."

Amber's imagery provided us with a kind of story. It's a story of a polluted river, which Amber and I agreed was her gut. It's a story of harsh, hostile parents who are not very loving. It's a story of being taken over by batlike creatures that are hard to combat. They seemed to represent inflammation to us—at least, that's what our shared story came to say about these bats. Now that we had a story, ideas for treatments just flowed. The subtle complexity of the story led us to consider homeopathy. She thought of garlic, herbs to fight *Candida,* and probiotics to detoxify her gut. I suggested an anti-inflammatory diet, including some herbs, and suggested she join a drumming group and a healing circle. The drumming would drive out bad energy, including her parents. The healing circle would continue the dialogue we had begun in the imagery.

Next we invited all of Amber's friends and family to come to a meeting. The first step was to assemble the community. We learned about the disharmony in the relationships among Amber and her fiancé, father, and friends. We learned about Amber's anger at her father's new, Mexican bride. Through her struggles in these relationships, she had entered into increasingly greater loneliness and isolation. We next did a talking circle with her community to address the sources of disharmony and imbalance. The group agreed that Amber should try traditional Chinese medicine, yoga, ceremony, and imagery or meditation. Amber was part Tohono O'odham (Native people of southwest Arizona), but was out of touch with her heritage. She felt drawn to recover that Native side of her background. Step two involved inviting all of Amber's potential healers to a meeting with her community. We identified people who could provide these services and invited them to the meeting. The third step involved starting a conversation with these healers and the community. Next, a healing circle evolved to maintain this conversation. Over six months, the disharmony healed. A mysterious transformation had occurred. Amber was off steroids and managing with just an occasional puff of one inhaled medication (a beta-agonist). She was no longer being hospitalized. How did this happen?

Conventional medicine's typical response is to ignore unexplained healings like Amber's. The healing or cure didn't happen. If it did, it was accidental. What seems apparent to me from the stories in this chapter is that conversation resulted in the emergence of a story that held substance and could lead to a new physiology that did not include asthma. These stories permit and facilitate a reorganization of identity and behavior in such a way that the symptoms can disappear.

When we let the illness speak for itself, when we let it emerge as a character in its own right, and when we externalize it so that we can dialogue with it, a reorganization that leads to healing is more likely. An individualized solution unfolds that is unique to that person and circumstance. This solution cannot necessarily generalize, as conventional medicine requires of a good answer, so it is dismissed. Yet, the principle can generalize. The idea that each person needs a unique personal solution, different from every other person's, and arising from her context and interpersonal environment, can generalize, and that is what talking to illness teaches us.

8
Talking with Mental Illness

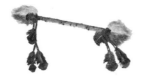

What's madness but nobility of soul
At odds with circumstance? The day's on fire!
I know the purity of pure despair,
My shadow pinned against a sweating wall.
That place among the rocks—is it a cave,
Or winding path? The edge is what I have.

THEODORE ROETHKE[1]

The context for all the suffering we can encounter—physical, emotional, and spiritual—is the social world into which we are born and in which we continue to interact. Ongoing interactions mold and shape us into who we think we are throughout our lives. These interactions comprise many small stories that we incorporate as stories about "self," an elusive and fragmented concept since we rarely have the opportunity to reflect upon all these small stories and integrate them into one bigger, coherent story. Therapy provides this opportunity for reflection, as do spiritual retreats, enforced periods of rest that come with illness or accidents, vacations, and retirement. These opportunities allow us to make bigger stories out of our many small stories and to reflect on the apparent contradictions between many of our smaller stories. Cognitive-behavior therapy is an excellent approach for demonstrating the contradictions between our internalized stories.

Stories organize experience into interpretive frameworks, but these frameworks are not necessarily "true." Their teachings can save our lives or make us more efficient at survival. The example of the many stories provided by the world's religions illustrates this, for more than one story argues that it is the only truth. Our break with established psychology and medicine occurs when we assert that all stories are suspect, that all may be capricious and arbitrary, that there are no privileged stories except those that work, when and where they do work. Within medicine, this means challenging the sanctity of the randomized, controlled clinical trial as the only valid way to obtain knowledge. It provides a fresh critique of what has been called "evidence-based medicine," from the understanding that acceptable evidence is itself determined by a story about the world that can be challenged. Our very perception is reduced to a story that tells us what to perceive, that tells us what qualifies as evidence and what qualifies as research.

Bipolar disorder is one of my favorite conditions for exploring the interfaces among mind, brain, body, relationship, environment, and spirit. But what is bipolar disorder? Is it a label without substance? Does it have a biological reality outside our culture and our creation stories about it? The conventional story about bipolar disorder is a consensual one, forged by psychiatrists and other mental health professionals in collaboration with patients, the media, and the pharmaceutical companies. It is developed through communication and dialogue. People have learned to recognize the signifiers of bipolar disorder within themselves and to present them to professionals. While bipolar disorder may or may not have an underlying biological reality, it is highly culturally laden, and there are alternate stories to the contemporary one.

People who suffer from bipolar disorder are thought to have pathological mood swings from mania or hypomania to depression, with cyclic patterns of exacerbation and remission.* Here is where culture

---

*Mania is operationally defined in the DSM-IV in terms such as grandiosity, hyperreligiosity, reduced need for sleep, boundless energy, excessive spending, suspension of good judgment over the consequences of one's actions, loquaciousness, inability to stop a behavior once started, inability to modify one's plans based on feedback from the

enters. What is mood? Mood is not objective, like a concrete thing. We must learn to feel the emotions that come to be characterized as mood. Different cultures recognize and enact emotions differently. Moods vary from family to family and from culture to culture.

The developmental psychologist Lev Vygotsky believed that we learn to reflect upon our emotional state by internalizing conversations we have with others and conversations others have about our emotional states.[3] Through repeating these conversations to ourselves, we come to think of them as our own.

I suspect that young children do not have words for feelings. They perceive an unbroken stream of experience. When they exhibit behavior that significant adults in their lives can interpret, a pointing or labelling process begins. A significant adult says, "Oh, so you're sad." Now the unbroken experience becomes organized into a concept called sadness; a category has taken shape. As children learn words and language, they label their internal states with some correspondence to reflect the way adults label their appearance. Different families define sadness in very different ways, as do different cultures. The languages of some cultures even lack words for sadness. Similarly, behavior can come to be labelled as excitement or as irritability. All of this is a sophisticated exercise in pointing. The adult points at the child and puts a name to what the child is doing and experiencing, and that name is sadness. Only after the word is learned and the child equates the word with the internal experiences associated with the word can she say that she feels sad or excited or irritable. A major project in negotiating love relationships is the collaborative mapping of what words for emotions mean to the individuals involved. The same word may have a different meaning in each of two different families. My sadness may bear little resemblance to yours.

Stanley Fish said that all the thoughts we "can think and the mental operations [we] can perform have their source in some . . . interpretive community."[4] The range, complexity, and subtlety of our thought; its

---

environment, and the like. Hypomania is defined more as persistent irritability or mild euphoria—in other words, a lessened and harder-to-recognize form of mania that oscillates with periods of depression. Both types of bipolar patients spend more time being depressed than high or irritable.[2]

power; the practical and conceptual uses to which we can put it; and the issues we can address all depend on how thoroughly we have been initiated into knowledge communities. Clifford Geertz said, "Human thought is consummately social: social in its origins, social in its functions, social in its form, social in its applications."[5] The thoughts and feelings that are labelled as bipolar disorder are initially social and socially derived.

Values, habits, emotions, manners at the table, and so forth are transmitted through social interaction. Erasmus, for example, wrote manuals of good behavior in order to codify social interaction.[6] Conversely, social interaction produces patterns of behavior.

Throughout our childhood, and perhaps even before birth, we begin a lifelong process of negotiation. Even six-month-old infants engage in conversations with their mothers and other caretaking adults, and through these conversations, create theories or stories about the world. Because their well-being depends on understanding their mother's language, both verbal and gestural, infants begin interpretive conversations with their mothers (and other caretaking adults) as soon as they can register and distinguish changes in physical attitude and gesture, tone of voice, and facial expression. And because a mother's well-being depends in part on understanding and adapting to her infant's needs, infant and mother are, to that extent, knowledgeable peers. Together they compose a unique but culturally crucial knowledge community whose members are learning from each other as they go.

Vygotsky described a scene illustrating this process of community composition and collaboration that involved a six-month-old infant. The infant saw an attractive object—a shiny spoon—and extended his hand to grasp it. The spoon was out of reach. For a moment the infant's "hands stretched toward that object, remaining poised in the air. His fingers made grasping movements." The infant appeared to be trying, at the most elemental level, to establish contact with a bit of physical reality. Shoved around by the physical world, he shoved back. He wanted a response from the object or a relationship with it that corresponded to his reaching for it. But the object did not cooperate in the effort to be known. Objects never do. For a moment, then, the infant reached and nothing happened. "Then something did happen. The object still didn't cooperate, but mother did. The infant's mother moved the object closer, so that the infant could feel it, look at it, and put it into his mouth."[7]

This brief, mundane scene provides a key to understanding knowledge and collaborative learning. When infants reach for an object, they do not merely reach. They send a message. When a caretaker gets the message and responds, infants learn indelibly the importance of this seemingly irrelevant side effect. Our first effort to grasp an object, Vygotsky tells us, is the first step we take in learning to point. Pointing, Vygotsky argues, "is an unsuccessful attempt to grasp something, a movement aimed at a certain object which designates forthcoming activity. . . . When the mother comes to the child's aid and realizes that his movement indicates something, the situation changes fundamentally. Pointing becomes a gesture for others. The child's unsuccessful attempt engenders a reaction not from the object he sought, but *from another person*."[8]

Vygotsky tells us that knowing is not an unmediated, direct relationship between the self and an object. We need the involvement of others in order to know something. Other people are always involved in our learning processes. The infant in Vygotsky's illustration eventually learns to know and master the shiny spoon by learning how to make an adult respond and give it the spoon. Infants begin to "understand [their grasping] movement as pointing," Vygotsky says, when they understand that their "object-oriented movement" has really become "a movement aimed at another person, a means of establishing relations."[9] Learning involves relationships with other people. The experience is collaborative because, when they finally get the message and respond, the caretakers have understood the infant. They have learned a gestural word or phrase with which the infant is now able to converse. They have learned to expect some forthcoming activity from the infant. From the infant's point of view, they have learned to obey orders.

These moments in the lives of six-month-old infants contend seriously for the attention of college and university teachers, because the process implied can be traced from infancy through childhood to the learning of adults. Infant and mother learn what they need to know about each other by internalizing the language that constitutes their community, encapsulating the results of their ongoing conversations into conventions and routines. As infants grow and learn, becoming children and then adolescents and adults, they incrementally nest membership in that first, small, closed knowledge community of mother and child, expanding toward larger communities with which to pledge allegiance.[10]

Vygotsky described the actions of a four- or five-year-old child trying to take possession of a piece of candy by figuring out how to use some basic tools to advantage, in this case a stick and a stool. As the child worked, she talked through her solution to the problem. But she did not talk in a state of fantasy involvement with the objects that concerned her. She talked about them, and about herself, to *someone else*. Sometimes she talked to another person at hand. Most of the time, she talked to herself as if she were another person.

Vygotsky said that the child was using social speech instrumentally, to get something done. By the time she was four or five, much of her "socialized speech (which had previously been used to address an adult) *had turned inward*." Rather than appealing to the adult, she appealed to herself. He wrote, "Every function in [our] cultural development appears twice: first, on the social level, and later, on the individual level; first, *between* people . . . and then *inside*."[11]

Children and adults interact to shape and change each other's responses. Learning and understanding emerge as individuals create and accomplish interactive tasks in everyday conversations. Bamberg calls this "talk-in-interaction." We learn as we go. People learn to recognize and talk about their emotions through interactive dialogue. Knowledge about sadness cannot be separated from the conversation going on between the people involved. Knowledge is not separate from society. Instead, we see "trials of strength" in which knowledge, conversation, emotional involvement, and social relationships are inseparable. By exercising her native talent for linguistic improvisation, a young child translates and retranslates until she gets it correct. Membership in a community means that everything we do is unhesitatingly correct or incorrect according to specific criteria within that community. Correct means acceptable to the community in which the child lives.

As we mature, we internalize conversations about emotions as thoughts. "The fact that under stress, we tend to re-externalize thought as direct or indirect conversation (talk and writing) demonstrates the continuing relationship of thought and conversation in adult learning, even when that relationship ceases to be readily apparent. Stress occasions our talking to ourselves ('Don't let yourself feel so sad'). Stress occasions the rap sessions and endless dorm-room talk typical of adolescence and early adulthood."[12]

This digression into how children learn to categorize emotional experience, to carve it up from the unbroken whole, and how they learn to express emotions, returns us to the possibility that the state of being manic may be learned.[13] We may learn how to enact mania as a means of communication. Perhaps it also gets carried away with itself. Perhaps once learned, we cannot stop. Depression typically follows mania, with its accompanying loss of self-esteem, withdrawal, sadness, and even risk of suicide. I suspect we also learn how to do depression—when to label ourselves as depressed. We learn what useful functions depressive actions play in social life and how to be depressed.

Research on synesthesia is a basis from which to wonder about the role of culture and local practices in shaping the brain's abilities. Synesthesia is the mixing of two or more senses.[14] It's a sensation produced at a point other than the point of stimulation; for example, seeing a color as the result of hearing a certain sound. Synesthesia has been documented to exist based upon PET studies showing different cortical blood flow patterns among women with the condition compared to women without.[15]

British psychologist Simon Baron-Cohen has wondered if adult synesthesia arises from a failure of the perceptual system to differentiate beyond the undifferentiated phase of perception that is normal during infancy.[16] For me, this raises the possibility that our nervous systems are relatively plastic and that culture or other circumstances can influence the emergence of some capabilities at some times and not at others. Synesthesia, telepathy, and spirit communication may be abilities favored in some indigenous societies and in some people, but not in mainstream, globalized modern society. Thom Hartmann (author of *The Edison Gene*) makes a strong argument for the usefulness and adaptability of the genetic contribution to what we now call attention deficit hyperactivity disorder (ADHD). He suggests that we are now discarding these young people because our society no longer desires their special abilities.[17] Similar considerations may exist for all aspects of brain function.

Baron-Cohen's neonatal synesthesia hypothesis states that all babies experience sensory input in an undifferentiated way until about four months of age. "Sounds trigger both auditory and visual and tactile experiences. A truly psychedelic state, and all natural . . ."[18] The related cross-modal transfer (CMT) hypothesis, presented by Meltzoff and Borton, states that objects can be recognized in more than one sensory modality as a result of infants being able to recognize objects in an abstract form.[19] Evidence for this lies in the fact that babies are able to recognize visually an object that they have only touched previously.[20] CMT refutes Jean Piaget's claim that the sensory systems are independent at birth and gradually become integrated over time.[21] CMT lends support to the idea that inter-sensory equivalence is present at birth and that perceptual development is gradual.[22] These findings also support Vygotsky's ideas about infant development over Piaget's and others. Our interest in these ideas is to support the idea that social factors select brain attributes to strengthen and to atrophy. Various cultures may differently influence brain development so that perception and interpretation in these cultures is neurophysiologically different.

Adult synesthesia represents the persistence of neonatal synesthesia, which may be more likely in some social contexts than in others. There is an anatomical basis for neonatal synesthesia, including transient connections between the retina and the main somatosensory and auditory nuclei of the thalamus in the neonatal hamster. Kittens have similar transient connections between auditory, visual, somatosensory, and motor cortices.[23] For humans, but only during infancy, evoked responses to human voices are recorded not only in the expected area of the temporal cortex, but also in the occipital cortex. Widespread cortical responses to visual stimuli also exist in the first two months of human life.[24]

Psychologist Jerry Fodor believes that the sensory system becomes increasingly modular after initial synesthesia, because modularity leads to more rapid and efficient information processes, and is therefore more adaptive.[25] What may be underappreciated, however, is the question of adaptive to what context? Modularity is encouraged, but is that true in all cultures or contexts? Does the social context determine to greater extents than previously believed, the directions in which the brain develops? Emotional development is no exception.

We can even question the time-honored "developmental tasks"

and perhaps reconceptualize development as evolving through social interaction. People grow and change to become better matched to their physical, social, and spiritual environment. Growth and change occur as the by-product of our relationships with others and the ways in which we are changed through relating. As such, changes cannot be judged as more or less mature. Anthropologists previously thought indigenous people were less mature than European people. They were just different. Their ways of behaving matched their physical environment and social milieu quite well; it was just that these environments were constructed very differently from nineteenth-century Europe. Even adolescence as a social process didn't exist in the indigenous cultures of North America in the way that it is now constructed in our mall-rich society. Can we question the concept of "developmental stages" in which we have the task of creating an identity and maturing into an "adult"? What this progression leaves out is the continuous, ongoing process of growth and change that occurs throughout life and happens in dialogue with others.

Within a narrative perspective, these findings support our belief that people who become diagnostically labeled with psychotic disorders are talented people whose talents have gone awry. People who get this diagnosis have lost their ability to stay engaged in the social dialogue and to match the expectations of the physical and social environment. This is a more hopeful perspective than believing they are hopelessly defective based upon imbalances of brain chemistry. The more important point to consider, perhaps, is that psychotic identities cannot be understood outside of the context of the larger group to which the individual belongs.

The Conventional Story about Bipolar Disorder

Modern psychiatry's recognition of bipolar disorder dates back to 1921, when psychiatrist Emil Kraepelin applied the term "manic-depressant insanity" to cyclic episodes of mania alternating with depression, a syndrome which has been recognized in various forms for more than two thousand years.[26] The profession introduced the term "bipolar disorder" in the mid-1970s in a largely unsuccessful attempt to lessen confusion between this condition and schizophrenia.[27]

In the conventional story, bipolar disorder is a chronic disease affecting more than two million Americans at some point in their lives.* The DSM-IV describes two types of bipolar disorder, type I and type II. In type I, the person has experienced at least one full manic episode. In type II, periods of hypomania involve less severe manic symptoms that alternate with at least one major depressive episode. In the conventional story, bipolar disorder appears between the ages of fifteen and twenty-five, affecting men and women equally. The exact cause is unknown, but is believed to be a disturbance of areas of the brain that regulate mood. Chronic stress early in life in vulnerable persons is thought to predispose them to both bipolar and ordinary depression. There is a strong genetic component. The incidence of bipolar disorder is higher in relatives of people who have the condition.[29]†

The symptoms consist of alternating episodes of mania and depression. In the manic phase, we see an increase in goal-directed activities (either socially or at work), increased energy, distractibility, flight of ideas or the subjective experience that thoughts are racing, an inflated self-esteem or grandiosity, an increased involvement in activities that may be pleasurable but may have dire consequences (such as spending sprees), and a decreased need for sleep (for example, the person may feel rested after three hours of sleep). The patient may be more talkative than usual or feel pressured to speak. He or she may be easily agitated or irritated and lack self-control. Hypomanic episodes are similar but less intense. Delusions, if present, are congruent with mood (such as delusions of grandeur or a sense of special powers and abilities).

In the depressive phase, people experience persistent sadness and depressed mood; feelings of hopelessness, worthlessness, pessimism, and

---

*From 1.2 to 1.6 percent of the American population has been diagnosed with bipolar disorder, with the prevalence increasing.[28] The recognized incidence is thought to be an underestimate because of under-recognition and under-reporting of manic and hypomanic episodes.

†The approximate lifetime risk of bipolar disorder in relatives of a person with bipolar disorder is 40 to 70 percent in a monozygotic twin and 5 to 10 percent in a first degree relative, compared with 0.5 to 1.5 percent in an unrelated person.[30] Commonly cited studies show that 65 percent of monozygotic twins have concordance for major depression, compared with only 14 percent of dizygotic twins.[31]

"emptiness"; loss of interest or pleasure in activities that were once enjoyed, including sex; sleep disturbances; motor slowing or agitation; withdrawal; feelings of guilt and worthlessness; fatigue; overwhelming sluggishness; difficulty concentrating, remembering, or making decisions; loss of appetite and weight loss, or overeating and weight gain; and thoughts of death or suicide. If delusions are present, they are typically congruent with mood (such as delusions of worthlessness or accusing voices).

The construction of bipolar disorder as a biological and genetic disorder allows psychiatry to flourish. The accompanying idea that bipolar disorder can only be treated with medication allows the pharmacology industry to flourish. The costs of conventional psychiatric treatment of bipolar disorder are large. A 1991 report from the National Institutes of Mental Health estimated total U.S. costs for bipolar illness at $45 billion annually, a figure that is growing exponentially. The dominant discourse of modern psychiatry recognizes pharmacological treatment as the mainstay for bipolar disorder. People diagnosed with bipolar disorder who subscribe to the biological story can relinquish all need to participate in any conversations except about which medications to take. The conventional story involves other people only as support group members or in educational sessions about the illness. Larger communities are excluded from dialogue, except to educate family about "how to live with a mentally ill member," as one class is described at a hospital where I work. If bipolar is entirely biological and is entirely treated biologically, then no value comes from conversations among affected parties, except to educate them from the expert paradigm.

Conventional medicine usually hospitalizes people with acute symptoms so medications may be started to control the symptoms. These medications include antipsychotic drugs, antianxiety agents (such as benzodiazepines), and antidepressants. Mood stabilizers (such as lithium carbonate) and anticonvulsants (including carbamazepine and valproic acid) are started as maintenance therapy to relieve symptoms and prevent relapse. However, at best, only 50 percent of people with bipolar disorder improve on medication. The gold standard of American psychiatric research is the randomized, controlled trial. In various clinical studies of drug treatment regimens for bipolar disorder, including combinations of antidepressants, anticonvulsants, lithium, and placebo, the highest medication response rates barely topped 50 percent. In many of these studies, more than 25 percent of study participants reported good results with placebo treatment.[32] This leaves some room for a critique of the purely biological model. However, stories of medication nonresponders are rarely part of the conventional narrative. When biologically narrowed psychiatrists speak to the public, rarely do they point out the plight of the 50 percent of people who are nonresponders. Nor do they tell stories about the 28 to 32 percent of people who recover through use of placebos. These people embarrass conventional biological psychiatrists.

Swarthmore philosopher Ken Gergen writes, "enormous problems inhere in distinctly psychological modes of explanation."[33] The same can be said for distinctly biological modes of explanation. We could say that privileged explanations are usually inadequate. As one might expect, the biological narrative has even infiltrated the field of literary criticism; we are all embedded in the same larger culture and share a common history, whether psychiatrists or English professors. In writing about Virginia Woolf's mood swings (now called bipolar disorder), Thomas Caramagno demonstrated the effect of the psychiatric narrative on literary criticism. He says,

> [We must reconsider Virginia Woolf's] fiction in light of recent medical discoveries about the genetic and biological nature of manic-depression—findings allied with drug therapies that today help nearly one million American manic-depressives live happier and more productive lives. In the real world of the clinic, treatments using lithium, antidepressants, and antipsychotics have revolutionized psychiatric care for mood swings and produced miracle remissions for cases that thirty years ago would have been considered hopeless. But in the rarefied atmosphere of literary academia, many critics still cling to the Freudian model of this disorder as a neurotic conflict that the patient is unwilling (either consciously or unconsciously) to resolve.[34]

Proponents of the biological story argue its superiority over the previous Freudian story in that it describes people as unable to change instead of unwilling to change. What hasn't changed is the assignation of the "problem" to the individual, with an implicit judgment of inferiority. Freud's movement stole "mental problems" from the Church, turning moral inferiority into psychological inferiority. Biological psychiatry transforms this further to genetic inferiority.

What do medication nonresponders do within the biological narrative? Their lives are rarely studied. I have observed that they pursue a variety of courses; common ones include chronic alcohol and drug abuse as a self-medication strategy. Some use hidden talents and resources to excel in communities where their mood swings become attractive eccentricities. The stereotype of the leading lady of the 1940s had this kind of moodiness. Some pursue other types of healing, spontaneously lose their bipolarity, die, become soldiers, have spiritual transformations, and otherwise remain hidden from the dominant discourse. I will tell several of their stories later in this chapter.

I have tried to find references to what could be considered bipolar-like symptoms in writings about post-Columbus indigenous people, only to have failed. The closest I have come is the visionary healer or spiritual leader and the fabled warrior. Descriptions exist of those who experienced days of ecstatic visions only to collapse and sleep for days. This behavior was honored and supported. If it was "manic" or "psychotic," the person was protected during the ecstasy, because the visions were expected to be portentous, of great importance to the tribal group. When spirit left the person, as these descriptions commonly report, and the person collapsed, the community was present to nurse them back to health. If this was bipolar disorder, it had a completely different meaning and context in tribal society.

Perhaps the tendency of indigenous cultures to see problems in terms of whole communities and not individuals renders the bipolar label unintelligible in this context. Perhaps bipolar requires reduction to individualism in order to appear or exist. Within traditional communities, I suspect that affect is regulated differently than among members of modern Euro-American culture. When people live tribally, women menstruate at the same time, and probably other biological cycles synchronize. I suspect that the community modulates affect and provides regulation when the individual is unable to do so. Biological psychiatry's genetic drift hypothesis states that the most severely bipolar people would be isolated and alone, since they are too bizarre to maintain normal social relations. Of course, they would say this from their individualistic, biological story. An indigenous explanation might reverse this thinking and conclude that isolation and loneliness without community is harmful.

Alternative Stories about Bipolar Disorder

Betty Running Bear came to see me in the height of medication despair. She had been prescribed so many different medications for her bipolar disorder that it was confusing. She took Thorazine, Haldol, Depakote, Prozac, Klonopin, and lithium. I wondered how anyone could get so many drugs. Betty was half Cherokee, half African-American in origin. That weekend a yuwipi ceremony was scheduled with a local Native healer from the nearby reservation. Yuwipi means "they tie him up" in Lakota. The ceremony was given to Horn Chips in a vision on the top of Bear Butte, South Dakota, in 1868 with a purpose of curing "white people disease."

In the yuwipi ceremony, a ceremonial space is created in the center of an empty room. A rug is laid upon the floor, covered by a star quilt. Number 10 tin cans are placed at each corner, each holding enough earth to support a stick carrying a flag for one of the Four Directions (represented by the colors yellow, red, white, and black). Strung like the ropes of a boxing ring are 405 prayer ties—small pieces of fabric containing tobacco, all tied upon a cotton string. The windows of the room and the doors are covered with black plastic, so no light can be seen. As the ceremony begins, the healer's hands are tied behind his back, then together. Next his arms are tied, and then he is wrapped in a star quilt, which is tied around him. When he is completely tied up, the lights go out, the singing and drumming begin, and somehow, sometime in the darkness, the spirits untie him. When the lights go on and he is revealed to be untied, the healing of the sick commences. Lakota people half joke that the ceremony must have worked because smallpox has vanished.

Betty presented herself for healing in the yuwipi ceremony, and the medicine man took her home. He recognized her suffering and had her move in with his sister, whose husband had just died. Perhaps he recognized that Betty's pressured loquaciousness would offset the silent loneliness of a bereaved widow. Being a client of the mental health system, Betty had no place better to go. She lived in a group home in which the major activity was watching television. Connectedness among residents was minimal.

The moment Betty moved in with the medicine man's sister, she became part of a large, extended kinship network in which life could be completely contained. Between healing ceremonies, family obligations, and social activities, Betty needed no planning for any aspect of her life. She did help the sister with her household activities and was an avid house cleaner, which was appreciated in that family. Like the schizophrenic who was taken in by Melvin Grey Fox in *Coyote Healing*, Betty became another family member. Her life was regulated. One year later, she was on half the amount of medication she had used previously. Two years later it had been reduced to about a fourth. Four years later she was off medication completely.

An alternate story for healing had been substituted for psychiatry's biological narrative. In this story, embeddedness in community and participation in ceremony regulates mood quite effectively. The participants in this story would not even be able to enunciate it, for it is their life. Now a member of the medicine man's family, Betty's life revolved around ceremony, social obligations, reciprocal family relationships, and service to others. She had learned skills for self-soothing—notably ceremony and ritual, all of which serve to induce the kind of trance state found in hypnosis or meditation. The physical work of housecleaning, cooking for post-ceremony feasts, and the camaraderie of Native American women transformed Betty's life experience. When life experience changes, I argue, so does genetic expression and physiology. What a different story from the medication-for-life narrative.

Lauren came with a diagnosis of bipolar II disorder, currently depressed. Her mood alternated between depressed and mildly euphoric (what some people would call happy). Lauren had been participating in the medication story for more than fifteen of her forty-five years, but was increasingly unhappy with the side effects of the drugs. She was taking

Prozac, Zyprexa, and Depakote and had already started to reduce her dosage on her own.

I worked with Lauren, along with Will (an osteopathic physician) and Amy (a yoga teacher). My perspective with Lauren was that other daily practices needed to replace the daily practice of taking pills. Yoga is an effective daily practice. My colleague, Amy Weintraub, has written about the use of yoga for depression and has reviewed its positive benefits.[35] I offered Lauren the Chinese point of view that you can't very well evaluate whether or not something will help until you have done it for 101 consecutive days.

Lauren came to us from Louisiana with plans to stay for ten days. Each day would focus on skill building, on learning practices and tools that she could take home and use on a daily basis. We had collectively decided that her tools would be yoga, ceremony, and visualization. Will would help this process along by facilitating structural change in Lauren's body with cranio-sacral therapy, neuromuscular realignment, and whatever else emerged as potentially useful. I would teach visualization and ceremony.

I began by suggesting we banish the "bipolar word," as I often do. I suggested we enter an altered state of consciousness and let "what we were dealing with" define itself. Lauren agreed, and I began to lead her through and teach her meditation and visualization techniques. I began by focusing on breathing and staying mindful of the present moment, leading into deeper relaxation and letting go of thoughts and preconceptions. After about fifteen minutes of this, I suggested that the things that had brought her to me could organize themselves into their own entity. In the dreamtime (trance or altered state) they could take form and shape. That form and shape could have a voice, and that voice could communicate.

The connotations associated with the bipolar label, and probably other aspects of Lauren's story, too, began to coalesce into the shape of a character who called himself Take It Easy. I double-checked for gender, and he was definitely male.

I gave suggestions to go backward on the river of time, using Lauren's own desired mode of transport—steamboat, raft, canoe, powerboat, whatever she wanted—until the driver of her craft landed her at the place in the stream of time in which Take It Easy had been conceived.

We journeyed backward seven generations to Lauren's ancestral home in Scotland. Images arose of children being beaten to conform. The Scottish Protestant ethic was to "beat it out of them." A story emerged about many generations for whom "taking it easy" meant conforming—stuffing originality, protest, opposition, and other undesirable traits. Overthrowing Take It Easy meant rebelling against self-criticism, for the perspective from which the criticism could be made was a family culture of conformity that didn't match the story Lauren wanted to tell about herself. She wanted to be more outlandish, outspoken, even flamboyant. Being a little manic allowed her to flirt with these qualities, but always in a way that would leave her open to shame later, vulnerable to criticism from herself and others.

We developed a series of practices for her to use to oppose self-deprecation. These included daily yoga, daily ceremony, and daily meditation. My theme for her was, "It's all good. It's all fine. You don't have to change. In fact, don't do anything." This was a recipe against the self-critical perspective.

I encouraged Lauren to gather together everyone she knew who was interested in healing to meet on a weekly basis as a healing community. She did this, and it has proven to be an important part of maintaining her harmony and balance. Her example stands in stark contrast to the stories of the seriously mentally ill clients who populate the mental health care system and remain isolated without support, despite their plethora of medications.

These two stories are about people who have broken free from the biological psychiatric narrative. They spend no money on drugs. Their daily "meds" include yoga, meditation, and prayer, all embedded within community. These are alternate stories that would likely go unnoticed by the dominant paradigm. If noticed at all, these stories would be dismissed as quacky, so rare and resistant to generalization that they would be deemed either unimportant or evidence of misdiagnosis (since bipolar disorder is, by definition, a lifelong problem).

Sandy gives us a good example of emerging from an unclear medical diagnosis (she might or might not have schizophrenia) into a purposeful, self-created, alternative story that became an essential part of her healing.

Sandy was sixteen years old and had been hospitalized for what was clearly an acute psychotic episode, which began while she was away at camp. I was asked to meet with the family. Another psychiatrist was the attending physician and was managing the medication. The family consisted of the divorced parents, a sister, a stepmother, and the patient. Immediately an epic battle emerged between the two parents. Both daughters agreed it had gone on as long as anyone could remember. Whatever dad thought, mother didn't. They agreed on nothing. The attending psychiatrist was an invisible member of the meeting. He had diagnosed schizophrenia and was telling the parents that Sandy, the patient, would have to be on medications for life, and that they should lower their expectations for what she could ever do. In his guise of educating the family, he appeared to be enforcing one possible story of many.

Father liked this story. He liked the genetic story, because other members of the mother's family were on medications and were also "crazy." In his mind, this proved that Sandy suffered from a genetic disorder that came from his ex-wife's side of the family. Trained and working as an engineer, he liked the cleanness of this approach—genetic disorder, give a medication, all is fine. His new wife had clearly learned not to disagree with him—that was her new wife story. The battle even entered the courts with Sandy seeing she was being overmedicated, Dad insisting that doctors always know best, the psychiatrist insisting on high-dose treatment with the drug Zyprexa, and Mom demanding natural healing, acupuncture, and spiritualism.

Sandy had metaphors for herself—that she was an insect under glass, a butterfly exhibit, a pithed frog, and the like. She had no story to tell about herself. Her life had been spent in pursuit of excellence—in the classroom, in track and field, and in piano. She did everything perfectly, though she couldn't tell why. Now she was in tears because everyone was saying she was crazy and there was no telling why. She didn't want to be a part of her mother's world of sweatlodges, traditional healers, and holistic medicine, but she didn't want the world of drugs either, because the drugs were making her feel so bad. She told a story about a movie called *Mr. Jones*. She really identified with this movie. Whenever Mr. Jones felt happy, he did something to get him labeled crazy and sent to the psychiatric hospital, where he stayed for a long time. This included an episode in which he tried to conduct a symphony better than its own conductor, who rather resented the attempt. Sandy resented the story that she was defective, but like Mr. Jones, was lost in her search for understanding of what had led her to the psychiatric ward.

Eventually Sandy was discharged, but only after her mother took her out of the hospital on a day pass from which Sandy didn't return as agreed. Father filled out commitment papers, and the police came and dragged Sandy back to the psychiatric ward just when she was starting to feel better. High-dose medication was then applied (primarily to treat her delusion of believing she could live without medication). That was the end of her meetings with her father. She never wanted to see him again.

When she was finally discharged, she was not on court-ordered treatment, so her mother switched her care to me. I began to meet with this group of the family. I found that I needed to see Sandy by herself, then her mother, then both of them. We represented the other family members with a photograph on a chair; Sandy would have nothing to do with her father since he had committed her.

Sandy began gradually reducing her medication. She would have completely stopped it all at once if I hadn't begged her to take it slow. We were in a political bind, because her father would file commitment papers again if he knew she had stopped taking her medication. I was in a personal bind, because I didn't want to be seen as publicly opposing the former psychiatrist. On the other hand, I wasn't at all sure of the diagnosis, regardless of my disdain for diagnoses. I didn't have a clue as to what had precipitated her psychosis, nor did she remember or tell. Each week, however, Sandy seemed a little better as the medication dosage went down.

We began to talk about her experience of being trapped between two crazy parents. She began to follow my instructions to look for movies that were suitable for a person in her position. I told her my story of how I had left home. I encouraged her to interview others who had had impossible parents who were both crazy and to find out how these other people had escaped. Off medication, Sandy was a bit irritable and moody, but she had also recently turned seventeen, so it was hard to know what was what. "Is there something wrong with my brain?" she asked one day.

"Do you mean something beyond being trapped between crazy parents who can never agree?" I asked.

"Yeah," she said. "Beyond that."

"Beyond that your brain is fine," I responded. I told her the story of the psychologists who had arranged to be admitted to the psychiatry unit with made up stories about their insanity. After admission, they went about acting just like themselves. The research followed the extraordinary narratives of their insanity on the ward. It was published in *Science* and called "On Being Sane in Insane Places."[36] She laughed about that. We continued to seek alternatives for dealing with her "crazy mother."

"I don't want to go to church or sweatlodges or see healers or acupuncturists or take vitamins or eat weird or do anything strange," she said. I supported her self-determination not to be involved in such practices, despite my belief in the usefulness of these strange activities.

Meetings with her mother revolved around getting Mom to be less intrusive. Sandy didn't want her mother barging into her room, walking about the house naked, telling her negative things about her father, involving Sandy in her own crazy plans, or otherwise annoying her. Mother wanted the perfect daughter, the pre-psychotic Sandy.

I told Thomas King's story entitled "You're not the Indian I was looking for."[37] In this story, King, one of Canada's most celebrated Native writers, tells about growing up half Greek and half Cherokee in Roseville, California. He becomes a merchant marine, but no one will believe he is an Indian because he doesn't have the classic look defined by the photographer Edward Curtis. Despite his strong cultural identification, his "Indianness" is discounted because of his lack of classical features. I suggested to Sandy that maybe she wasn't the daughter either of her parents were looking for. Like in King's story, Sandy's parents had adopted a classic description of what a good daughter should do and be, which she did not fit. So how could she escape both of their expectations and find something fun to do?

Sandy began to brainstorm about what would be fun. She wanted to be sponsored for track and field, but that seemed less likely since her hospitalization. She wanted to win a piano scholarship, which was also receding from her grasp. I reminded her that neither of these approaches would work, since they would please her parents. She then started fantasizing about working at a ski resort and earning her lift tickets. Then she could run cross-country there in the spring and summer.

Over time, Sandy began to reconstruct a story of herself as a typically rebellious teenager who was being tortured by two very crazy parents who had literally driven her mad. She began to collect new friends who supported this worldview, which, of course, I supported as well. We were successful in finding books and movies about teens whose parents had driven them mad and how they escaped. Eventually she enrolled in a college that was next to a ski resort and studied half time and skied half time. She's doing reasonably well, is a year from graduating, and sends me e-mails from time to time. She completely overthrew the defective brain story.

We structured Sandy's experience into an alternative narrative, one that had a beginning, middle, and ending, that, like an Arizona highway, stretches far and straight into the distance, going somewhere.

All of these stories represent a kind of underbelly of American psychiatry, but perhaps also a repository of potential transformation and help for the 50 percent of people who do not respond to treatment with conventional medications. They give us a glimpse of alternative approaches that offer solutions in addition to medication—or instead of medication, as the case may warrant. Such solutions would perplex modern psychiatry, for they are postmodern—meaning that they are part of a philosophical movement that rejects single explanations and absolute truths. Each individual has his or her own path to reduced suffering. The solution develops out of the affected community, not the professional expert.

Psychologist Carolyn Kagan says, "Western social psychology views people very much as individuals, separate from others, responsible for our own successes and failures, our own health and well being—albeit in interaction with others." She compares this to Bantu sayings that translate as, "a person can only be a person through others. It is through you that I am who I am, and do what I do—for which I thank you."[38]

9
Talking with Cancer

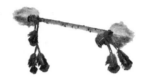

I like nonsense, it wakes up the brain cells. Fantasy is a necessary ingredient in living.

DR. SEUSS[1]

Cancer is the most feared disease of our contemporary world. Despite the numbers of people who survive or live well with cancer, many people view the diagnosis as a death sentence. I have been interested in collecting stories of people who heal from cancer. At lectures I give, usually 20 to 30 percent of people present know someone who healed in spite of a bad prognosis.

How does a person heal despite dire medical predictions and outright pessimism? How do we move from the middle of the statistical distribution to the tail where the outliers live? We do so by beginning a conversation, which starts when people question the pronouncements of the prevailing medical model and wonder if they could get well. Through this questioning and through conversations with other people who have had cancer, current cancer patients, healers, and health care practitioners, it is possible to invent a story of possible healing, of how it might look to get well. The particulars of an individual's story about healing can vary dramatically, from macrobiotics to Chinese medicine to spiritual healing, but, like all conversations, the story needs an audience. When people talk with each other, they generate an emergent process in which healing is one side effect. Through the enactment of the new story, transformation occurs. Some transformations involve healing and curing.

I have collected many stories of remarkable cancer survivors. These stories inspire me because my medical education tells me these people shouldn't survive. A survival model with a normal distribution would predict that some people with cancer, even metastatic cancer, should die very quickly and some should live a very long time, but the medical model assumes that everyone behaves like the mean. I call these stories miraculous because they inspire me with wonder and awe. They seem miraculous because I have been taught that survival is next to impossible. Remarkably, the stories seem more ordinary to the people who live them. What seems miraculous to me is ordinary for the story's characters. Perhaps only through the transformation to ordinary can healing take place.

In a recent workshop for medical librarians in Phoenix, a self-proclaimed cynic told me her physiology professor husband asserted that miracle stories could be attributed only to incorrect diagnosis. I assured her that in all of my stories, the cancer had been confirmed histologically. Pathologists had studied slides of the tumors and declared them cancers. Patients had often received chemotherapy and radiation therapy in addition to other forms of treatment. To answer her, I struggled to find a more postmodern or indigenous approach (assuming either would lead to a novel response). I found myself saying that these healings had happened, though one possible response to my stories would be to dispute their veracity. While it is possible that the stories are not true, it seemed like a trivial way to respond, because almost everyone I meet has at least one story to tell of an acquaintance that lived despite a dire cancer prognosis, despite the insistence of physicians that the patient must die.

It reminded me of a story about a white raven I heard from the Haida people of Queen Charlotte's Island, British Columbia. While very uncommon, the white raven lived. The black ravens chased it away from their community, so the white bird lived amid the giant stumps left over from logging, and the people in the village fed it. To argue that this bird did not exist, when many people had seen and fed it, would end all further dialogue on the subject.

The more interesting questions to ask, I proposed to my cynic friend, are how frequently these stories appear (and I don't know) and whether they are due to chance. The argument, I suggested, hinges on whether or not people with cancer can affect their position in the survival curve through their own efforts and efforts made by others on their behalf. The resolution to this question is largely rhetorical, I suggested, and not intrinsic to the stories themselves, which stand on their own merits. Postmodernism proposes that all interpretations are equally true, that we can't prove anything. "So," I said, "you are welcome to conclude that these stories are all well and good, but actual survival is randomly distributed and people's efforts don't matter. The storied approach to researching that question would be to assemble stories of people who have died on schedule for comparison with stories of people who have lived longer than expected. I have done that, as has Alastair Cunningham (immunologist and psychologist of the Ontario Cancer Center[2]), along with multiple others. We have all concluded that people's efforts do enhance the duration of their survival. But you are welcome to claim the opposite."

My cynic then told a story about a friend of hers who had ovarian cancer. This friend, she said, was the most optimistic person in the world. She insisted she would be well. The only conventional medical treatment she had was surgery. She went to Mexico for coffee enemas. She visited some of the great spas of the world, and she died seven months after diagnosis.

"That's a good story," I responded, "because it helps us illustrate a point. I don't think optimism prolongs survival. I'm not proposing that being positive makes a difference in survival. Actually, both Alastair Cunningham and I found that a realistic appraisal of one's situation was more common in stories of survival than an overly positive attitude. I'm proposing that each story of cancer survival stands on its own, that there is no common theme or thread, that the essentialist argument that certain factors make people live longer or die sooner is incorrect." Each person's story is unique, I suggested. Each person is what we call "an N-of-1 trial," meaning they represent a clinical study that includes only one subject. A collection of stories can teach us something about survival, but survival is an emergent property, a result of a reorganization of many systems and levels, and not the result of a linear increase or decrease in one factor or another. "It's not simple linear algebra," I said. "It's quantum physics.

"I'm proposing," I said, "that we refrain from premature interpretation of stories and should remain much longer in a state of contemplating the mystery of it all. We should acknowledge more often the state of our own ignorance."

"That's interesting," she said, "because my friend insisted on everyone being positive and talking as if she was already cured."

"That's not my experience of what the traditional healing elders do," I said. "Their prayers go something like this: 'Creator, Spirits, Ancestors, we are just little people without any power. We can't do much of anything on our own. That's why we're here, crying out to you for help. Please, have pity on us, and on our friend here. You know what's wrong with him. You know he has this illness. And we don't have the power to heal him. And he doesn't either, because he's just a little person like the rest of us. So we're asking you for help. We know you're more powerful than we are. So, if it's possible, and if you'll allow it, we sure would be grateful if our friend here could be with us still next spring when the grass turns green. We sure would appreciate that.'"

"That's very different from my friend's attitude," said my cynic.

"That's my point," I said. "The elders would never even ask for cure. They'd just keep extending the time frame. If spring came and the patient was still alive, then they'd pray for their friend to be still with them by the time the leaves fall. If that worked, they'd extend the time frame to snow fall. They'd just keep extending the time frame indefinitely until eventually everyone agreed that the person was well, and they'd never take credit for the healing. It would always go to the spirits and the Creator. I think that illustrates accurate appraisal and awareness of what little power we do have, unlike the New Age ideology that, in my view, exaggerates the power of the individual to demand change and healing."

We ended our discussion with my suggestion that biomedicine lacks the tools to study healing. Biomedicine's tools are linear and additive, especially its sacred randomized, controlled trial. Healing is nonlinear and definitely not additive. As an emergent property of a quantum field state, healing arises or doesn't arise, and its arrival is not predictable based on any one factor or even a simple addition of several factors.

Thus we see that the story itself does not heal. The treatment does not heal. Transformation alone alters the world so that cancer no longer exists. Transformation comes from a reorganization of the elements of involved and participatory systems (organ, human, family, community, cultural) and how they communicate (or converse). Healing is an emergent property that we cannot fully understand because it seems to arise from nowhere. It emerges in communication patterns among organs and people as the individual's health status changes.

Elena's story exemplifies this transformational process. Elena came with metastatic colon cancer. She wanted a spiritual retreat because she believed she had achieved the maximum benefit conventional medicine could provide. She had multiple small tumors throughout her liver. She wanted them to coalesce into a large tumor that could be surgically removed. Over ten consecutive days, we meditated, we did yoga, we did imagery, and we did ceremony and ritual.

In one ceremony, we saw a woman's face in the clouds. Elena recognized it as St. Theresa of the roses. This was part of her story, since none of us were Catholic. She seemed transformed in that moment and found an unexplained peacefulness. Upon her return home, she found that her goal had manifested. She now had only two tumors—large enough that they could be surgically removed. I explain this as an emergent property of transformation. An internal and external reorganization or shift had occurred, coinciding with the tumors merging to become operable.

Here is a story I told Elena to help foster her transformation. I chose this story because the trials and tribulations of its main character matched those of Elena in many ways and could transport her to a new way of thinking about cancer as a healing journey. I heard this story from Norman, the Haida physician I met, and it comes from his people.

One day Raven fell deeply in love. This was curious, because Raven had created the differences between the sexes in the first place by mating the delicate lips of the chiton with the curious long muscle of the clam, all for a joke. But that's another story, and best told by an old woman on Queen Charlotte's Island. She'll tell you how that joke still has its repercussions and has even turned around to bite Raven in the butt.

Raven fell in love with a stream. He met her when she was dallying on her private beach in the form of a young woman. Her nails were pure, solid copper. Live hummingbirds nuzzled in her hair. She carried a stick adorned with the carving of a frog, also known as the crab of the forest. Raven assumed his most respectable form and asked her to marry him. She accepted. After the marriage feast, he built her a fine house made entirely of water. She lived for many years there, until she was driven underground by clear-cut logging of her watershed, but that's another story—one that is still going on. No one knows what the outcome will be, but it is known that creek women do not take insults lightly.

The story begins as a parallel to Elena's life. She did fall in love with a man who was virtually absent for most of the twenty years of their marriage. It was a bit like Raven falling in love with a stream. The chemotherapy and other medical treatment were a lot like clear-cutting and had driven her almost underground.

Many years later, a young woman from the mainland found herself lost in the forests of the islands. She was a long way from home. She had been tramping for many days in the forest. Her hair was matted, her clothing torn, her feet bloody and muddy and blistered and sore. She still carried her regal speech and bearing. She sported a dogfish tattoo on her back. A young man found her and brought her aboard his canoe. He took her to the house of his parents, where she was bathed and fed.

Elena was also a long way from home. In a spiritual sense, she was as lost as this dogfish woman. She didn't know where to turn or what to do next, which is why she called me. We had to help her construct a story that would reorient her. Her previous story of being the dutiful housewife who repressed her feelings but was actually enraged didn't seem to be helping. It wasn't correlated with wellness.

Once the young woman had rested and been refreshed, she told her story. Her family had owned a powerful hat in the shape of a double cormorant. When a dancer wore it, the earth would quiver under his feet and he could dance for days. The hat had to be worn after ceremonial preparation and only when ritual required it. One day her brother wore it fishing. Several days later, he came home without the hat and without his three friends.

I always made sure Elena was rested and prepared before we worked. In a sense, she had a hat.

What happened is that the hat kept falling off the brother's head. In anger, he threw it into the water. He and his friends caught trout, cooked them, and laid them on skunk cabbage leaves. A copper-colored frog hopped out of the bushes onto the brother's fish. He threw the frog back into the bush, threw away the fish, and cooked another. The same thing happened again. The third time it happened, the brother threw the fish, the frog, and the skunk cabbage leaves all into the fire, put on more wood, and fanned the blaze.

The frog sat in the flames a long time, glowing like a coal until it suddenly exploded, putting out the fire. All night long the boys heard the eerie voice of a woman crying about her lost child. The next morning, they passed a woman standing on the shore. She wore a hummingbird in her hair. Her walking stick was covered with frogs. She was crying, "Where is my child? What have you done with my child? Where are his clothes?" The boys were frightened.

Further on, they passed a man on the shore whose face was painted red and black. The man said, "You will die." He pointed at each of the boys in turn, one by one. He told the brother that he would die only after telling his tale. Everything happened the way the man said it would. One by one, the boys died. The brother died only after reaching home and telling his tale.

I thought of the frog as Elena's chemotherapy and the red and black painted man as her doctors giving her dire prognoses. We had to address this. We couldn't just let it go.

Then the hummingbird woman came to their village. The elders predicted trouble. Her grandmother hid the young woman in the latrine. A few days later, the earth shook and a huge fire burned down the village. Nothing was left when the fire went out. All the homes, all the carvings, everything had turned to ash. No one lived except the girl hidden in the latrine. All she could save was a small stone bowl.

Once she was sure the fire was out and the hummingbird woman had left, the young woman started walking. She walked until she collapsed in exhaustion on a beach. A young hunter found her and carried her back to his village. The chief of the village had just lost a daughter. He had planted a mortuary pole in front of his house. The crest on that pole was the woman's own crest, the dogfish. So the chief adopted her to replace his lost daughter. A potlatch was held and her fame and reputation spread. When she reached marriageable age, a man came from the mainland and took her back. She lived. She had children. And one day she told her children this story of the Haida Gwai islands.

We were metaphorically adopting Elena, as did the people in the story.

One day the woman's youngest son said the other children were teasing him for not having any relatives, saying he was a foreigner and an orphan. This made her resolve to visit her family. Her husband provided gifts and provisions and canoes to carry them to the islands, in order to make amends for the insults of his people.

She returned to the islands. She learned that her parents were dead. Her adoptive brother was now the chief. All went well, until her eldest son took to sleeping with the chief's wife when his uncle was hunting. Eventually the uncle heard about this. The chief announced that he was going on a hunting trip, got his gear and left, and returned that night early to surprise his wife and his nephew in bed.

I used this event in the story to stand in for general adversity, which the cancer surely was. I wasn't sure if the story had another connection with Elena's life, as they often do when I am intuitively called to use them.

The chief placed his nephew in a large wooden chest, closed the lid, caulked it shut along the seam with spruce gum, and tied the lid down with cedar bark line. He set the chest adrift on the falling tide. The young man bobbed and floated for many days, starving and feverish. Eventually he felt the chest become stationary. He heard a woman saying, "He's mine. I'll take him home."

He awoke in a handsome six-beam house. The woman who rescued him from the box had claimed him as husband, and he was now invited to sit beside his wife. She introduced him to her father, the chief, and her grandmother. Eagle skins hung all along the walls. Eagles flew through the smoke hole, took off their skins, and looked human. He met the chief's son. He had come to a village of eagles.

What is important here is that the nephew prevailed against overwhelming odds. In the face of certain death, he was found by eagle women and nursed back to health. He even goes on to become a productive member of their community.

Eventually he grew tired of watching the others fly off to hunt and demanded that he be allowed to go along. The chief gave him a skin and a warning: "Do not hunt or touch the giant clam. It is stronger than we are." The first day of hunting he caught a salmon. Before the end of the month he brought home a seal, a sea lion, and a killer whale. Again the old woman warned him not to hunt or touch the giant clam. The next day he caught two killer whales.

The day after that, he saw the clam. He forgot the warnings and thought he was stronger than the clam. He grazed it with his talons and was suddenly stuck fast to the clam, unable to pry loose. He struggled. Others came to pull him off and got stuck upon him and upon the others, until a great, long chain of eagles had formed. All the brothers, uncles, chiefs, and princes of the eagles, each with talons in the others' shoulders, were slowly being dragged under the water by the giant clam.

This mirrored the way Elena had gone through a series of rescues and relapses throughout her treatment.

The old grandmother realized what was happening, put on her eagle skin, and flew off stiffly. She grabbed the highest, last eagle in the chain and raised the entire pillar of eagles out of the water. She did this by singing a song. The last skin was empty. The rescued young man had remained in the sea with the giant clam. The song could not save him. His wife was inconsolable. Her grief was so bad that the old grandmother formally asked the chief to resuscitate the girl's husband, lest she die.

The eagle chief entered the corner of the house, opened a large stone box, and uncovered a hole to the sea. He put down his net and sifted through everything ever lost in the ocean. At length, he found all the bones of the young man and reassembled his son-in-law. He wiped all the bones clean and laid them out on a bed of fresh seaweed. He leapt over them, back and forth, to and fro, for four days. On the second day, new flesh came to cover the bones. On the third day, movement began. On the fourth day, his son-in-law stood before him.

I thought this would parallel the ceremonies that we would be doing for Elena at night with the Yaqui healer. Elena heard this story and understood that she needed to speak to her cancer. She needed a sense of a helper spirit. I started to tell her how important it was to relax and open her mind to the possibility of an encounter with her cancer. "You can allow the cancer to set the stage for the meeting. You can allow the cancer to come to you. This is not creative imagery in which you do the imagining. This is like going to the movies. We're just going to invite the cancer to create an environment in which it would like to speak, to take a shape and a form, to find the opportunity to have a conversation with us."

Mainstream culture teaches us that we cannot talk to cancer. It doesn't have a consciousness. It doesn't have a mind. It's just a playful game of the mind to imagine that cancer can talk to us. This is the metaphorical approach. I'm interested in cultivating a more direct approach, as if cancer is real, as if it has a spirit, as if we can talk to it. Perhaps we can. This approach is more similar to aboriginal thought and knowledge. If we want to know about cancer, we must talk to cancer. We must interrogate it. We must begin a dialogue with cancer that will reveal its secrets—its weaknesses, its preferences, its origins, its desires. In my view, we do talk with cancer. It does have a spirit. We can engage in this communication. Probably it works just as well for the person to think it is metaphor, but I believe the work is more powerful if we can step out of the metaphor and into the literal.

Trance is important. How deeply relaxed a person is matters a great deal in the process. We must be able to step outside of our ordinary minds. More importantly, we must step outside the preconceptions and constructions we have made. I continued to encourage Elena to slow her breathing, since that would also slow her heart rate and her mind. She could slowly but surely stop thinking so much and so fast. She could begin to drop down into that state of mind from which dreams arise. She could have a dream but still be awake. She could see images just as she would as if she were asleep. I continued this line of talk to encourage a deepening of her state of mind. I imagine that our ancestors learned to master their minds so completely that they could enter a deep trance immediately. Modern people need more assistance. I often remind them how quickly they lose themselves at the movies, suggesting it's possible to go ahead and do that now. I told Elena she could lose herself just as completely in the images that would arise in her mind.

I began to talk about mist, how I love the mist as it rises above the river, how thick the mist can become, so thick you cannot see through it. The world dissolves as the mist thickens, so there is no world outside of the mist. Only the mist remains. In fact, we could be transported any-where and not even realize it. I suggested that a silent canoe could come through the mist for Elena, a canoe that would take her through the mist to the land where the cancer waited to meet with her. I talked about how drastically the land might change from where she entered, as if she were walking into the mist and coming out into another world. "The cancer is waiting," I said. "Let it take a shape. Let it take a form. Allow it to emerge as it wishes. Perhaps you will have to walk a bit to find it. Perhaps you will have to explore the land before the cancer is willing to appear. Perhaps you will have to track it, to follow its footprints in the sand until it emerges and is willing to talk."

Eventually the cancer did emerge. Elena was able to describe it from her trance state. It was a dark figure covered with a cape and a mask, almost a Zorro figure. At first it scared her. She worried that it had come to take her life. It was imposing, impressive.

"We could take your life," it said. "But we will not. We have enjoyed our time with you. You have fed us well. We have eaten so much better with you than with anyone ever before. We love the vitamins you take, and the herbs."

I suggested some questions. "Where did you come from? How did you get here? What was the purpose of your coming? How have you helped me? How have you hurt me? Where are you going? What would make you want to leave, to move on?"

"Before we came," the cancer said, "you didn't feel loved. You didn't feel that you had the right to ask for love from anyone. We changed your whole perspective on life. We shortened your time frame. We made everything seem so much more immediate. We helped you transform your view of yourself. Now you know you deserve love. You know you deserve help. Now you will ask your parents for help. You will ask other people for help. You tell yourself a different story now, that you are valuable and loveable, that you deserve to be loved—by your parents, your family, by a man in your life. We came to teach you that. Now that you know, we can leave. But we warn you. You must continue to live in this way. We will be back if you return to your old ways. You must never do that."

She found herself asking the cancer where it was going to go. "We will transform," it said. "We will die in this life and return to the Creator. We will stop being cancer and become something else. We've had a good run.

"Take the chemotherapy one more time," it said. "Let the doctors think they killed us, rather than tell them we died by choice. Let them take the credit like they always do. Our departure will be more believable that way."

Elena found herself getting back into the canoe and gliding through the mist again to return to the present. I began to talk about how she had probably felt like the young man, trapped in the cedar chest, but obviously for very different reasons.

"Perhaps you have felt sick, you have felt feverish, nauseated, and unable to help yourself. Cancer has a way of doing that to people, if not directly, then through the treatment. Perhaps you also need a helper spirit to keep you strong. Perhaps you need a rescuer, the same way the young man needed to be found and brought back to life. And like the story shows, we get more than one chance. The young man ignored the instructions about the giant clam and went ahead to hunt it. He was destroyed, but he got another chance. Even though his father-in-law didn't want him to have another chance, his wife's grandmother interceded, and he got one. We all need intercession from time to time. Who will intercede for you? Who is your helper?"

Elena began to describe the spirit of a horse, her horse, the horse who had been the salvation of her childhood. "I would have died without that horse," she said, "and now it's here for me. The horse will help put me back together." She struggled to describe the joy, love, and protection she felt from that horse. Words are never sufficient for these moments. The feeling of the horse's presence was so much stronger than could be described.

When we were finished, Elena was sure she could cope. Her cancer was leaving. It was willing to transform and to cease to exist as cancer, to become something else. The horse, her helper, would see her through the process.

One more idea came to my mind. I am reminded of this idea whenever I fly in a jet plane. The jet creates a vacuum before it into which the plane is sucked. I think of the future as sucking us into it from the past. We are pulled into the future by the future. I explained this concept to Elena. "Let yourself, if you will, begin to imagine a cancer-free future," I said. "Let yourself feel the future pulling you toward it. See the cancer leaving. It's going, going, gone. It's gone. You're well. See yourself as completely well. Let that wellness pull you forward into it. Let that wellness be your beacon, drawing you steadily onward. See yourself loved and well. Let yourself believe that this has already come true."

This conversation felt like our turning point, though we had many more. Elena continued to work with her helper spirit, her horse. She even acquired a few other helpers. In doing this, she fell into a long-standing tradition of the people of North America. Cultures vary in how they define ordinary medicine powers as different from shamanic powers. The Chipewyan had only two classifications, while the Choctaw had a complex system of fifteen different types of shamans.[3] Perhaps it doesn't matter. What matters is effectiveness.

I have helper spirits, too, and I saw my helper spirits aiding Elena as we worked. What are we to call ourselves, those of us who work in this way? Shaman is too pretentious. The word has become so pregnant it is about to burst. The feeling–sense of the word is important, but as a noun, it has become too grandiose. I prefer to think of myself as a collaborator, collaborating with people who ask for my help in whatever way I can. I am interested in accumulating power to help. I would like to be able to attract the most powerful spirits possible to help people. But so little is up to me. The person who asks for help decides if she wants the help of the spirits. They must be asked. Something we are doing must relate to them sufficiently for them to find a way to help.

I understand that in days gone by, families controlled spirit power that could be passed from generation to generation or to other family members. I see my grandparents in this way, though in the form in which they come to me, they might not even be my grandparents. They could be spirits completely unrelated to my actual grandparents who present themselves to me in this format because it's familiar to me. I have cultivated these relationships over a lifetime of attending ceremony and doing healing work with people, but still I don't know how helpful this power is, or not. So much is uncertain, indeterminate, and unknown. Yet we must always do what we can, and the spirits help. Sometimes I see them adjusting people's brainwaves to change the present. Is this really happening? Is it my imagination? Regardless of what I prefer to believe, experience unfolds and must be acknowledged.

Donald Hines writes that the recipient of power has to ask for the power.[4] Receiving it is contingent upon the spirit's approval. If the power is satisfied, it will help. If it is not, it won't. My approach is consistent with the idea that anyone can "catch" a power spirit or spirit helper. Any human can access the state of consciousness in which we contact power spirits. I use ceremony, stories, and guided imagery to accomplish this process, though it can be done in many other ways. Perhaps today people are being asked to move beyond the search for powerful healers to seeing all of us as capable of becoming powerful healers. I do frequently see and consult with my helpers and ask them to help others as Michael Harner describes,[5] but I also try to facilitate each person's ability to do that on his or her own. If we can help everyone do this, the hierarchy of powerful shaman and weak patient dissolves into a collaborative framework in which everyone is engaged in the dialogue. As Fred Allen Wolf said, "Who needs trance mediums to contact the spirit world, when it's something we can all readily do?"[6]

I suspect that the more we all fast, dream, and have visions, the more we will be connected with this power. One purpose of the spiritual retreats I lead is to help people connect with the source of the power and continue to cultivate relationships with helper spirits long after the retreat. Imagery provides one means by which to dialogue with spirit power. Ceremony is another. Perhaps this fusion of aboriginal culture with modern life will allow us to step outside of superstition to a more modest relationship with spirit power that is always for the good. In this way, we will all become medicine people. We will all manifest spirit power—so necessary for eliminating cancer.

Culture changes. Aboriginal healing practices evolve. Anthropologist Marlene Brant Castellano describes how indigenous knowledge is a part of a dynamic cultural system that is continually moving toward something new.[7] The people who consult with me are evolving knowledge of healing through the dialogues we generate in our work and ceremonies. At least we are evolving my knowledge, which is influenced by indigenous thinking but is not an indigenous knowledge system, except in the sense that it comes from my experience. What makes it nonindigenous is that I am not embedded in an indigenous community, although I have been involved with aboriginal culture since birth. As Thomas King says, "I'm not the Indian you were looking for." I'm not the romantic ideal of the shaman–healer, but I've been evolving ways to help people become their own shaman–healers. This seems eminently more practical for today, since it is so hard to find healing elders and there are so many cultural barriers.

My sense is that new times bring new spirits. We are all amalgamations of the various cultures and belief systems with which we have contact during our lives. I sometimes find Christian spirits appearing in my dreams, visions, and ceremonies. I'm sure spirits from other religions would also make an appearance if I knew more about them. We are becoming postmodern by default, immersed in diversity. Despite this, it is important to preserve generic knowledge from multiple indigenous knowledge systems about how to dialogue with spirits. I want to deepen our belief in the reality of this realm, this conversation, and the advice obtained in this way, though it requires social confirmation, as has always been true in indigenous communities. New spirits bring new medicine powers along with new means for calling their use into play, which in turn generates new power ceremonies.

I believe we all need our personal ceremonies as well. These will differ, because different spirit powers come with different sets of instructions. The ceremony facilitates the continued contact with the spirit powers. In Elena's case, I wanted her to continue to dialogue with her spirit horse and anyone else who appeared. The deepening of these relationships would build her power to heal.

Later in the week of the spiritual retreat, Elena found a stone that looked like her horse. She became convinced that she could do a ceremony to turn this stone into a robe for her horse spirit to enter when it came to visit. A strong tradition exists for the idea that spirit power can be concentrated into individual objects that can be used to help with the healing. This is the concept behind power objects. The fusion of object and power is created through prayer. The spoken word shapes reality.[8] The power of mind and prayer facilitates the help of spirits. Any object has the potential to be a power object, even Elena's stone—especially Elena's stone.

I assisted Elena in designing and carrying out a ceremony to put medicine power into her stone so that she could wear it. We talked about "feeding her power object," or putting more intent, prayer, and consciousness into her object from time to time. This was to be done in a prescribed, ritual manner. Her focused attention on the object is what keeps it powerful. Sacred objects should also be kept free from contamination. They are cleaned periodically with sage smoke. I have learned to store them in corn meal and tobacco, but this is by no means the only way to keep them. It is not the objects themselves that count but the human consciousness that has been imparted to them. Power objects must be cultivated and kept alive.

We did a sweatlodge for Elena two days later. The sweatlodge and other purification ceremonies help us cultivate humility to make sincere prayers to change reality. The heat and the darkness cause thinking to stop. Internal dialogue ceases, deepening the trance state and facilitating spirit contact. After the sweatlodge, the leader used his eagle feather fan to "wipe off" any bad energy, including the cancer, from Elena's body. He then spit onto some cedar bark, covered it with cornhusk, and waved this around Elena's body four times. Then he walked off into the east, where he buried the cedar bark.

The next day we taught Elena a song for calling her helper spirits. This would become her individual song, her private property. The following night was her night for vision questing, for sitting out in nature for the night and fasting. In traditional practice this was done for four nights, but our retreat format of one week generally only allows for one night, unless the person is really motivated to do two nights. Vision questing is another way to consolidate the entities with whom we have made contact and assure continuity of the dialogue. Elena picked out a place for her vision quest that she thought would be particularly conducive for communication with spirits. These are sometimes called power spots or sacred places.

The next day we made a mask for her and a mask for her cancer. When we wear these masks it makes us more able to feel connected with the spirit or energy represented by the mask. For Elena wearing the mask made it easier for her to let her cancer go.

Of course, no one really knows what a "spirit" is. We are left only with our concepts, since spirits may not be knowable, at least in our European sense of the term. Michael Harner says that spirits are all-knowing beings, though that has not been my experience.[9] In my experience, spirits are not all-powerful beings. They too have their limitations.

Elena and I continued to work together. She eventually did die, though she outlived her oncologists' predictions by eight years. Is that a success? I think so. Whenever a family calls me and thanks me for the difference we made in a person's life, I feel as if the work was worthwhile. We can't predict life or death. We can only do our best and let it take us where it will. What this distills to is the idea of transformation.

Cancer or any disease or challenge is an invitation to transform. Doing so is always helpful—sometimes to miraculously live, sometimes to die well. What happens emerges as an outcome through doing the work. It can't be predicted. All that's certain is that we will find more meaning and purpose and our quality of life will improve.

10
Making Meaning for Diabetes

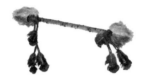

It is ever more clearly a struggle between . . . a para-
digm that perceives life as a means to accumulate [things]
against [a paradigm] inspired by indigenous peoples who
perceive life as an end and all else as means to protect and
promote it.

Manuel Rozental[1]

I consider diabetes to be a social illness that manifests in an individual's biology. Type 2 or adult onset diabetes has been called a disease of colonization. It did not exist in North America to any significant degree prior to European contact. Type 2 diabetes results primarily from receptor insensitivity to insulin, rather than an inability of the pancreas to make insulin, as in type 1 diabetes. Type 2 diabetes arises more from how people live and from their relationships with others, from a general lack of meaning and purpose, than from genetic defects. It makes sense within the story of each person's life. This "sense" may not always emerge in questionnaire research, though many studies do link lifestyle and stress with glucose levels.

Questionnaire-based research has failed to capture the richness of how mind and body work together in health and disease, because these inter-workings are storied and unique to each person. Meaning is lost when sophisticated stories are reduced to the simple "yes–no–somewhat" categories of written questionnaires. People often have difficulty relating to the stereotypical questions typically asked on psychological scales and inventories. This is because people manage their views and experiences through dialogue that involves a sense of constant change, depending upon who is talking.

Once upon a time, I had an enlightening experience during research involving questionnaires. As a data collector, I naïvely thought it was important to engage the people in dialogue, to understand their interpretation of the questions, and to respond to their questions about the meaning of individual items. I saw myself as part of a larger process of enabling people to tell their stories. When I innocently revealed what I was doing, I was asked to leave the study because I was "corrupting" the data. The belief was that the human respondent had to interact alone with his questionnaire, with no other human influence, in order to provide accurate responses. As I was inspired to consider this point of view, I realized that it too invalidated the findings, since the purist researchers actually had no idea of the true variance in how people interpreted their questionnaires. Questionnaires cannot capture the richness of stories.

When I spoke on diabetes for the San Carlos Apache tribe at a conference held in their casino, Apache Gold, the walls outside the room were lined with photographs of famous and ordinary Apache people from the nineteenth century, including Geronimo, Cochise, and Mangus. Other photographs showed a host of mothers, children, and grandparents. None were overweight. No Apache had diabetes in the nineteenth century. Geronimo could run further in a day than a horse could. The people were fit and lived lives of meaning and purpose. When they had food, they ate well. Simple sugars and trans fats were unknown.

Today Apache people are chasing the Pima for diabetes prevalence. What changed for these people? Both were moved off their land onto useless patches of dirt. The Pima had worked centuries to create irrigation systems and to develop agricultural practices that made their land responsive to their food needs. That land and those irrigation ditches were quickly covered with buildings. The city of Phoenix overran them and their land. They were moved to land that lacked game to hunt, infrastructure for irrigation, plants to gather, or any meaningful activity. They sat on bare dirt, unmodified by the centuries they had spent molding their homeland to their needs. Their lifestyle had changed to sitting in box houses, eventually gaining televisions to watch, and eating government food (high in starch and sugar). Without the capacity and opportunity to feed and care for their people, they lost all meaning and purpose. Their activity plummeted. No longer could they run for hours. Diabetes appeared, along with a host of other illnesses.

I used this story to ask the Apaches at the conference what had changed about their lifestyle. Diabetes had only come to the people in the 1940s. Before that, it had not existed. What had changed? "We no longer hunt our food," one said. "We eat crap from the convenience store," said another. "We don't walk anywhere. We don't ever run. We just sit around." The answers poured forth.

Then what could we change now, and how? We can change it by living the way our ancestors did, people responded. By eating what they ate. By walking how they walked. By following in their footsteps.

The unmistakable message I heard was that there is wisdom in the stories passed down to us from our ancestors. Within aboriginal knowledge systems, the ancestors have sent us messages about how to live. We simply have to engage them in conversation.

Melissa was a Cree woman with diabetes. She had recently had cardiac bypass surgery. Nothing was working for her, and her sugars were high despite a regimen of medication and insulin. She had originally come to me for the diabetes, with an "oh, by the way" story about feeling chest twinges when she walked up and down hills and stairs. The story sounded suspiciously like angina. A stress test confirmed that she was on the verge of a heart attack, so she went to bypass surgery. Now we were meeting in her hospital room.

While Melissa's personal story is unique, the broad brush strokes could apply to millions of people around the world, indigenous and modern alike. Melissa had diabetes for years. Her self-care was marginal. She took her medicine when she remembered. She raised her children and helped with her grandchildren. She made beautiful jewelry to support her family, though not as well as she wished. Her husband worked as a carpenter and was always improving their house. On the surface, Melissa's life was good, even though she had her stressors.

Melissa's father had molested her daughter, awakening her own memories of being molested by him. She tended to deal with that pain through eating. She had gained 110 pounds over the past ten years. The incest situation had been resolved. Her daughter was thriving, but bitterness remained between Melissa and her mother. No charges had been filed, but Melissa kept the girls away from their grandfather, and her mother refused to forgive her for that. Her mother couldn't accept the story of the molestation. In her mind, it simply had not happened and would not be discussed.

During this period, Melissa had withdrawn from her husband. He had an affair while working on a construction site some distance away. He had been spending his weekdays at the site and his weekends at home. He had stopped the affair, but Melissa's anger had never been discussed. It too was ignored.

Before her surgery, I asked Melissa to bring everyone she knew to a talking circle with an elder to prepare for the surgery. The Cree elder and I met beforehand to settle on a plan for the talking circle. We would begin with my agenda of posing specific questions to everyone present. Then he would do a ceremony to doctor Melissa and to build the power of prayer for her. While this circle was decidedly aboriginal in flavor, the concept is general and can be created within any culture.

The simple beauty of the talking circle is that people must take turns speaking, which keeps them from blurting out the first thing that enters their mind and paves the way for the power of uninterrupted speech. Each person can speak only when holding the talking stick (or whatever object has been chosen to serve this ceremonial purpose). When each person must stay quiet until it's his or her turn, the likelihood increases that people will actually listen to what others say, along with the possibility that those words will change the listener, altering what he or she will eventually say. When I participate in talking circles, I rarely say what I thought I was going to say when it's my turn. The power in the stick and the group process transform my thoughts into better words than I could manage on my own.

A talking circle can be done with or without a leader. It can be done within any religious tradition, from Hawai'ian to Islamic to Christian. The basic idea is to begin with a prayer and pass a beautifully decorated stick around the circle of people. Ideally, the stick has previously received prayers and blessings to aid the people in communicating and it carries that intent, though I've done many powerful talking circles without the correct props—for example, using a fork as the talking stick, because that was all we could find in a conference hotel setting. I tend to start the circle with a prayer and a question, and then pass the stick. My prayer was for Melissa's highest good and for the healing of her heart, her community, and her family. My question was simple: "On all possible levels, why is Melissa's heart hurting?"

Some time after her surgery, Melissa joined a week-long spiritual retreat that I was coleading. We began with an opening ceremony and guided imagery. I started by saying *ta'nsi,* which literally means "how?" and is used in a similar way as the English "hello, hi, how are you, how are things?"

Melissa responded in the traditional way, *m'on-na'ntaw,* which is the response to *ta'nsi* and means "fine" or "hi." She added, *"Kiyama'ka?"* which means, "and you?"

"Peyekwan," I said, which means "just the same." I am slowly learning Cree; I've found that a small effort makes a world of difference in communication.

After the opening ceremony, I used my words and voice to help Melissa enter into an altered state of consciousness from which she would be completely absorbed in what we were about to do.

Mihaly Csikszentmihalyi, chiefly renowned as the architect of the notion of flow in creativity, asserts that people enter a flow state when they are fully absorbed in activity during which they lose their sense of time and have feelings of great satisfaction. Csikszentmihalyi describes flow as a state of complete involvement in an activity for its own sake. Nothing else matters. One's ordinary sense of time changes. We feel a sense of connection between each moment. The sense of flow comes from the way one moment follows the next.[2]

Once Melissa was relaxed, I invited her to let a countryside appear in which she could track down the diabetes spirit and get to know it. She found a rocky coastal countryside, not unlike her homeland in the north. There were dirt roads, small churches, marshes, and sea birds. It was the height of summer.

"We need to find where Diabetes is hiding," I told her. "What prints does it leave? What are the clues to its presence?"

From her youth, Melissa recalled her grandfather's tracking abilities. She remembered a young man who had wandered into the bush and gotten lost, and how her grandfather had led a search party that had found him. In similar fashion, she saw footprints in the wet sand. "He's got reptile feet," she said. "He's like a vertical reptile. He's cold-blooded."

"Alright," I said. "Let's follow the prints to see where they go."

"They follow the trail along the lake," she said. "I'm following him. I know it's a him. The tracks are leading into a church. It's a small, one-room Catholic church, like the one I had to attend as a child. The prints are fresh. They go up the wooden stairs. The water's not even dry."

"Let's offer some tobacco in our mind's eye, for protection," I said. "Let's make sure we're totally safe before we go in there."

"Okay," Melissa said. "I'm doing that."

"Go inside," I said. "I'm right behind you."

"I'm inside," she said. "It's dim. Candles are burning in the rack. There's a shadow guy by the altar. He's coming toward me. It's not Diabetes. It must be one of his helpers. He looks like the hunchback of Notre Dame from that Disney movie."

"Stand your ground," I said. "Greet him."

"I am," she said. "He's telling me that Diabetes is gone, but he was here. He comes into the messages of shame that I grew up with. He's telling me that Diabetes came to us through the Catholic Church. He came with the priests. That's what made my father sick and his grandfather before that. It made the people feel bad about ourselves and our ways. That's what started all this."

"Great," I said. "Now we know how it got here, but how did it get into you?" I asked.

"Through the Church and my father," she said. "When he did what he did, it came into me."

"What does it eat?" I asked. "How does it survive?"

"It thrives on shame," she said. "It likes self-hatred. It's cold-blooded. It makes your heart freeze. When the heart freezes, icicles build up on the walls and the ceilings. Pretty soon there's no room for the blood to get through."

"I guess we're going to have to warm up your heart," I said, "or the same thing will happen to your new blood vessels all over again. How are we going to do that?"

"I better ask the hunchback," she said. "He's been living in this church for a long time and has seen it all. He's seen priests come and go." I'm silent while she asks. "Forgiveness and love is what he says. I need to practice forgiveness and become better at loving everyone in my life."

"What about your dad?" I asked.

"Him I can forgive, but I don't have to forget."

Following the conclusion of this imagery, I decided to tell Melissa the Dene story of what happened after Coyote stole fire from Fire Mountain. Little did Coyote know, his actions had unintended consequences. I told Melissa that all utterances, all communications, reflect directly or indirectly upon the people who make them. Coyote was perpetually learning that. We communicate and converse to influence each other. Stories have many effects, some of which are to promote values compatible with group survival. Traditional stories encourage generosity, cooperation, restraint, and sacrifice. Melissa actually had enough of those qualities. What she needed was to take better care of herself and to let her community also take better care of her. In a sense, she needed to hear the story, so that she could appreciate her role as recipient of the community's concern. This Coyote story, like others, has been repeated from generation to generation, making its influence felt across time. Like all traditional stories, it provides people with the wisdom they need to live well, and without diabetes.

In contrast, University of Arizona anthropologist Kathryn Coe points out how our modern culture's stories encourage individualistic or self-serving behavior.[3] Noted physician and student of salesmanship Spencer Johnson writes that, "one skill all great salespeople have is the ability to tell compelling personal tales that illustrate the points they wish to make" and persuade people to buy what they are selling.[4] In courtrooms and elections, the best story wins.[5] Stories are powerful ways of influencing human behavior. We should use them wisely. This is why I tell stories and why I told this Coyote story to Melissa.

When he was running down the mountain, a burning branch tied to his tail, Coyote didn't even notice that he was setting the mountain on fire. He was too busy dodging the arrows of Fire Man. Coyote was leaping from bush to bush. He was aware that his usual zigzag pattern would not work, because it would slow him down enough that the ties that bound the burning branch to his tail would burn away, and he would lose the fire. He didn't know that he was setting each bush he passed on fire as he went by.

Watching the ever-increasing number of burning bushes, Fire Man chuckled. He knew that stolen gifts often cause more trouble than they're worth. He knew that soon Coyote would be cursed for stealing fire because no one would know how to put out the blaze. They would soon have more fire than they would know how to handle. So Fire Man put away his arrows and went back to Fire Mountain.

Little Wind Boy loved the sparks and embers. What wonderful new toys! For every fire Coyote lit, Little Wind Boy lit three more. As Little Wind Boy continued his dance, soon the entire mountain was ablaze and a wall of flames was heading toward the homes of the people.

The people were so excited by Coyote's gift that they didn't notice the fire coming toward them. They were gathering burning coals and taking them into their homes to light fires for heat and cooking. They didn't see the smoke billowing so high it obscured even Fire Mountain. They couldn't hear Fire Man laughing about the sweetness of his revenge upon Coyote and the people.

It was Cardinal who first noticed the blaze. He came to warn the oblivious people. "Look," he shouted. "Look at Fire Mountain! It's burning and it's coming for you. It's out of control. Look at me. I flew so close to the fire that it turned my feathers red."

First Woman heard Cardinal and sounded the alarm, since the people always listened to her, even if not to Cardinal. She thanked Cardinal for his sacrifice, for caring so much for the people. She gave him a new name. "From now on, you will be known as Firebird, since you sounded the fire alarm for the people."

The people were frightened. They blamed Coyote. "He shouldn't *have stolen something he didn't know how to handle. It's his fault that our homes are going to be destroyed." Coyote was ashamed. He felt misunderstood. Of course, he hadn't known how to handle fire. He had no experience with fire. But someone had to get it and bring it to the people or they'd still be suffering in the old ways. Someone had to take the first step and take a risk. That was Coyote's job, he thought proudly, to go boldly where no one had gone before and change the world. Having fire would certainly change the world. But, right now, it was burning out of control, and that wasn't good.*

First Man chastised Coyote. "You should have thought this through more carefully," he said. "From now on, when people carry fire, they will cut a reed that has grown under the water, split it into four parts, cover those parts with moss, and then carry the burning coal on top of that moss. The wet reed will not burn, and the moss will keep the coal glowing for a long time." And, even today, that is how the people move fire from place to place.

"Well, now we have to put out this fire," said First Woman. "How are we going to do that?" Unfortunately, none of the people had a clue. They had never dreamed that they could have fire in the first place. It had seemed so unattainable on top of Fire Mountain, and not only unattainable, but dangerous. Now they knew they were right. Fire was dangerous and not even worth seeking. Coyote knew they were wrong. Someone had to dream the impossible dream and start some action, and that was Coyote. Now it was up to the people to figure out how to manage this new gift.

First Man proclaimed that water would put out the fire. "But how are we going to get water out of the deep lakes and rivers and onto the slopes of Fire Mountain?" the people asked. "We could carry it there, but we could never get on top of the flames to put them out, and we would be cooked trying. And we could hardly carry enough water in our hands or our mouths to make a difference, could we?"

First Woman announced that she would make a container to carry the water. She went to the marsh and wove reeds into a vessel. She covered those reeds with clay. This she filled with water from the lake.

Then she fastened a rope of twisted water lilies so that the container could be carried. "Now," she asked, "who will carry this basket full of water to Fire Mountain and drop the water on the fire?" (Coyote was hiding from the people, who were out to get him for creating a new problem, but he was proud. He knew that new problems create new technologies and solutions, and from now on the people would be glad to have baskets and basket making. It would serve them well for years to come, and it arose all because Coyote had stolen fire, thereby creating a need for new inventions. First Woman had risen to the occasion and given a true gift to the people.) First Woman looked toward the Bird People, to see if they would help.

Mockingbird was the first to agree to carry the water basket, but the amount of water he could carry was limited. While baskets were a wonderful idea, they apparently were not the solution to this problem. They could not carry enough water to make a difference.

Not being one to give up too soon, First Woman went to the water-dwelling animals. She approached Hosteen Beaver, Hosteen Muskrat, Hosteen Weasel, and Hosteen Mink, asking them to use their great engineering skills to divert the waterways to the base of the mountain so that the fire would not spread all over the Earth. "What do we care?" said Hosteen Beaver. "We live in the water. Our homes are protected by water. The flames will never reach us." First Woman was saddened by their selfishness as she walked away.

Then First Woman approached the waterfowl to see if they would help. In turn, she went to Hosteen Duck, Hosteen Goose, Hosteen Gull, and Hosteen Loon. Hosteen Gull expressed the sentiments of the waterfowl by saying, "What does this matter to us? We can wait out the fire, bobbing up and down in the middle of the lake. Regardless of what burns around us, we have plenty of food swimming beneath us in the lake. This is not our problem."

First Woman was saddened by how much selfishness had already crept into the Fifth World. She had not expected the water dwellers to be so callous about the plight of the land animals and people. Finally she struck a compromise. Those who lived at the edges of the water in and around the marshes still had much to lose from a fire. The heat and the

flames could destroy their homes, despite the proximity of water. That led
her to Hosteen Frog. She presented her case to him, suggesting that the
Frog Nation could fill up their expandable cheeks with water. If she could
find birds that would fly the frogs up above the fire, they could let all this
water loose onto the hillside and put out the flames.

Hosteen Frog had many excuses as to why the Frog Nation could not
do this, but as the flames steadily came closer, his excuses evaporated
and he agreed to do what First Woman asked. Hosteen Crane stepped
forward, and offered on behalf of his nation to carry the frogs up above
the flames to let go of the water. A veritable army of cranes and frogs rose
up out of the marshes of the Fifth World and let loose a huge barrage of
water. The water they released cut streams into the side of the mountain
and great clouds of steam rose up into the sky. The fire was out.

As a result of all this steam, something had changed in the world.
Clouds were created and did not go away. They sat above the mountains
wondering what they should do. They asked First Woman, who considered
the question. "Frogs and cranes are not a convenient way to put out fires
or prevent them in the first place," she said. "You clouds could be a little
more helpful. Why don't you collect water from the lakes, rivers, and
oceans, and bring that water to the dry areas and let it go. We will call
this rain. You can prevent and put out fires in this manner and make sure
that all the people and animals share in the gift of water."

This pleased the clouds, and all over the world, it has been that way
ever since, except when the clouds sulk and cause droughts. This is usually
the result of incomplete or insufficient prayers to the clouds, so honoring
ceremonies must be done to bring the clouds and rain back.

Over time, through references back to this story, I helped Melissa link
the idea of dryness to diabetes and of rain to insulin. This has some physiological relevance, since hyperglycemia results in a kind of dehydration
or internal "dryness." Insulin allows glucose to go from the bloodstream
into the cells where it is needed and end this metaphorical dryness. Insulin,
in this respect, resembles rain. We focused on the dryness within the
landscape of Melissa's body and the way that metabolic fires (oxidation)
could burn out of control. She needed water (insulin and antioxidants) to

put out the fires. She needed a collaborative effort with others in her life, just as First Woman needed the help of the frogs and the cranes to put out the fire. We developed this story about resuscitating her with the help of frog and crane, and eventually building an army of clouds to regulate her sugars. Similar to the story, not everyone had Melissa's best interests at heart, just as not all of the animals that First Woman approached wanted to help put out the fires. Those in her life who didn't care about her health and well-being we called waterfowl, beavers, minks, and weasels. Like some of the people in Melissa's life, some of the animals only cared about themselves and their own well-being. If helping Melissa didn't benefit them, they weren't going to do so.

Over time, Melissa's diabetes began to improve. We were able to find people who would take her for walks, especially her daughters who had been student athletes. That made a world of difference. We were also able to negotiate a better relationship between Melissa and her husband, cooling the "smoldering embers" of their previous "forest fires." I continued to use the "water putting out fire" metaphor for several aspects of Melissa's life, consistent with the story I told her. During a talking circle, Melissa's daughters were able to tell her that they resented her apparent judgment in telling them how to live their lives. A productive, circular discussion ensued in which Melissa responded that she thought she was offering her daughters wisdom and counsel and they revealed how annoying they found her efforts. She had thought that they needed her continual worrying about them and frequent offers of help and advice. They, on the other hand, wanted to run their own lives without her micromanagement, though they welcomed her presence so long as she didn't meddle quite so much. I reflected that culture changes, and the degree to which Melissa was trying to run her daughters' lives was probably appropriate for her own mother, but not for her daughters, given the change in how people lived today. The tight-knit matriarchal family of the reserve had become larger and looser.

As Melissa became less involved in micromanaging her children's lives, her stress levels decreased and her diabetes improved. Consistent with the improvement in her relationship with her husband, Melissa began to sell more jewelry and her financial stress lessened. An elder who helps me told me that the bad medicine that had surrounded Melissa was lifting. One could see this statement as metaphor or reality—the end result is the same. Over six months, Melissa's LDL cholesterol normalized. Over one year, her glycohemoglobin (a measure of long-term glucose control) dropped into the normal range. Her pleasure in life, the quality of her relationship with her husband, and her enjoyment in being with her daughters all improved. Her diet improved a bit, as did her walking, but the dramatic changes could clearly not have been attributed just to diet and exercise. Her quality of life improvements paralleled and reflected her diabetes improvements. In short, her story about herself and her role in her family and community had changed. As that changed, so did her diabetes.

11
Talking with the Universe

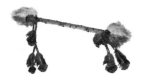

*Nor again must we in all matters demand an explanation
of the reason why things are what they are; in some cases,
it is enough if the fact that they are so is satisfactorily
established.*

ARISTOTLE[1]

Conventional medicine and psychology tend to think and behave as if
humans are separate from the Universe, as if nature consists of a series
of variables that exist independently of each other and us. The alternate point of view is that of inseparability. We are the Universe and the
Universe is us. The moment we say this, however, we become aware of
scale. The commonly cited metaphor is that of smaller boxes within
progressively larger boxes. The box metaphor, however, assumes sepa-
rability. A better metaphor might be the different levels of organizations to which we belong—family, community, city, province, country,
the world. Within an indigenous worldview, the organizations or entities
to which we belong have spirit or consciousness and can also engage in
dialogue, as do the very large entities—God, the Universe, Earth. How
do we dialogue with these larger beings?

Physicists converse through experiments. Astronomers interpret
light and radio waves. Shamans use trance and ritual to interact with

nonphysical entities. The message that returns from all of these methods is that we are all connected and there are no isolated, local environments. Entanglement and embeddedness have replaced independence and control.

How do we talk to larger entities, beings whose scope encompasses our world? What knowledge systems can guide us? Some indigenous knowledge comes from spirits and may be received in ceremony and ritual, through dreams, or in ordinary life. Materialist philosophies teach disdain for people who say they communicate with spirits, but some of their questions are valuable. How do we know we are not imagining the conversation? Historically, tribal people required multiple sources of confirmations for information provided by spirits. The message had to make sense within the context of nature. It had to be confirmed by several people. An entity larger than the receiver of the message had to consider the information and agree it was worth acting upon. The idea of one person emerging from a trance and telling other people what to do was not traditional, though it happens in the movies.

Within the indigenous cultures of North America, we send prayers and messages to Creator, but typically smaller spirits, including our ancestors, mediate this communication. In teachings from my elders, I have learned there are many layers of sacred beings, or spirits. Some are closer to us and can relate to the difficulties associated with physical existence. Others are farther removed and may have never experienced life on Earth. They may even need spirits closer to us to interpret our needs and wishes. Without the experience of physical existence, these beings cannot so readily answer our prayers. The best way to understand the practical uses of communication with spirits is through a story.

Elsa was a Native Hawai'ian woman whom I saw during the year I spent living there. She had been diagnosed as depressed and tried on multiple medicines, without success. Her children had left for better paying jobs on the mainland. One lived in Las Vegas with Elsa's grandchildren, another lived in Los Angeles, and a third lived in Seattle. Her youngest lived in the San Francisco Bay Area. Elsa had recently recovered from rheumatoid arthritis—the condition had actually disappeared. But she now felt isolated and alone. She kept to herself. She saw few people. She had become a recluse.

I began by asking Elsa about the spirits a Native Hawai'ian would ask for help. Who were her spiritual ancestors? To whom did she owe allegiance? If we were going to pray, whom would we address? Elsa responded that she vaguely remembered the old stories, but not in enough detail to be true to the story. I asked Elsa if she would be willing to get a story for our next meeting. This would force her to approach an elder or at least immerse herself more deeply in her culture of origin. I asked her to find out what spirits might respond to her needs. She agreed to accomplish these tasks.

Eduardo Duran, an aboriginal psychologist, would link Elsa's condition to colonization.[2] In the past, she would have never been so alone. She would have had grandchildren who needed her wisdom. She would have had a ceremonial life with others in the community. She would have participated in transmitting knowledge to the youth. Only in "modern" society was she rendered isolated and alone. In the modern value system, which many of us share, getting the best job is more important than being close to family. Getting the best job often requires mobility, especially in the United States, where the ladder to success often involves a series of lateral transfers, slashing a zigzag pattern toward ultimate rewards.

When we met a week later, she said, "I remembered parts of some stories, and I went to see my aunties, who filled in the blanks for me." "I brought the story of Keaomelemele. It's a good story for me because it's the name of my street. I knew I remembered what that street was named for, but I just couldn't recall. Now I know." I asked her to tell me the story.

Keaomelemele is the daughter of Hina and Ku, two of our sacred beings. She was raised in Nu'umealani by her ancestor, Mo'o. When Keaomelemele was about to be born, a spot of blood appeared on the crown of her sleeping mother's head. Mo'o took this blood and wiped it on Kealohilani, a star that rises in the night of Maui in the month of Welo. As the star rose, the blood was smeared across the sky, and Keaomelemele was born.

Mo'o named the child and took her home so that she could be properly raised. She asked the many varieties of clouds to guard the child.

Today we see Keaomelemele when a yellow cloud appears. She gives us signs and omens and teaches the kahunas *and* kapunas *how to interpret them. She and her sisters became the first hula dancers and chanters.*

"That's what I know," Elsa said. "Is that a start?"

"Yes," I answered. "The story gave me questions. I wondered about your sisters. Where are they today? Did you dance the hula with them? What was it like when you were a child?"

These questions prompted Elsa to tell me about her childhood. Her alcoholic mother had been in and out of sobriety. She and her sisters had gone through a parade of foster homes. Some had been abusive. She had spared her own children the effects of colonization, buffering them from the forces that had tortured her life. Her children were successful, but she had paid a price. They had become so successful they could leave the island for better jobs on the mainland. Though Elsa had healed a debilitating physical illness on her own, she had not yet healed her spirit.

"I don't know what spirits Hawai'ians pray to," I told her.

"Neither do I," she said.

"Then let's try something," I said. "Since it's the best we can do, let's pray in my way with any modifications you'd like to make, to both my spirits and your spirits. They can sort it out."

"Fine with me," she said. So I started the Lakota prayer ritual. I burned sage and smudged us. I sang a Four Directions song. I invited the spirits to notice us. And here I specifically mentioned the spirit of her story—Keaomelemele, the yellow cloud. We asked her for a sign. We asked her for her teachings. We asked her for support for Elsa. In addition to the Four Winds, the Sky Spirits (Wakantankan), the Earth Spirits (Ni'kun Si'kun), and all the relatives, we also honored Kealohilani, the star that related to Keaomelemele's birth. We asked the Hawai'ian spirits to tolerate our presence and come to Elsa, who wished to reconnect with them, to return to the roots of her traditions. I offered tobacco and taro leaves, to cover both cultures, and we sat quietly to listen.

After a while, Elsa spoke. "They spoke to me," she said. "I saw Keaomelemele. I live on her street. She knew me."

"Did she give you any instructions?" I asked.

"She said to pray with her and to learn hula," Elsa said. "She said the healing of the people is always present in the hula, and it will heal me as well. It will take away my sadness, loneliness, isolation, and grief. It will make up for my children's absence. It will show me the way to the future."

Elsa knew women who taught hula. She would go to their classes. What made this simple idea profound was how deeply affected Elsa was by her encounter with a spirit, by receiving information from a spirit. I could have said, "Take hula," and my advice would have had minimal impact. Seeking guidance from the spiritual realm and the message provided in response were much more meaningful than ordinary human talk. This provides some confirmation for its reality.

"What else did it say?" I asked.

"To pray every day," she said.

"Do you know people who could teach you the Hawai'ian way to pray?" I asked.

"I do," she said. "There are kahunas and kapunas in my family. I can go to them." Our next step was for her to make commitments to learn hula and reach out to the traditional Hawai'ian healers in her family. The best I could do was model prayer and ritual for her by doing it with her. We prayed together, and her spirits came.

I didn't know any Hawai'ian stories, so I told Elsa a Dene story I had learned in Arizona. I told her that the story was about finding and planting seeds and nurturing them until they grew. This story paralleled the way in which I wanted Elsa to plant seeds to cultivate her own happiness and well-being. She needed to collect more seeds, since she had given all of her seeds to her children, leaving nothing to plant for herself. I mentioned this parallel to her. "You have lost the seeds of your ancestors," I said, "just as the Dene people left their seeds in the Fourth World. Just as First Woman did when the people began to settle in the Fifth World, which is this world, you must go around and collect your seeds. You need to reclaim the seeds that have been lost or left behind. Then you can plant them and stop being spiritually hungry. You will need some help to regain all these seeds, so I'm going to tell you this story, which will tell you what to do. Its spirit will enter into you the way the spirits of stories do, and it will guide you through the process of recollecting your seeds. That's what a sacred story does. Its spirit mingles with your spirit and inspires you to do what you need to do to heal."

When the people scattered about in all different directions to build permanent homes [the way Elsa's children had done], they sought locations near water—creeks, rivers, streams, lakes—and also near wood, often at the base of mountains, so that there would be ample supply for building and fires. After building their houses, the people began to wonder how they would get food. In the past, they had gotten their food wherever they traveled, by hunting and gathering nuts, berries, fruit, grasses, and seeds, but now they realized they would have to start growing food, the way the Pueblo people did. Otherwise, they would run out, since they couldn't move on.

The people created irrigation ditches to bring water to the fields they planned to plant. When they were ready to plant, First Woman called them together, asking them to bring all the seeds they had. First Woman especially wanted corn, beans, squash, and melon, for they were the most nutritious. When the people assembled into a circle, she asked what seeds they had brought. Lo and behold, they had no seeds.

This was Elsa's state when we first met. She had forgotten her heritage. She had lost the seeds of traditional Hawai'ian spirituality.

"How is it that we have no seeds," First Woman asked, "when the Stone House people have plenty?"

"It is because of Turkey," the People said. "Turkey brought seeds from the Fourth World, but Turkey went to live with the Stone House people and took all his seeds with him."

I know this was true, for I have visited the homes of the Stone People in Bandelier, New Mexico, and seen their turkey pens.

First Woman wanted to find out if anyone else had brought seeds from the Fourth World. She sent a messenger to inquire if Ant had any.

This was similar to the way we had gone looking for spirits to speak to Elsa. She had gone to her relatives and asked them for seeds (stories and the names of spirits to which to pray).

Ant had brought some seeds, though they were not the ones most desired by First Woman. Ant gladly gave First Woman her seeds of grass and saltbush. First Woman was glad to have these seeds, for they would grow where there was little water and would benefit the people. In exchange, she gave Ant striped yellow jasper for her house.

This reminded me of how we had prayed to my spirits in order to find Elsa's spirits; I told Elsa how this part of the story reminds us to always give gifts in exchange for what we receive—tobacco, taro leaves, cloth, and other offerings.

The people were glad, but also disappointed, since these seeds would not nourish them through the harsh, cold winters of the Fifth World. First Woman agreed with them and went to see Hosteen Squirrel, who lived in a hole in a tree on the other side of the mountain.

When she got to Squirrel's house, he was peeking out the door, and she asked him if he had brought any seeds from the Fourth World. "Yes," exclaimed Squirrel, bouncing up and down on the tree limb, excited he could contribute something to the quality of the people's lives in the Fifth World.

"Go get them, Hosteen Squirrel," said First Woman. "Let us see what you have brought." Squirrel proudly returned with four sacks to show First Woman. He emptied each sack in turn before her feet.

"First Woman," said Hosteen Squirrel. "I have pinon nuts, sweet acorns from the white oak, and burr oak acorns."

First Woman smiled tenderly at little Hosteen Squirrel. "You have done wonderfully well, my friend," she said. "You have brought amazing gifts for us from the Fourth World. But these will not do for our fields. They will grow into trees, which are not what we want in our fields. You plant these seeds for your people. We will use these foods too, but they will belong primarily to the Squirrel Family, and we will show respect to you whenever we take these things for our use."

Hosteen Squirrel smiled sheepishly. He was touched by First Woman's praise, but saddened that he could not be more helpful to the people. "I have already planted these seeds on the mountain slopes," said Hosteen

Squirrel. "They are growing in many places to furnish nuts for our autumn harvest."

"You have done wonderfully well, Hosteen Squirrel," said First Woman again. "In appreciation of that and to honor you and your family, I give you these two black, woven tassels to wear on the tips of your ears. In this way, all the people will be made aware of the gift of the Squirrel Nation to life in the Fifth World."

When First Woman returned to the people to tell them what Squirrel had done, the people were overjoyed. They knew what good use they could make of the seeds Squirrel brought. They spoke about roasting acorns and grinding the nut meat to make flour for baking. They spoke about crushing the oily pinon nuts with grass seeds to make cakes for baking on flat stones. "Every fall," they said, "when the frost opens the oak burrs, we will go to the mountains to harvest acorns and pine nuts."

At this point of the story, I mentioned to Elsa that she was in somewhat the same situation. What she really wanted was her children to come home, but that option wasn't available. However, she could take advantage of what was available to her—her relatives, her culture, and hula, just as the people would take advantage of Squirrel's gifts.

First Man, however, was not so enthusiastic about Squirrel's gifts. "But we still do not have any seeds to plant in our fields," he said pensively.

"We will look further," said First Woman. First Man and First Woman began walking beside the river, looking for clues as to where to find seeds. Then they saw Mrs. Quail eating pin cherries that grew there, staining her beak and vest red. They greeted her warmly, asking her if she had brought any seeds with her from the Fourth World.

"Yes," Mrs. Quail said. "I brought four kinds of seeds that I have already planted on the banks of the creeks and the river."

First Woman asked her what these seeds were. Quail answered that she had brought seeds for all the wonderful berry bushes that sustained her. She had chokecherry, pin cherry, gooseberry, and raspberry seeds. She told First Woman that she had planted these seeds when the mountains were first being formed, and already the bushes had grown and were producing berries. The ripe ones would sustain her all summer, and the ones that dried on the limbs would keep her going all winter.

First Woman thanked Quail for her efforts on behalf of the people, announcing that the people would follow her lead and eat ripe berries in the summer, drying berries to preserve them for eating in the winter. In honor of her contributions and to remind the people to always show respect to the Quail Nation for bringing berries to the Fifth World, First Woman presented Quail with three white feathers to wear as a crest upon her head.

When First Woman told the people about the berries, they were glad. "These berries will go nicely with our seed cakes in the winter, but we still have no seeds to plant in our fields," they said.

"I will go looking for more seeds," First Woman said, as she left the people beside the river eating pin cherries and chokecherries. "I will go visit Hosteen Crow at his home in the high cliffs to see what seeds he may have brought from the Fourth World."

"Who calls me?" Hosteen Crow demanded when he heard First Woman's voice wafting upward from the base of the cliff below, where she stood calling his name. Hosteen Crow invited First Woman to come up the cliff and sit with him in his house, but she could not, having no way to climb the steep, sheer wall that marked the foundation of his home. Instead she asked him from below if he had brought any seeds from the Fourth World.

Hosteen Crow ran into his house and returned with a spiral basket filled with four types of seeds. He proudly announced to First Woman that he had brought the seeds of the crow onion, the wild turnip, the white potato, and the wild parsnip from the Fourth World. He told her to tell the people to plant these seeds in their fields and water them and they would be well worth the trouble. He had already planted enough of these delicacies in the meadows at the base of the mountains to feed the Crow Nation, and did not require any further seeds.

First Woman was confused. "Why should we plant these in our fields?" she asked, "when we can just harvest them from the meadows in *the same manner as the Crow Nation? Why should we bother to do all that extra work?"*

Crow answered that the plants that grew in the meadows would be hard and small, the way crows like them. Those planted by people in the fields would be large and sweet, the way people like them. Then First Woman understood and thanked Crow for his gift. She offered him sharp flint to wear on his beak, to make it easier for him to dig in the hard earth for the roots he gathered for food. She promised that the people would honor him whenever they planted and harvested these foods, always leaving some for the Crow Nation. The shine of the flint would remind them to show respect to the crows.

When First Woman presented these seeds to the people, they were grateful, for they finally had something to plant in their fields, but they were disappointed because it was not enough. "While these foods are good," they said, "they will not sustain us all winter long. We need more than this."

"I will look for more seeds," said First Woman. "But I will have to be very careful about where I go next."

"Quack, quack," came the sound of Hosteen Duck, diving in the marsh of Muddy Lake for pollywogs. Hosteen Duck could hardly speak, for her mouth was full of moss and frog eggs. But she brought out four sacks of seeds from the Fourth World—wild rice, wild millet, wild barley, and sugar cane.

When Hosteen Duck finally swallowed her lunch, she told First Woman how she had planted these seeds in all the marsh areas she visited in spring and autumn, so she would have food to take with her wherever she wished to go for summer and winter. First Woman wondered if those seeds would grow in the fields of the people, but all Duck would say was the word water, over and over again. First Woman finally understood, saying, "She means they will grow if we provide them with enough water. Thank you, Duck, for these gifts, for which we will always show you respect when we plant or harvest or eat them."

First Woman then said, "I give Duck two curly feathers to wear in her tail to show the people's appreciation." To the people she said, "Plant these seeds in your fields where you can provide them with plenty of water, and you will never go hungry, not even in the winter. Dig out all the weeds that would choke their growth."

"We will do so," said the people, and they worked hard all spring, summer, and fall, growing and gathering food from the seeds provided to them.

Late that next winter, the people came to First Woman, complaining, "Our lives are better, but we work hard for small amounts of food. The Pueblo people are much better off with their corn, beans, squash, and melons. They have three winters worth of food in their storehouses, while we barely have enough for one. They are not as lean and hungry as we are, and they don't work nearly so hard."

"Why don't we send an emissary to the Stone House people to ask for seeds?" said First Woman. She wondered who could go. She spied Blue Lizard sunning himself on a rock, decked out as he was in a cream colored vest and a long coat that sparkled in the sun. "Will you go to the land of the Stone House people and ask them to give us seeds?" said First Woman. Anticipating his objection, she added, "I will ask Spider Woman to make you a sack, which will grow larger as needed and accommodate as many seeds as you are able to get." Anticipating his next question, she pushed on by saying, "And I will send you with a fine necklace of pink coral that I brought from the Fourth World. The Stone House people will admire this and most likely accept it in trade for their wonderful seeds. I will hang it around your neck loosely, so as not to disturb your pleasant voice."

"I have no choice but to make this journey to the South," said Blue Lizard, leaving that very moment on his journey, which would take a day and a night.

"Who is this who comes so early in the morning carrying an empty sack?" said the Stone House people.

"It is I," said Blue Lizard, "bringing you a beautiful necklace to exchange for some of your seeds."

The Stone House people ridiculed Blue Lizard, saying, "Whoever heard of a necklace of worthless pink coral being offered in exchange for lovely farm seeds!" They told Blue Lizard to go home and tell the Dene to be satisfied with their roots and nuts. They said they might consider a trade for white shell beads, which would be of some value, not worthless pink coral.

"Then let us make a white shell bead necklace," said First Woman, telling Blue Lizard to keep the pink coral necklace, which he wears around his neck to this day. "Who can bring me white shells with which to make this necklace?" she asked.

Without further discussion, the animals scattered about to bring the necessary materials to First Woman to complete the necklace. "Thank you, Crane," she said, when Crane brought her white shells from the riverbank. "Thank you, Ant," she said, when Ant shaped these shells. "Thank you, Locust," she said, when Locust drilled holes in them. Since she couldn't find Blue Lizard again, she asked Roadrunner, "Will you take this necklace to the Stone House people who live near the river called Father of Waters? Surely they will fill your sack with seeds when you show them this lovely necklace."

"I can't go," said Roadrunner, who did not want to go. "I have no way of carrying this sack once it is full of seeds."

"I will give you a carrying basket," said First Woman. "This is a magic basket made by Oriole, which we will tie to your back. It will not grow larger and larger like Spider Woman's bag, but anything put into it will grow smaller, so the basket will hold everything they give you without any added space."

Having no more valid objections, Roadrunner accepted the basket, and First Woman tied it to his back. Roadrunner traveled all day and night over dusty paths toward Father of Waters, arriving early in the morning. "Who is this who comes so early in the morning with an empty basket on his back?" asked the Stone House people. "It must be a messenger from the Dene. He looks tired and dusty, as if he has been walking all day and night."

They wondered what the Dene could possibly want. Roadrunner answered them, "I have brought you a fine necklace of white shell beads to exchange for some of your wonderful seeds. We would like to grow corn, beans, squash, and melons in our fields." Roadrunner waited outside the village while the people had a council meeting to discuss his request for seeds. He could hear them talking. Everyone admired the bead necklace, but no one wanted to relinquish a basket of seeds for it. Finally he heard the people agree that they would offer a mixture of seeds for the necklace. The council broke up and a spokesperson came to trade corn with Roadrunner for the white shell bead necklace. Roadrunner excitedly ran home all day and night, bringing the seeds to the feet of First Woman, announcing his wonderful trade.

"These are lousy seeds," proclaimed First Woman as she examined them. "They smell like mice have been chewing on them."

Likewise, the bean, squash, and melon seeds were wormy. When Roadrunner heard this, he ran into the bushes and hid for shame. The people had compassion for him, for they knew he did not know he was getting a bad bargain. "What can we do to get the seeds?" asked the people. "We could send someone big and strong to take them, but we do not want to anger our neighbors and start a war all of us will regret. Perhaps we could secretly raid their fields at night and carry off as many plants as we can to harvest seeds from. Perhaps in time we will have enough seeds to feed all the people."

This last idea inspired Hosteen Packrat with an idea of his own. He came forward and explained his plan to the people. First Woman was skeptical. "I doubt your plan will work," said First Woman, "but there is no harm in trying, and those people certainly owe us a basket of seeds for that white shell bead necklace. Go ahead, though I doubt your luck will be any different from the others."

Hosteen Packrat returned to his home to examine all the objects he had collected over the past several years. He chose four large red cactus apples and started out on his journey to the Stone House people in the South.

Late that night he arrived at a pueblo and crept into one of their storehouses, where he left the four red apples, taking four baskets of different colored corn. The next morning the Stone House people were so happy to find the cactus fruit they never noticed the missing baskets of *corn. On the second night, Hosteen Packrat brought four yucca bananas to exchange for four baskets of beans, and again, the people did not notice anything missing. On the third night, Hosteen Packrat left a basket of ground cherries and took four varieties of ground fruit: gourds, pumpkins, squash, and melons, and again, the Stone House people noticed nothing missing. On the fourth night, Hosteen Packrat left a basket of acorns and took celery, bee weed, mustard, and sunflower seeds. Again, nothing was noticed missing.*

When he was done, Hosteen Packrat distributed his newfound cache to all the people. No matter how they clamored to find out how he had traded for all these wonderful seeds, he would only smile, and to this day has never told the story of how it happened.

The conclusion Elsa and I drew from this story was that she should trade for what she wanted in the manner of Packrat and in the manner of her ancestors, who had gone to sacred places and left offerings wrapped in taro leaves, taking objects they found there to put in their homes. I had visited waterfalls and sacred grottos in Hawai'i where these offerings abounded. Elsa was going to make pilgrimages in the same manner, dance the hula in these sacred spots, and leave her offerings, taking peace and contentment home with her in exchange. She would also send little mysterious gifts to her children and grandchildren, she decided, until she could afford to visit them in person. Each week she was connecting more strongly to her ancestral spirits and the spirits of the places she visited. The hula was strengthening her. Her depression was only a wisp of a memory, like fog on a pond in the morning.

Spirit communication is common in Indian country. Growing up the way I did, I find it hard to imagine not talking to spirits or getting their advice. It must be lonely and isolating to lack ancestors with whom to talk. My grandparents remain with me. I smell my grandfather's cigars. I smell my grandmother's lilac bushes. A story about a ceremony for three women will help illustrate the way in which indigenous people maintain their connection with spirits.

Within Cherokee culture, contacting the spirits to ask them to

explain the cause of an illness is important. We need their input to proceed with the correct approach to curing. Ceremonies exist to facilitate
this connection. I was called upon to do this ceremony for three sick
women. I couldn't find anyone older or more experienced to do it, so I
had no choice but to do it myself.

I began by burning sage. The smoke of the sage removes any bad
energy we bring to the ceremony. Then I burned cedar to fill the holes
left when the bad energy departs. I sang a Four Directions song to ask
the spirits to take notice of us. I asked for their help. I told them about
the three women and described their "diagnoses" in conventional medicine terms.

As I began the ceremony, I felt the presence of spirits immediately.
They were listening. They could decide whether or not to help. Sometimes
they make snide remarks. Sometimes they joke. Sometimes they give
heartfelt speeches. They do whatever they want to do. I recognize their
voices, because their voices are not mine. I don't talk or think the way
they do. They are clearly "other." Meditation is required to hear them.
We must still our minds in order to listen. This is why so many modern
people fail to hear spirits—because their minds cannot stop thinking. We
do not hear the spirits whispering if our minds are going at full speed.
We must stop the world and listen.

When I do ceremony, certain spirits are likely to come. These include
my grandparents, Hazel and Archie; the Big One, whom I first met in
Arizona (he is twenty feet tall and gives me the hiccups); Big Nose, the
main helper of one of my previous teachers (though I recognize that
he may not be the same spirit my teacher sees); and one of the Christ
spirits (I'm told there are many, because so many people are believing in
and praying to Christ that it takes more than one to respond to all the
requests). Others come sporadically, but the ones I just mentioned are
the most common for me.

At the ceremony for the three women, I expected one of my usual
spirits to come, but suddenly I heard singing over my right shoulder. I
became aware of a group of spirits sitting around a fire, singing sacred
songs, behind me to the right. I knew where they were—on a jut of
land along the river near the retreat center. Just then one of the women
announced that she could see some Native men singing and that they

were going to come doctor us. She described her image, and it was the same as mine. The spirits came and I felt a deep inner relaxation, a deep inner peace. I dropped down into a deeply meditative space, waiting for them to clear, as if they were their own pleasurable storm.

They told me that they were visiting from the future and they had come back to a past when they were Indians, before first contact. They were on holiday. Though they had initially resented the disruption in their holiday, they were willing to help us. They gave me accurate diagnostic information for these three women, details that I had not known. About the first woman, they said she had excess fire in her liver—too much heat. Inflammation was the word that came to me. They said the heat was rising into her brain. Her mind was feverish and needing calming and cooling down. This fit. She had hepatitis C and had been previously diagnosed with a variant of bipolar disorder. They said she needed to pray and meditate and sit on the Earth itself to become more grounded. They thought yoga or t'ai chi could help, because she needed to learn how to situate herself between Earth and sky.

They told me the second woman had kidney problems, in the metaphorical sense of Chinese medicine. The toxins that were accumulating in her body were affecting her eyes. She needed to detoxify on all levels, including emotional and spiritual. Juicing would be good for her. She needed to believe that she could be well, and then she would be. She needed to paint, they said. If she would paint, her eyes would be fine. Later I learned from her that she did, in fact, have an eye problem and that she was a painter. When she painted, her eye problem tended to disappear. When she stopped painting, it reemerged.

For the third woman, they were more concerned. They said she had a condition suitable to growing things like tumors. They wished she could find a way to enjoy life more, to lighten up, worry less, have fun. They compared her energy to a pessimist waiting for disaster to happen. She's either had a tumor or is getting ready to have one, or both, they said. She needs to learn how to prevent this. The woman later told me that she had had a breast tumor, which had been removed. She was deeply depressed and had no fun. She mostly stayed home and worried.

They suggested individual herbs for each of the three women. They made recommendations for further ceremonies. Then they asked if they could go back to their vacation. Would we leave them alone? We did.

We spent the rest of the week implementing what these spirits had suggested. In this way, we had followed the traditional procedure of asking the spirits what to do and then doing it. They knew. We were, in essence, having a dialogue with the Universe through the spirits to find out what needed to be done. This is much simpler and more productive than trying to figure it out on our own.

Aboriginal worldviews teach the importance of conversing with the components of the Universe that are not human. Most aboriginal knowledge systems recognize that the world arises through a continuous interaction among the rhythms of various beings in relationship with one another. In Elsa's example, the beings she described are still active and alive and present to the Hawai'ian people. It is not enough for us to talk to each other and to the spirits of illnesses. We must also talk to the ocean, to the clouds, to the rivers, and to the spirits that move upon the winds.

Many cultures and peoples believe that creation was a gift.[3] If so, our lives are also gifts. Within that context, our obstacles can be seen as gifts. Indigenous knowledge systems teach that one way of knowing about ourselves, our lives, and our afflictions is to ask the spirits directly. We can also inquire directly to nature. We can do so in ceremony or we can diligently observe nature to learn about its balance, purpose, peace, and harmony.[4] Many elders believe that we are obligated to learn from those beings created before us, especially the animals, as I described in the story about how the people learned to build houses.[5] Because we have freedom of thought and are storytellers, we are meaning makers. Therefore, we are entitled to gain knowledge through dialogue with the universe.

Elders consistently view proper human relationship with nature as a continuous, two-way, transactional dialogue. Within the aboriginal view, spirituality is embedded in all elements of the cosmos, because we are primarily spirit and secondarily matter. We are all cells in the body of the Universe, which remains constant as the Largest Being, Greatest Spirit, Biggest Possible Entity. We need to be in dialogue with other spirits. We need to be in dialogue with the natural world to sustain harmonious relations with it. We need the input of spirits to properly inform our beliefs and values. We need to communicate with the dynamic, ever-changing forces of the Universe in order to be part of a holistic, integrative system with a unifying life force. We need to dialogue about the unfathomable mysteries of the Universe—mysteries that mere humans can never fully comprehend. In this way, we open ourselves to become part of larger, transpersonal conversations, dialogues that enclose and engulf us and can potentially heal us.

12
Creating a Roundtable of Healing

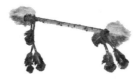

When thinking about poetry
I get lost between the poem and myself—who perceives it.
Is it possible to grasp the boundary between us, or not?
Poetry is like wind: it's not clear where it comes from,
It's not clear where it goes. And it's not clear what it
   means.
What a strange, naive thing—a snare for the wind!
How much fabrication and cunning in the movements of
the one who set it!

KORNELIJUS PLATELIS[1]

Confronting the assumptions of contemporary medicine and psychology can be a disturbing experience.[2] We must challenge the idea that facts are independent, neutral, objective, and verifiable.[3] We question the notion of an objective science of human biology independent from the milieu (social, geographical, cultural) in which we live. University of California at Santa Cruz psychologist Theodore Sarbin wrote, "The search for [the] causes of conduct, central to the mechanistic doctrine, ha[s] not been successful. To approach the complexity of human conduct, [we must] . . . cast a wider net and make sense of persons' actions through discovering how they emplot their lives."[4] This means we must examine the actions people take to get from the beginning to the end of their story. We need to reintroduce medicine to the ideas of story, to individuals' stories, and to the storied nature of human conduct. Similarly, medicine has not been able to predict who will get sick and why. Despite tremendous effort from epidemiology and other disciplines, we cannot look at a person and reliably expect an illness or expect health. As with psychology, we must cast a wider net.

Sarbin believed that the acts of individuals could be understood only within a primarily social landscape. Perhaps this is also true for the health of individuals. The state of our physical body is not separate from how we conduct our lives. Psychosomatic medicine failed to grasp what Sarbin called the narratory principle—the idea that "we live in a story-shaped world."[5] This principle suggests that illness must be understood in the context of the story we are living. The illness is part of the plot. At best, it can be poorly predicted by adding up risk factors. All of our experience, all of our memories, our entire lives are part of stories. Our dreams and nightmares, our crises at work, our family relationships, our spiritual lives, and our physical maladies are part of stories. If they weren't, we could not readily remember or describe them. Virtually the only experiences that are not storied are psychotic experiences for which the person has no words.

Sarbin's narratory principle involves both plot and action. Plot arises from the ways in which we link seemingly unconnected events together to tell a story. Action refers to what people (the characters in the story) actually do within the intentional, goal-directed context of a story. Sarbin believed that every story also has a moral dimension that permits the listener to consider and evaluate the motives of the characters. It is by reflecting on the moral of the story that we give meaning to the action(s) detailed within that story. What Sarbin and other psychologists missed, because it was outside their field, was that illness can be understood only within the context of a person's story. It is impossible to fully understand any illness outside the person's story, which is why so much research on the causes of disease has failed to provide real insight. Causes make sense only as intentions of characters within stories, and stories contain much more information than we can articulate.

This is why we must challenge the limitations of strictly biological diagnoses and ideas about cure. There are no objective diagnoses, causes, explanations, or cures independent from the stories in which they function as plot and action. Even surgery, the purest external cure, happens to a person who lives a story. The outcome of the surgery hinges upon its place in the unfolding plot and action of the story. External therapies (drugs, surgeries, and even healers acting upon passive recipients) depend for their efficacy upon their place within the plot of the stories people are living. Even in extreme examples—someone who dies from a high dose of poison or is saved from choking by the quick insertion of a pocketknife through the cricoid cartilage in the throat—there is a story about how the person came to be poisoned in the first place or what caused the person to choke.

If illness is storied, we cannot proceed without considering the culture of the person who is ill. I observed the truth of this statement in a dramatic way during my psychiatric work with the Native people of northern Saskatchewan. Psychiatric conditions are different there. People respond differently than they did in southern Arizona. Psychiatry has no one-size-fits-all therapy. Therefore, we must abandon our arrogance and invite the world's indigenous peoples to join our dialogue. After all, most of the world is indigenous. These less colonized cultures have different stories about health and disease. Stories from other cultures can help us see our blind spots and our hidden assumptions. They can show us what we lack or have forgotten. They can inspire us with novel ways to move toward health, better than taking plants from the Amazonian rain forest and turning them into pharmaceuticals.

The stories that colonized indigenous cultures have told about Euro-American medicine have largely concerned imposition. Red Cloud, a chief of the Blood people in Saskatchewan, said in 1890, "Don't send us your white medicine. We don't need it. We need medicine that walks."[6] He meant that food was more important for keeping people healthy than white people's medicines. In no uncertain terms, he announced that his people's own traditional medicines were adequate to treat their sickness, and that no medicine would work in the absence of food.

We must bring a similar sense of social justice back to medicine and psychology and, in the process, create space at the table for other systems of healing (including aboriginal healing) that hold different assumptions and values than conventional medicine. These ideas represent an alternative strategy to current institutionalized power relations, in which conventional medicine rides on top of the hierarchy. We are looking for a more egalitarian reciprocity and moral respect among all of the world's stories about disease and health (or getting sick and getting well).

We need to view stories no longer as merely true or false, but as more or less preferable for the given context and people. Of the multiple explanatory stories about health and healing that compete for our attention, including traditional Chinese medicine, ayurveda, and North American aboriginal medicine, all are equally true, but some may be preferred in specific contexts and purposes, depending upon local conditions. The occasional need for emergency medicine is obvious, but a potentially life-saving chest tube for a tension pneumothorax is only desirable in that situation. A ruptured spleen caused by a motor vehicle accident is best treated with surgery. In a case of life-threatening hemorrhage, stopping the bleeding is imperative, but hypnotherapist-obstetrician David Cheek told stories of using hypnosis to stop postpartum hemorrhage before he had time to administer medications. He could offer a hypnotic command in a few sentences, which took less time than was required for a nurse to draw medication into a syringe, inject it, and for the medicine to begin working. Situations arise in which the choice of therapy is urgent and obvious. Depending upon the circumstances, some stories are more practical than others or more aesthetic to our sensitivities.

Considering the multiple stories about health and disease, we must ask which stories we value most. Which ones do we want to integrate? We must ask, what is integration? Is it a process of increasing our tolerance to diversity through dialogue with multiple perspectives? This leads me to a story, which I invite you to interpret for yourself. For me, it's about restoring balance and harmony in the face of tragedy. It's about finding new allies as we work to create a new way of talking about health and healing. It's what we are trying to do with narrative medicine as we attempt to rise above the oppression and discrimination experienced by indigenous peoples all over the world.

When spring finally came to the country, Bear awoke from hibernation. She got out of her den and said, "The spring has arrived again." She went for a walk to the place where most of the snow had melted so that she could eat berries. She left her children behind where they were still asleep. After she had finished eating, she went back to her den and took a nap. While she was sleeping, her cubs woke up and saw their mother's mouth was purple from eating berries.

One cub said to the other, "Look, what's that in Mother's mouth, sticking to her teeth?"

The other replied, "Berries, I think. Let's get them." So they picked the berries out of Mother Bear's teeth and ate them. The wind hovered above them.

The first cub said, "These berries are very good. Let's follow Mother's footprints and see if we can find more." Their mother's footprints led to a patch of berries, where they ate their fill of berries and then went home. When they had nearly reached their den, they heard their mother making desperate cries, but it was too late. A greedy monster had killed their mother and was eating her. This monster knew there were cubs around because he had seen their footprints in the snow. He was excited because he knew baby cubs are very tasty and tender to eat. He smelled the cubs and started running after them. The wind made a great howling sound.

The cubs, meanwhile, had taken off running when they heard their mother's cries. After running for what seemed like a long time, they met Grandmother Porcupine along the trail. They said to her, "Grandma, please let us pass. We are running away from someone who has killed our mother. Will you try to stall him so we can get away?"

"I will," she replied. "You have another grandmother who can kill this monster. You will find her if you follow this trail." She pointed to the path ahead, where the cubs ran. Shortly thereafter, the monster reached Grandmother Porcupine.

The cubs could hear the monster through the forest. He said to

Grandmother Porcupine, "Please move out of the way, Grandmother. I'm looking for my grandchildren. They have run away from me."

Grandmother Porcupine said, "I will not move out of the way unless you can do what they did for me."

The monster replied, "What did they do?"

She said, "They built me a fire and they rubbed their faces on my tail."

The monster replied, "Oh, that's easy. I can do that for you." He built her a fire, and was very happy thinking she would soon let him pass. After he finished making the fire, he rubbed his face on her tail. As he did, Grandmother Porcupine swung her tail very hard on his face. Quills lodged all over his eyes and mouth.

"Now I will move out of your way so you can pass," she said to the monster. The monster passed, but had to stop to pull the porcupine quills out of his face. After he had finished picking the quills out, he was on his way again.

He saw the cubs' prints on the ground, still following the trail that Grandmother Porcupine had shown them. They finally reached their other grandmother's house. This grandma was a giant seagull. The cubs said, "Grandma, we are running away from someone who killed our mother. We are afraid he might try to kill us too."

Grandmother Seagull said, "Don't be afraid. I have killed this kind of monster before." The cubs were no longer afraid. She said, "I will take both of you across to a place you can stay safely." She took them across the water in her boat. She let them off on an island across a bay.

The cubs asked the seagull, "Will you kill this monster, Grandma?"

"I will," she replied. She got back into her boat and crossed over to the shore of the mainland. Then she painted the boat with dirty, smelly fish.

When the monster reached the crossing place, he called out to the seagull, "Grandma, please come help me get across!" She paddled her boat to the monster. "Did you see my grandchildren?" the monster asked. "I have been running after them. I was thinking of eating them, because they are still very tender."

Grandmother Seagull said, "Yes, I have seen them. I took them across. Would you like to go across too?"

"Yes," said the monster. And he got into the boat. When he got in the boat, he couldn't stand the smell of it.

Grandmother Seagull said, "If you can't stand the smell, hang your head over the side instead." The monster did so to avoid smelling the stinking boat. Meanwhile, the seagull took a huge knife out from beneath some blankets and cut his head off. It fell into the water.

After she had killed the monster, Grandmother Seagull went back to the bear cubs. "I killed the monster that killed your mother," she said. "You can both stay here, and I will make you toys to play with." The bear cubs played with their boat on the river, and they had a lot of fun. They stayed there forever and founded a new clan on that island that is still there today—the Bear Clan.

For me this story illustrates how we can find new allies in unexpected places, helping us to forge new solutions that draw on multiple points of view. Like the bear cubs in the story, we must ask for help and must respect the assistance that is offered.

It's hard for conventional medicine to abrogate its position as the superior voice, so convinced it is of its evidence-based superiority. Practically speaking, how would we proceed if we considered biomedicine just one of many points of view? Kit, who had a mysterious eye problem, will help us understand how. Her eye disease was inflammatory and not infectious. She'd already lost her right eye, but the continued inflammation posed a threat that she could lose the socket, too, and that the inflammation could extend still deeper into her skull. Her doctors feared that the inflammatory process could move into her brain or her remaining eye. Kit also had had chronic low-back pain for the past two years.

We wanted to create an opportunity for talk-in-interaction in which multiple viewpoints on health and disease could be entertained. Through an ongoing dialogue, participants can decide which perspective(s) they prefer, based upon their own unique decision-making process, which might be very different from what happens when doctors do a literature review to find currently available scientific evidence to support particular treatments. Nonmedical people don't tend to make decisions this way, but rather go through a process of social interaction and consensus building. In this context, biomedicine simply offers one interesting description of health and disease and how to manage it, which is as legitimate as ayurveda or traditional Chinese medicine, for example.

With deference to conventional medicine, we started with Kit's ophthalmologist. He was too important and busy to come to a roundtable. We had to go to him. Equal conversations with conventional medicine rarely happen, since medicine dictates its terms for encounter (the individual appointment in a small examining cubicle, taking place at a convenient time for the doctor). Several of us traipsed to an appointment in a small, sterile room into which we could barely fit.

Immediately upon entering the room, the doctor showed a deep discomfort, I presumed because of all the "extras" accompanying his patient. I imagined his defensiveness about saying the wrong thing and being sued. I tried to put him at ease in his own lair. The only unique attributes of the room were some photos of airplanes in the sky, taken from close up. "Are you a pilot?" I asked him. He nodded, with what was later described by Kit as the most enthusiasm she had ever seen him show. "Do you have your own plane?" He pointed toward a photo of a particularly elegant-looking two-engine plane on the far wall.

"That's mine," he said. I heard the pride in his voice. This airplane was where his passion went.

"Wonderful looking plane," I said. "You must have some great times in it." I knew we would get further if we showed respect for him as a human being. In his white-coated world, he could safely display very little of his personality or individuality. The exception was his airplane, which he loved so much that he put it on the wall, despite the fact that personal effects in exam rooms were not encouraged. I was hoping my questions would link us to his real passion and thereby get us more of his full attention, and my intention paid off.

"Great times," he repeated. Now he was smiling for the first time.

We got down to business. Dr. Larry Morgan didn't have a clue why Kit's eye was eating itself away. He'd read about problems like this but hadn't ever seen it before, which was saying a lot, because he was head of the opthalmology department at the university's college of medicine. "I don't know what to do," he said, "but just to be safe, I think we should do more surgery to debride the socket and get out more of whatever is in there." This reminded me of a saying we learned in medical school: "When in doubt, cut it out." The doctor was standing by the head of the exam table, while the rest of us sat on stools or stood around the pull-out desk.

Kit responded immediately. "No," she said. "I don't want to do that. If we don't know what it is, how can we know that surgery will cure it?" Dr. Morgan nodded sympathetically. At least he was taking us seriously.

"You're right," he said. "I'm just playing the odds, but you probably have other things in mind, don't you?" He looked apprehensive.

Kit nodded. "Don't tell me about them," he said, his smile wry now. "I might have to disapprove, and I don't want to do that." Paradoxically, his smile indicated care and concern to me, even as he told Kit that he didn't want to know her plans.

"Fine," said Kit. "I won't tell you."

"But I will tell you if they're working," said Dr. Morgan. "See me again in two months. We'll take another look at your eye then."

As conventional physicians go—especially surgeons—Dr. Morgan seemed relatively supportive. He didn't want complicit knowledge of Kit's use of alternative treatments, so no one could accuse him of condoning or supporting them, but he wasn't hostile about Kit pursuing her own course. I intuitively felt that he genuinely cared about her from his own vantage point.

I then began to assemble a meeting of all of Kit's other health practitioners, who would come even if her physician wouldn't. In preparation for this meeting, Kit and I, her friends and family, and some of the practitioners did a sweatlodge ceremony together to pray for guidance on how to approach her eye. "Gently," came the answer. I was urged by my spirit advisors to keep the lodge mild. Be kind and compassionate, they said. I had already put twenty-eight stones into the fire, though the afternoon's temperature hovered around 104°F (40°C). It was 7 p.m. and I was sure the temperature outside had dropped down to nearly body temperature (98.6°F, 37°C).

We've already met my spirit advisors. Their voices don't sound like mine. They give me guidance when I go into the sweatlodge before the ceremony and offer tobacco. They tell me what the theme of the lodge will be and how I should approach it. They tell me how to approach specific people and what to worry about. Despite my intentions to keep it mild, this lodge was hotter than most. We took longer breaks than usual and opened the back door to create a breeze between rounds of heat. We brought in seven stones for each round, using the entire twenty-eight, though I poured less water than usual. Cathy, a friend of Kit's, began to have an erratic heart beat. We had to shorten the third and the fourth rounds to accommodate her. That didn't displease Kit or her friend Tina, who had driven more than two hours to come.

After the sweatlodge, I wanted to talk to the spirit of Kit's eye disease. I wanted to get to know it better. I thought it might help inform us how to proceed toward healing. Approaching this spirit was difficult. Kit had many preconceived notions about health and disease. She was widely read and had trained her skeptical, doubting side. I used hypnosis techniques for Kit, as I often do in this context, to help people step out of their preconceived ideas about what should happen so they can have unscripted experiences. I try to engage people so that the images speak for themselves. I want to dialogue with the entity behind the image. The elders speak of the image as a mask. We want to communicate with what lies behind the mask, with what we can't see. To do that, we must speak with the image or the mask. We really want a dialogue with the energy or essence of the illness.

Kit's image of the entity behind her eye problem was a shadow figure, almost a caricature, like a character from the 1960s cartoon *Spy vs. Spy*. This shadow figure had stalked her family for generations. It chose to hide in dark places. It disliked vision. It hated light. It had no good feelings for her or anyone and was just intent on doing what it wanted. It had no sentiments to which we could appeal. It was dour and mirthless. It told a story of relentless pursuit and indolent, smoldering misery. Kit reflected that this reminded her of how it had felt to live in her family for years now.

The shadow figure dared us to try to remove it. "Give it your best shot," it taunted. "I'm not going anywhere. I'll stay here and quietly destroy you until you're dead," it said, "and then I'll move on to someone else in your family."

Several of Kit's supporters participated in this exercise. The next day, we had a community meeting to address what Kit should do. The cast of characters included her brother (who flew there from Montreal), her partner, five female friends, me, a family doctor who was also an energy healer, a naturopath, a massage therapist, a yoga teacher, a traditional Chinese medicine doctor, a chiropractor, and a therapist. We began with the usual talking stick procedure, in which the stick is passed around the circle and whoever is holding it is allowed uninterrupted speech. I asked people to reflect upon Kit's illness, what worsened it, and what made it better.

People present at the imagery exercise thought that the "creature" thrived on strife. They noted that Kit was an overachiever. They proposed fighting the creature by lightening up, relaxing, and having more fun. Kit remarked that she had already discovered from her venture into this collaborative process that she was approaching her eye in the way she would approach a graduate class. As successful as that approach was in the academic context, it was failing when it came to her eye. She was open to a different approach. The various practitioners each described how their modalities could help her eye. She was drawn to yoga because it provided flexibility she lacked. She liked the naturopath's proposal for high-dose antioxidant treatment and even intravenous vitamin C to quell the inflammatory process. She liked a proposed root and green vegetable juice fast designed to alkalinize her and thereby decrease the inflammatory response. She liked my proposal of a homoeopathic remedy with meditation and ceremony surrounding that remedy. She wanted to sit on the earth an hour each day.

Eventually an approach grew out of the talking circle interaction of Kit's family and friends, coupled with the input of the practitioners who were willing to be involved. It did not include pharmaceuticals or surgery. Over the past two years, Kit's eye has healed. The practices she accepted gradually changed her life. She found herself drawn to Mayan shamanism, which was readily available to study in her community. Her back pain disappeared. She eventually went to the Yucatan to study with local healers. Her ophthalmologist never changed. Although he confirmed Kit's improvement, he never wanted to hear what measures she had taken to heal herself. As he said, "it was none of his business." In short, he didn't want to be part of a roundtable of dialogue.

Here's another story about collaboration and recovery that unfolded with a family over the past eleven years, representing a collaborative approach to medical care as a way to overthrow conventional medicine's tight control and privileged position as arbiter of what is healing and what is quackery. It came as part of my effort to restore aboriginal and traditional medicine's validity as a bona fide healing approach, a story existing on its own merits in parallel to the biomedical story.

Jim's family thought he was already dead. Recently diagnosed colon cancer had already spread to his spine, traveling up to his neck. Upon hearing the news, the family wept. Jim was told that the cancer was extremely aggressive, inoperable, and could only be delayed in its inevitable progression.

Jim's experience was completely within the expert-based medical model of diagnosis and treatment. It was consistent with medicine eliminating all other treatment modalities than its own preferred methods— radiation, chemotherapy, and surgery. All else is considered adjunctive or "complementary"—the basis for the term *complementary medicine.* The emphasis is on addition and whether the addition is useful or not. A debate that includes other stories about how to approach cancer cannot be imagined as anything else but quackery.

It's hard to imagine a world in which experts are not in charge. Physicians have great difficulty deferring to stories about the world besides their own. The preferred story we are trying to create brings together all the possibilities for Jim. What allows this is our developing understanding that conventional medicine can only study what works within its paradigm. In our developing narrative paradigm for medicine, we realize that biology is entangled with community, family, spirit, and more. A simple biological paradigm that ignores other factors is inaccurate except in narrow ranges where people conform to the social culture of medicine (accepting medicine's expectations for when to die, for example, from a particular illness). The paradigm breaks down when people become increasingly different from the social culture of medicine's practitioners.

Our struggle is to get conventional medicine to understand that its predictions are more self-fulfilling prophecies than they are the natural history of disease. We are arguing against a natural history of disease since disease cannot be understood by reference only to the natural world. Since conventional medicine only studies what it sees as important, it cannot see these other factors.

We want to sit at a table at which no one story about health and disease has preeminence. This is hard for everyone, because we all have preferred stories. I prefer the story of spiritual transformation leading to amazing disappearances of tumors and patients outliving their doctors. Unfortunately, regardless of how many of these stories I can accumulate, I can't produce results like this on command. They are not reliable or predictable. The effects of radiation or chemotherapy are somewhat predictable but ignore these miraculous stories.

We must take stock of the resources available in the local community. This is the set of possible approaches for Jim. He could also travel to foreign lands for exotic treatments, but someone has to introduce them to him and this is a local person, even if it's a friend surfing the Internet. I invited all the people who had resources for Jim to consider to a meeting. I invited everyone who had a stake in Jim's health. Everyone's perspective is valid. All the stories about potential cures are worth consideration.

Jim listened to the various ideas and decided to take more chemotherapy followed by radiation therapy. The cancer continued to spread through his bones. Eighteen months later it was still spreading. A new, more radical chemotherapy was proposed, following which the cancer spread even more rapidly. Seven months later he had another series of radiation treatments, after which the doctor said, "There's nothing we can do to get rid of the cancer or stop it from spreading at this point. We can just help reduce the pain and try to slow it down."

Unsatisfied with this prognosis, Jim's family wanted another meeting. I met with the core of the family, consisting of Jim, his wife, and a very involved daughter. I proposed that we schedule another meeting of all the possible helpers that they could imagine useful. We talked about a list of people who thought outside the box about cancer. Jim's wife and daughter were interested in diet and nutritional supplements. They had tried some things on their own, but Jim had a difficult time taking pills and changing the way he ate. They wanted to deepen their spiritual life and had already set up an altar filled with objects of importance and meaning to Jim. They were already trying the style of meditation described in Jon Kabat-Zinn's book *Wherever You Go There You Are.*[7] Jim, however, found it difficult to meditate. He wasn't as interested in meditating as his wife and daughter.

I invited the practitioners that Jim's family wanted to consider for a meeting the following week. People tend to come to my meetings because they get referrals and because the meetings are actually fun and we all learn something. It's so different from the boring treatment team meetings that I attended during my training. Treatment goals for psychiatry consisted of "take all offered medications," "verbalize why medications are good," "express three alternate coping skills to using alcohol," "verbalize a no-harm contract every shift," "avoiding falling down," and so on. These meet with Board of Behavioral Health expectations. I'm interested in a more stimulating level of discourse.

I invited the family doctor/energy healer again, who had studied with shamans in the Yucatan. I included a cancer survivor support group leader and another man who had healed from metastatic colon cancer. I included as many others as would come—a naturopath, a holistic medical doctor, an herbalist, a traditional Chinese medicine practitioner, a yoga teacher, a Hawai'ian healer, a Yaqui medicine man, a minister, and a chiropractor. I included a colleague in our meetings who was a more typical family doctor, whose job was to advocate for the medical model since its true believers didn't believe our meeting was important enough to attend. Jim's family brought all three adult children and their spouses or partners, Jim and his wife, and some close family friends. The number of people at the meeting was close to twenty-five.

I start these meetings with a talking circle format. We begin with a prayer for the meeting to serve everyone's highest good and for us to be guided to the best possible path for the best possible outcome. As the talking stick goes around the circle, whoever holds it speaks as long as desired without interruption. Cross talk is forbidden. We talk only when we hold the stick. Otherwise, we listen. My first question was to ask for everyone's perspectives and thoughts about Jim's cancer.

As the talking stick began its first trip around the circle, I began to hear stories about a two-week vacation the family spent in a beach cottage in Tahiti. During this trip, the family reflected upon the reasons for the cancer and its meaning in Jim's life. At that time, motivated by his doctors' bleak prognosis, Jim made a decision to start doing some of those things on his list that he had never done. He wanted to make sure that the family got together regularly to continue the discussions they had started. I marveled at how the family had already initiated the very process we were doing without anyone having told them what to do.

I used to be interested in the question of why people thought they had cancer. Previously I thought the answers to these questions would shed some light on what to do. Now I realize that this line of thinking is still part of the problem-based system typified by the medical model. From my conversations with cancer, I realize that the cancer will tell us what we need to know to help us evict it or gradually help it to transform or move out if possible, and that people's stories about how they got cancer are only important in the sense that they may still be living these stories and these stories may be cancer promoters.

On the second pass of the stick around the circle, I invited everyone to consider what might be useful to Jim. On the third pass, we wondered what his life would look like if he healed from cancer. On the fourth pass, I asked everyone to state what they could do to assist Jim in healing.

From this "healing circle," concrete plans emerged. Jim decided to pursue conventional treatment, but not endlessly. He recognized the toll it had on his body and heard some of his friends who told him that the oncologists never know when to quit. Jim and his family were especially enthusiastic about natural medicine, including diet and supplements. We agreed that regular meetings with the naturopath would be valuable. Jim wanted to explore Christian Science, the religion of his mother. Having previously scoffed at it, he thought it might have new possibilities. He wanted to join a support group. He was not particularly interested in traditional Chinese medicine, chi gong, yoga, or the more esoteric practices. He was curious about the energy healing of the Yucatan and wanted to do that. The family collectively requested a sweatlodge, which I agreed to lead. We invited everyone who had attended our "planning" meeting.

Over the course of several hours, a plan emerged for what the group would pursue and what each person would do. Some were dismissed, like the Chinese medicine practitioner. Others scheduled appointments for further consultations, including the herbalist and the naturopath. A healing circle was emerging that would meet weekly. Regular retreats for the family were also desired. Jim joined the cancer survivor support group and expressed a desire to talk further with the man whose colon cancer had disappeared.

The following week, we did a sweatlodge ceremony together. What I appreciated about that lodge were the heartfelt prayers for Jim's highest good and the strength and endurance family and friends showed to sit inside the lodge for Jim's benefit. Their community was already growing stronger.

Later that year, when Jim saw his doctor because of abdominal pain, the cancer was found to have spread to his liver. The cancer in the bone had also spread to more places than the year before. It had gone to his shoulders, hips, and leg. The doctors were not very hopeful in their prognosis. They said they had done all they could and could now only help with the pain, to make Jim more comfortable. They reaffirmed that he was in the "later stages" of the disease. During one appointment, when Jim was out of the room, his wife made the mistake of asking the oncologist how much more time Jim had left. The radiologist answered, "Could be as soon as a month, or as long as six months, but no more than that."

During the chemotherapy, Jim used fentanyl patches for pain, with oral oxycodone as a backup. He stopped eating because of his constant nausea. All his food tasted as if ashes had been sprinkled over it. For Jim, the loss of taste was worse than the pain, because he was something of a gourmet. As time passed and he became weaker and more upset about his nausea and lack of taste, he became more open to suggestions made by the naturopath and herbalist. He added a super-nutritional drink every day. He drank more water and took vitamin C to flush toxins out of his system. He began walking to increase circulation.

As in the story about Kit's eye I told earlier, Jim's medical doctors were uninterested or even hostile about the efforts he was making with nutrition, exercise, and spirituality. If asked, they told him that none of those things mattered. It was unimportant. The healing circle became very important to Jim in supporting his explorations and keeping alive his other unconventional pursuits.

Jim descended into the illness and almost succumbed. However, Jim mysteriously rose up again from this descent into near-death with a renewed motivation to live, stronger than any we had seen before. He turned in earnest to taking Essiac herbal tea, a packet of immune-enhancing and antioxidant herbs prepared by the herbalist, and daily zinc for his taste problems. He was able to go off pain medication through his use of meditation and Christian Science practices. He drank a half gallon of water a day to help flush out toxins. He drank only filtered water to avoid adding impurities. When he was nauseous from the chemotherapy, he drank nutritional powder mixed with nonfat milk that was either organic or free of added hormones. He drank an electrolyte drink, stopped eating red meat, and cut down on sugar and dairy. He took regular daily walks and began taking vitamin E. He said "The Scientific Statement of Being" every night, which is a Christian Science motto. I believed that his practicing Christian Science was helping him connect with the spirits of his mother and grandmother.

During this time his attitude shifted. He became much more self-directed, peaceful, and confident in his healing ability. Was it the miracle of prayer? Did the energetic healing practices help? Was it the nascent community of love and support that had developed around him? Was it his new ability to abide with the process of death and not shrink from the feelings that brings?

One of Jim's daughters sent him a book, *A Ring of Endless Light,* by Madeleine L'Engle, which his wife and another daughter read to him during the bleakest month of his illness.[8] This book is about a grandfather dying of leukemia who goes to stay with his son and son's family one summer. It is an exploration of the many levels of meaning and experience in sharing the death process.

During this time, the healing circle proposed a ritual in which Jim wrote down what he wanted to give up. He burned it in the fireplace, asserting afterward what he wanted to keep and nurture in his life. They helped him set up an altar at home and inaugurated his "meditation center." Every morning the family meditated together. Sometimes members of the healing circle also meditated there. One day they did a ritual in which Jim shared his hopes and fears. He wanted to live to see his granddaughter, who was then three, attend junior high school. His wife's women friends used the healing circle to do a hands-on healing with him on the table. The family continued daily hands-on healings with Jim lying on the dining room table. They sang the chant, "purify and heal us, heal us and free us."

During this time the energy healer and Jim's daughter continued to do sessions with him. Spontaneously Jim decided that he wanted to be given a new remedy in which a bullet of radiation called Strontium-99 is injected and makes its way into the bones to zap the cancer. The doctors thought it was ineffective, but said they were willing to try it if he wanted. One of the radiation oncologists delighted everyone by saying he had never had a success with it. A younger colleague, however, announced that he had seen several successful cases. Jim wondered to his healing circle if it was the doctor's attitude that made that result. He said that attitude and the placebo effect might be a big part of the success of any treatment. "If that is the case," he told them, "if I do have it done, it will not be with the doctor who has never had any successful cases." The doctors humored him when he announced observations such as this. The healing circle stood steadfastly behind Jim in demanding his Strontium-99.

Nevertheless, he never received the Strontium-99, so his daughter and his healing circle helped him visualize what the treatment would have done to the cancer cells had he taken it. Energy healing also continued. He imagined zapping light into the cancer cells and dissolving them. He also imagined a large hypodermic needle injecting light into the bloodstream to dissolve the cancer. The energy healer reported that she could feel this happen. When the oncologist saw fewer cancer lesions on the bone scan after the treatment when compared to the previous year, he said, "I'm not kidding when I tell you that I have never seen anything like this happen before in someone with as advanced stage cancer as you had." As surprised as he was, he still had no interest in the other approaches Jim was taking.

After three years of thinking he would not live past the next Christmas, Jim began to feel better. A bone scan the next March showed that most of the cancer lesions in the bones had disappeared, also something that the doctors had never seen before. Jim had lived through metastatic cancer for over three years now.

Jim told us that his Christian Science practitioner, who he had begun meeting with shortly after our first healing circle, had seen a team of angels and deceased relatives around him, sending him love and healing and egging him on. They supported his ongoing slow but steady spiritual transformation.

It has been eleven years now since Jim was diagnosed with metastatic colon cancer. His healing circle has been ongoing, and he continues the practices he learned during his time of crisis. There is concern now about his heart, but he is eleven years older and will be eighty years old soon. He thinks back fondly on his healing adventure with cancer. "Of course," he says. "I might not have been so fond if I had died. You never know."

What I hope the story illustrates is the difference in a community-based approach to cancer versus an expert, medical-model approach. After the first meeting, the community approach was largely directed by the extended family and the healing circle. Unbeknownst to the conventional physicians, the healing circle was evaluating their proposals and assisting Jim in deciding what to do and what not to do. The healing circle met every week and sometimes more often during Jim's worst times. Various practitioners who worked with Jim (the herbalist, the naturopath, the Christian science practitioner, the energy healer, me) came either regularly or irregularly to the healing circle and participated as equal members. Expertise and privilege were not recognized. All voices were equal.

From this story, we can construct multiple stories to explain Jim's recovery. All have equal claims to truth; some are more aesthetic than others. I prefer the story of community mobilization leading to the development of a healing system in which unexpected properties emerged through the ongoing dialogue and communication of the members of this group. These properties included physiological change.

We can't deny the disappearance of tumors. That happened. Medicine would prefer a linear path that provides a prescription of certainty for how to remove tumors. That can't exist. All that Jim's experience tells me for the future, for other people who have cancer that I might meet, is that community matters and healing is possible. I don't know how it will happen, but I trust that it can happen when we put the community together and set it loose. Ideally the community should include multiple repositories of knowledge, including multiple practitioners and varying systems of healing.

What will this do to professionalism? I hope it will erode and destroy it. I hope we people who are paid for our experience and skills can step down from our thrones and privileged positions to be one of the people. Our knowledge does not necessarily give us wisdom, for wisdom arises from the collective mind of the community, which one person or even several people cannot generate. Paid providers of health-related services need to live in harmony as community members with providers of other services (teachers, plumbers, carpenters, mechanics). We can honor expertise without affording privilege to some professions at the expense of others.

With some notable exceptions from the field of public health, which typically lies outside of medicine on most university campuses, medicine has concentrated on achieving an increasingly narrow focus of concern—molecular, biological, and genetic processes as they impact human health and disease. The focus of conventional medicine on organs has been even narrower than conventional psychology's focus on individuals. Just as psychology ignores the larger context of the individual, medicine has taken a smaller box in the Chinese puzzle and ignored the individual within which the organs dwell. In their focus on the individual, medicine and psychology both ignore the role of the meaning that people and families and communities give to events and illnesses. Michel Foucault has already told the history of how this came to be in Western Europe and North America in *The Birth of the Clinic.*[9] What concerns us now is how to create a new story, a new history—one that looks forward with a different perspective inclusive of aboriginal cultures and multiple perspectives on health and disease. This new medicine is as concerned with day-to-day life within communities as it is with second-to-second enzymatic reactions within organs. Let us learn to respect the aboriginal perspective that connects the two. Equality and justice will emerge as important in the health and wellness equation.

CONCLUSION
Revising Our Stories about Health Care and Healing

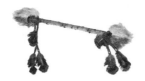

There is a light in this world, a healing spirit more power-
ful than any darkness we may encounter. We sometimes
lose sight of this force when there is suffering, and too
much pain. Then suddenly, the spirit will emerge through
the lives of ordinary people who hear a call and answer in
extraordinary ways.

MOTHER TERESA[1]

What can health practitioners and health care consumers do immediately to change health care? Stories are the best way to make a point, so
I will answer my question by telling a story. For me, this story is about
how difficult it is to change the status quo. It takes a person who refuses
to accept the conventional wisdom, and it takes a good story. This one
comes from northern Canada.

Once upon a time, a long time ago, before there were many people upon
Earth, the best fish and game were found in the far north. The people
journeyed there every summer and stayed as long as they could, but the
North Wind was ferocious and beat them back for many moons of the

year. In those days, North Wind was greedy and wanted to control the whole world. He wanted to make every nook and cranny of the world frozen and icy. North Wind fought with South Wind every chance he could. South Wind was kind and gentle and compassionate toward the people. Wherever South Wind walked, flowers bloomed. South Wind's steps could be traced by the blossoming of prairie roses and woodland violets. He seemed to walk on a trail of wildflowers across the country.

Rather than apologize for equating North Wind with the conventional, I should point out that North Wind traditionally brings us strength and endurance, and that opposing the conventional does make us stronger and forces us to get very clear about what we propose and what we do. As is said in Lakota prayers, "May you look your enemy in the eye and shake his hand." For me, this story is apropos because conventional thinking has become too hard and rigid, like ice. It needs a gentle warming. It needs the power of the South Wind: love, kindness, forgiveness, and compassion.[2]

The power of South Wind seemed greater than that of North Wind. Without so much as casting one blow, South Wind's presence chased North Wind away. Under his influence, melons blossomed, corn grew tall, bean plants spread their leaves to catch the sun, and squash grew large and ripe. Corn, Bean, and Squash are the Three Sisters, so beloved by the South Wind, who nurtures them and helps them thrive for the benefit of the people. The warmth and joy of summer flows from South Wind. The people dance, celebrate, and give thanks to South Wind all summer long.

South Wind, unfortunately, had limited energy (just like us). As he walked across the Earth, he got tired. Eventually, he became so tired he had to sit down. Upon sitting, he got out his sacred pipe, and began to smoke a mixture of tobacco, sage, chokecherry bark, and bearberry. The smoke rose as a gentle haze and spread over the surface of the Earth. The wind grew still. All was well until he finished smoking, at which time he fell asleep. That was when the North Wind took over. It happened every year. To his credit, South Wind's presence died away slowly, and it took time for North Wind to overcome all that he had done, but the job was inevitably completed. South Wind needed a long sleep to recover all the energy he had spent.

One year, the people had particularly good luck with game. South Wind had stayed awake longer than usual, and had only recently succumbed to his weariness. The temperature was dropping and the hunters were preparing to leave, to journey south with their cache of meat and furs. One man, however, refused to go.

Often it only takes one person who refuses to follow the conventional program to change everything.

This young man said to his friends, "I can manage North Wind. I can make him bow down to us, the people." His friends thought he was crazy. If South Wind always became tired and fell asleep, how could one measly human think he could defeat North Wind?

"I can do it," said the young man. "I have studied North Wind for some time, and I know his weak points. I will build a sturdy lodge and cut enough wood to keep warm. He cannot get me in there. When I go out, I will dress warmly and I will beat him. He cannot stop me. When you come back next spring, I will have the greatest supply of fish and furs and meat that anyone ever dreamed. You will see." His friends begged him to reconsider. No one survived the fury of North Wind. But regardless of how they begged him, he would not renege. The more tearful and pleading his friends, the more stubborn and set in his ways he became. Finally, when they could bear the cold no more and their tears froze on their cheeks, his friends reluctantly departed and headed south, sure they would never look upon his face again.

Weary of their dour looks and pessimistic projections and grateful for their departure, our hero immediately went to work. He split more wood than seemed humanly possible. He collected herbs to make his winter smoking mixture. He prepared his trap lines and snares, chose the spots where he would make holes in the ice, and readied himself for a nice long winter. He was looking forward to North Wind's arrival.

We must make our preparations, even as our friends and colleagues expect us to fail.

The young man was not disappointed. North Wind was gleefully flexing his muscles, wondering if he had finally defeated South Wind for good, when he noticed our hero. How strange that a mere human would dare to challenge him. He would freeze this little man with one whiff of his cold breath. He blew around the young man and whiffed, but, to his surprise, nothing happened. The man happily hummed along and went his way. North Wind tried harder and harder to get the young man's attention, but failed at every step. Finally he turned himself into Grandfather Winter and blocked the young man's path.

"Hello, Grandfather," said the young man in greeting. "How nice to see you. Would you care to join me for some tea?" North Wind was nonplussed. No one had ever treated him so kindly before. He felt compelled to accept the young man's offer and did.

This is how we must approach the authorities that enforce the conventional paradigm.

When they were seated inside the lodge, the young man threw log after log onto the fire, and North Wind got increasingly warm and uncomfortable. Then the young man served him steaming hot birch bark tea. North Wind was expected to drink it and did so. He started melting. He was scared. Nothing like this had ever happened to him before. "Grandfather," said the young man. "You don't look so well. Perhaps you'd like to lie down."

Imagine how to translate this into a confrontation with representatives of conventional medicine or psychology. We should aim for complete politeness, invite them into our territory, and kindly show them where our strengths complement their weaknesses.

"No," stammered North Wind. "I'd best be getting home. I do feel a little peaked, but it's nothing that a good nap won't cure."

"Alright, then," said the young man, "but please visit any time."
North Wind agreed.

The next time North Wind came upon the young man, he was not
so kind. "How dare you invade my world," North Wind shouted. "I will
destroy you. I am going to freeze you to death. You will be sorry for staying
here. I will make you pay for this transgression."

We can expect the opposition to become progressively more antago-
nistic the more we persist.

"I'll bet you won't," challenged the young man. "I don't think so."

We must stand our ground.

North Wind was so angry with this young upstart that he knocked him
down. The two began to wrestle. But hard as he tried, North Wind
could not defeat the young man. He turned into Grandfather Winter
to wrestle. That was his most physical form. But the more he exerted
himself, the weaker he became. He was actually melting. Then, to his
horror, he noticed that the exertion was keeping the young man warm.
No matter what he tried, North Wind was no match for this heat.
Before he should melt away completely, he announced defeat and the
young man let him go.

See what I told you; the fight will make us stronger. It sharpens
and refines our wit and our skills. It allows us to demonstrate with our
appropriate collection of stories, sometimes even statistical stories, that
what we do works.

"You haven't seen the last of me," muttered North Wind as he skulked
away. He didn't stay long enough to hear the young man's retort. The
cold spell passed that way. Whatever challenges North Wind threw at the
young man, he accepted and overcame.

Remember the lesson from the I Ching: Perseverance furthers.

Finally, North Wind had a new plan. He offered to meet the young man in a gesture of truce.

Expect to be co-opted when it appears we will succeed.

The young man agreed. North Wind came to the young man's lodge and was invited in. Again, he felt the heat. Again he started to melt. "Now come with me outside," said North Wind. "Honor me before the stars." The young man did so, and immediately they began to wrestle. North Wind planned to take the young man this time. He planned to put him under the snow once and for all. They fought furiously all night long, but the North Wind could not defeat the young man, nor could the young man make North Wind melt. By daybreak, both were exhausted. "I suppose you want me to agree to let people live here," North Wind said.

"Exactly," said the young man. "We need game all year around."

"I suppose I have to let the people pass peacefully," said North Wind.

"Yes," replied the young man. "You must let them pass."

"But I get to freeze any that disrespect me or show me contempt," said North Wind.

"You may do so," said the young man. "You may have those who are too foolish to show you proper respect."

This is how our current state of affairs came to be. When the young man's friends returned, they were amazed and ecstatic to see him alive. He explained to them that the people could live in the north all year long now. He had struck a deal with North Wind. Not all believed him, and they went south. But those who did believe him live in the north now, working the trap lines, fishing through holes in the ice, and hunting wild caribou.

And this is how we will change conventional medicine and psychology. We must prepare thoroughly, train ourselves to survive, maintain our composure and civility, expect a fight, and engage the enemy even as we shake his hand and look him in the eye. We must eventually strike a deal, knowing we must maintain our respect for the enemy and our skillfulness, ethics, kindness, and compassion. If we get sloppy or disrespectful, the enemy will devour us.

Grandfather Winter is the coldest, most conservative, most entrenched character ever. We must be like this young man, and draw conventional medicine into a dialogue with us in which we cannot lose, as he did with North Wind.

One way we physicians can change medicine is to promote a new understanding of the people who consult us. We must endorse the idea that people are active agents in their lives. Meaning drives people's actions; behavior is governed by plots, people live in time and create interpretations for their experiences. Even those who seem most defective when regarded through the medical model become competent within this narrative model. They construct their own stories, seize opportunities, and maximize resources in ways they can communicate to us if we physicians will listen.[3] Our culture must advance an appreciation for how the settings in which people operate are socially mediated and how setting defines and restricts the roles that people enact.[4]

The narrative approach concretizes the idea that the next step for medicine is to understand that health and disease cannot be seen separate from the plot and action of the story in which they appear. This simple concept would revolutionize medicine to focus on real people, moving about in everyday life, interacting and living, outside the realm of laboratories, hospitals, and clinics. It would generate a new science that could make sense of health and healing by studying how they operate in people's lives.

If we physicians understand that people are active agents in their own lives, we automatically give them more respect than accrues to the word *patient*. We will recognize that people with whom we interact do make things happen. They initiate goal-directed behavior. They have purposes in mind when they act, even when they do things we don't like (smoke, drink excessively, ignore their diabetes). They make choices, even if their choices are severely limited. From this point of view, we will come to see that our role as physicians is to increase the range of choices that people can make. Our job is to increase their sense of agency, also known as empowerment. Our job is to collaborate, not order.

I am attempting to change medicine's perception of "the truth." Michel Foucault wrote, "Truth is to be understood as a system of ordered procedures for the production, regulation, distribution, circulation, and operation of statements. Truth is linked in circular relation with systems of power, that produce and sustain it, and to the effects of power, which it induces and which extends it."[5] He called this a regime of truth production. Today, we might replace "truth" with "knowledge." Conventional medicine produces an enormous mass of knowledge every day. The question becomes how relevant and useful is that knowledge if it is never questioned within the regime of that knowledge production? This question is as political and economic as it is scientific.

Medicine must change the way it produces knowledge. This means recognizing that what we call knowledge and what we call truth arise from a social process achieved through interaction, not simply the output of a scientific laboratory. It means promoting the recognition that we cannot separate biological response from the milieu in which it occurs. We must expand medicine to explore the lives of *real* people, the telling of *real* stories in *real* contexts. To the extent physicians have this understanding, the way they practice will change.

Narrative medicine says that story-making, storytelling, and story comprehension are fundamental concepts for understanding and treating physical diseases and for addressing the physical health of the body. The focus on narrative is a viable alternative to the current medical paradigm of today in which we try to fit one treatment to everyone with the same diagnosis. Changing medicine means making new stories, telling these stories, and appreciating the stories of others. What this means for psychiatry is that we must oppose the massive outpouring of money for drug research and the ensuing production of a "truth" revolving around brain chemicals, and counter the view that other forms of inquiry are unethical, frivolous, or irresponsible. What it means for medicine is that we must leave our clinics and offices and go out into the world to see how people live and how it affects their health. We must move beyond merely providing medications.

Foucault said we cannot escape power.[6] Everything we do is concerned with an aspect of the production of truth, which is the exercise of power. When we create a mutually respectful discourse, the power exercised is positive. When we bully people and force our will upon them, that power is negative. When we disempower people in the name of maintaining our position of superiority, we abuse power.

Power is a statement about transactions among people, and it is recognized through its results. How much power you have is directly determined by how able you are to influence others to agree with your truth. Power and truth are almost synonymous. Regimes of power produce truths, and regimes of truth exercise power. Our task in the field of health is to overthrow the exclusive claim of conventional medicine to truth and to introduce other stories into the arena of health and healing.

As a culture, we need to retract our tendency to put values on everything. My work in assisting people to revise their stories is an exercise of power, because I am involved in the process of changing their stories. That seems reasonable if a person does not like his or her story, but I'm still exercising praxis—taking action in the world—to produce a story about changing existing stories to ones I prefer, and am attempting to convince people to change their stories. I have any number of rationalizations about why my stories for you are preferable, including reducing the risks of imprisonment, improving health, or maintaining adequate public standing. However, the fact remains that I cannot act in the world without engaging in story production, which is an exercise of power that may or may not have positive effects, with outcomes I can discover only when I see how influential my productions are. To interact is to influence, and to influence is to exercise power. By becoming aware of this, perhaps physicians can learn to exercise power in more constructive ways.

We will be more effective in treating mental illness among certain populations if we can disentangle the prison system from the mental health system. I have tried to point out the hidden assumptions behind the concepts of "treatment" and "therapy." A similar movement exists to point out the faulty assumptions behind locking people in prison— the widespread belief that it teaches them to be better people, satisfies a need for revenge, or otherwise improves society, none of which it actually does. I am not saying that there are no people who should be separated from society at large, but I am suggesting that we should take such measures for our safety, not to punish or exact revenge.

We must continue to walk the spiral toward an integrated understanding that all is connected. We must offer options for relieving suffering that are more varied and humane than the impersonal gaze of conventional medicine. We need to oppose the disempowerment of people and focus upon what people can do to help themselves. So much of what psychiatry and medicine purports to treat is really the result of poverty, homelessness, racism, isolation, and resultant substance misuse. We need to address the roots of suffering, rather than the symptoms.

How can we support communities to pursue and further develop their own local healing practices with legitimacy? The mainstream, licensed health professional system is already largely alienated from the local practices of indigenous communities. In Canada, however, local healers are being recognized by their communities and put forward as deserving of pay by Health Canada. In Winnipeg, at the University of Manitoba Aboriginal Health Unit, traditional healers are sponsored by the medical director, Judy Bartlett, and are credentialed for their services, which are covered by Health Canada. Since their training is entirely traditional, this represents an important assent and recognition by the community and the medical staff.

I suspect we need to deregulate the practice of healing to some degree in order to return power to local communities. I find the coach metaphor to have a certain appeal. Communities can be facilitated to come together to decide upon the structure of their health care and who should provide it. More variability is needed in training and credentialing, so that communities can set their own standards that are appropriate for their locality. This could be accomplished without any loss of quality. Some degree of de-professionalization and deregulation may be needed to create genuine collaborations among people of multiple and diverse backgrounds. Many ancient healing practices that are considered "therapeutic" today were not seen that way by the communities in which they evolved, because the concept of "therapeutic" hadn't been invented yet. Instead the goal was to restore harmony and balance for everyone. The healer was never separate from the outcome or exempt from the accountability that was required.

We need to resist attempts to turn the narrative perspective and approach into an algorithm, a technique, a series of steps to follow. We can take lessons from indigenous knowledge studies on this topic. The narrative perspective is broad and all encompassing, like some aspects of elders' teachings. There are principles of healing, education, and social relationship with which almost all elders would agree. The implementation of these principles varies widely with local areas.

Thus, as we consider the practice of narrative medicine and how to be maximally helpful to people of all cultures, several ideas emerge that are inspired by Saskatchewan First Nations' philosopher, Eber Hampton:[7]

> Health practitioners must be concerned with spirituality, at the center of which is respect for the relationships that exist between all things. We must nurture these spiritual relationships and allow them to work on us.
>
> Health practitioners must be concerned with service. We must serve the people who come to us. This ideal must hold sway over our own individual status or desire for advancement.
>
> Healers must show respect for diversity, which requires self-knowledge and self-respect, without which respect for others is impossible.
>
> We must respect different cultures' ways of thinking, learning, teaching, and communicating.
>
> Health practitioners must maintain a sense of history.
>
> We must maintain continuity with the traditions of living cultures.
>
> We must participate in relationships of personal respect.
>
> As healers, we must be relentless in our struggle for that which honors life and against that which does not.
>
> We must recognize and nourish the powerful pattern of life that lies hidden within personal and group suffering and oppression.
>
> We must recognize the conflict, tensions, and struggle inherent in life and between cultures.
>
> Health practitioners must recognize the importance of a sense of place, land, and territory. From this point of view, it is clear that we must promote involvement in community, rather than isolation or segregation.
>
> We must recognize the need for transformation in relations among all people, as well between the individual and society.

We are going to struggle in narrative medicine with multidimensional maps in which conventional medicine is just one vantage point, and not always a correct one. This book has addressed how we begin this struggle to transform ourselves, our illnesses, and the field of medicine. We do so through immersion in a diverse world of stories—those of the world's many cultures and their healing practices. We do so through honoring the many different paths to wellness and by understanding that healing is not necessarily rational. It lies more within the new quantum physics than classical mechanics. It can be unpredictable and not replicable, but nevertheless valid. Its reality is contained in the stories we tell.

Notes

Introduction:
Awakening to Narrative Medicine

1. Oliver Sacks, *An Anthropologist on Mars: Seven Paradoxical Tales* (New York: Vintage, 1996).

2. National Center for Health Statistics, U.S. Department of Health and Human Services (DHHS) *Publication No. 88-1232* (Washington, D.C.: Public Health Service, 1988); National Center for Health Statistics, *National Vital Stat Rep 49*, no. 12, October 9, 2001.

3. Leon Gordis, *Epidemiology*, 3rd ed. (Philadelphia: W. B. Saunders, 2004).

4. Daniel Callahan, *What Price Better Health? Hazards of the Research Imperative* (Berkeley: University of California Press, 2003).

5. Susan L. Johnston, "Native American Traditional and Alternative Medicine," *The Annals of the American Academy of Political and Social Science* 583, no. 1 (2002): 195–213.

6. Kim Anderson, *A Recognition of Being: Reconstructing Native Womanhood* (Toronto: Sumach Press, 2001); Kim Anderson and Bonita Lawrence, *Strong Women Stories: Native Vision and Community Survival* (Toronto: Sumach Press, 2003); see also http://www.uoguelph.ca/atguelph/06-01-11/ (accessed 16 January 2007).

7. Michael Bamberg, "Talk, Small Stories, and Adolescent Identities," *Human Development* 47 (2004): 366–69.

8. Wendy Levinson, "Doctor–Patient Communication," *The Journal of the American Medical Association* 284 (Aug. 23/30, 2000): 1021–27.

9. N. Ambady, D. La Plante, T. Nguyen, R. Rosenthal, N. Chaumenton, and W. Levinson, "Surgeons' Tone of Voice: A Key to Malpractice History," *Surgery* 132 (2002): 5–9.

10. Lewis Mehl-Madrona, "Native American Medicine in the Treatment of Chronic Illness: Developing an Integrated Program and Evaluating Its Effectiveness," *Alternative Therapies in Health and Medicine* 5, no. 1 (Jan. 1999): 36–44.

11. Wade Davis, *The Clouded Leopard: Travels to Landscapes of Spirit and Desire* (Vancouver: Douglas and McIntyre, 1999), 122–23.

12. Kathryn Coe, *The Ancestress Hypothesis* (New Brunswick, NJ: Rutgers University Press, 2003).

13. Leon Gordis, *Epidemiology,* 3rd ed. (Philadelphia: W. B. Saunders, 2004).

14. A number of studies show the wide variability in survival. The following study found the longest duration to relapse with a specific treatment was 23.5 years with 18 percent of those relapsing doing so later than ten years after diagnosis: R. B. Weiss, S. H. Woolf, E. Demakos, J. F. Holland, D. A. Berry, G. Falkson, C. T. Cirrincione, A. Robbins, S. Bothun, I. C. Henderson, and L. Norton, "Natural History of More Than 20 Years of Node-Positive Primary Breast Carcinoma Treated with Cyclophosphamide, Methotrexate, and Fluorouracil-Based Adjuvant Chemotherapy: A Study by the Cancer and Leukemia Group B," *Journal of Clinical Oncology* 21, no. 9 (May 2003): 1825–35. Another study from Norway shows the uselessness of quoting median survival rates given the long survival of some patients: L. E. Rutqvist, A. Wallgren, and B. Nilsson, "Is Breast Cancer a Curable Disease? A Study of 14,731 Women with Breast Cancer from the Cancer Registry of Norway," *Cancer* 53, no. 8 (April 1984): 1793–800.

15. Claire V. Edmonds, Gina A. Lockwood, and Alastair J. Cunningham, "Psychological Response to Long-Term Group Therapy: A Randomized Trial with Metastatic Breast Cancer Patients," *Psycho-Oncology* 8, no. 1 (1999): 74–91.

16. Lewis Mehl-Madrona and B. Chan, "Faith Plays a Role in AIDS," *Alternative Health Practitioner* (December 1999).

17. Lewis Mehl-Madrona, "Success of a Biologically Inactive Treatment for Autism: The Pygmalion Effect" (forthcoming 2007). Manuscript available from Dr. Madrona by e-mail request to narrativemedicine@gmail.com.

18. Raymond J. Demallie, ed., *The Sixth Grandfather: Black Elk's Teachings Given to John G. Neihardt* (Lincoln: University of Nebraska Press, 1984), 28.

Chapter 1:
The Roots of Narrative Medicine

1. Alfred North Whitehead, *Essays in Science and Philosophy* (New York: Philosophical Library, 1948).
2. HealthGrades Quality Study, "Patient Safety in American Hospitals July 2004," http://www.healthgrades.com/media/english/pdf/HG_Patient_Safety_Study_Final.pdf (accessed 19 January 2007).
3. D. Graham, D. Campen, R. Hui, M. Spence, C. Cheetham, G. Levy, S. Shoor, and W. Ray, "Risk of Acute Myocardial Infarction and Sudden Cardiac Death in Patients Treated with Cyclo-oxygenase 2 Selective and Non-selective Non-steroidal Anti-inflammatory Drugs: Nested Case-control Study," *The Lancet 365*, Issue 9458 (2003): 475–81; Wikipedia, "Rofecoxib," http://en.wikipedia.org/wiki/Vioxx (accessed 19 January 2007); Defective Drugs, "Vioxx Heart Disease," http://www.adrugrecall.com/vioxx/heart-disease.html (accessed 19 January 2007); Science Daily, "Heart Risks From Vioxx Happen Much Earlier Than Believed," http://www.sciencedaily.com/releases/2006/05/060504081246.htm (accessed 19 January 2007).
4. Parker Waichman, "Injury from Paxil?" http://www.yourlawyer.com/topics/overview/paxil (accessed 19 January 2007); Dean Fergusson, Steve Doucette, Kathleen Cranley Glass, Stan Shapiro, David Healy, Paul Hebert, and Brian Hutton, "Association between Suicide Attempts and Selective Serotonin Reuptake Inhibitors: Systematic Review of Randomised Controlled Trials," *British Medical Journal* 330 (Feb 2005): 396; Alliance for Human Research Protection, "Can a Popular Antidepressant Cause Teenage Suicide?" http://www.ahrp.org/infomail/03/08/06a.php (accessed 19 January 2007); Alliance for Human Research Protection, "Coroner Calls for Withdrawal of Paxil, http://www.ahrp.org/infomail/0302/13.php (accessed 19 January 2007).
5. Lewis Mehl-Madrona, "Successful Treatments for Autism," *Mothering Magazine* (Jan–Feb 2006): 39–43.
6. W. C. Willet, J. C. Koplan, R. Nugent, C. Dusenbury, P. Puska, and T. A. Gaziano, "Prevention of Chronic Disease by Diet and Lifestyle Means," http://files.dcp2.org/pdf/DCP/DCP44.pdf (accessed 19 January 2007).

7. Highmark Blue Cross Blue Shield, "Dr. Dean Ornish Program Substantially Reduces Health Care Utilization for Heart Patients," November 7, 2003, Pittsburgh, PA, https://www.highmark.com/hmk2/about/newsroom/pr110703 .shtml (accessed 19 January 2007).

8. This story also appears in William Reid and Robert Bringhurst, *The Raven Steals the Light* (Seattle: University of Washington Press, 1984) and is summarized by Tad Beckman at Harvey Mudd College, available at http:// www4.hmc.edu:8001/humanities/beckman/western/raven.htm. Another version of the story appears in John R. Swanton, "Types of Haida and Tlingit Myths," *American Anthropologist* 7, no. 1 (1905): 94–103.

9. Argyris Arnellos, Thomas Spyrou, and John Darzentas, "Towards a Framework that Models the Emergence of Meaning Structures in Purposeful Communication Environments: Application in Information Systems," www. syros.aegean.gr/users/tsp/conf_pub/C34/C34.doc (accessed 28 January 2007).

10. Shankar Vedantam, "Patients' Diversity is Often Discounted," *Washington Post*, 26 June 2005.

11. J. H. Flaskerud, "Ethnicity, Culture, and Neuropsychiatry," *Issues in Mental Health Nursing* 21 (2000): 5–29; I. Nachshon, J. G. Draguns, I. K. Broverman, L. Phillips, "The Reflection of Acculturation in Psychiatric Symptomatology: A Study of an Israeli Child Guidance Clinic Population," *Social Psychiatry and Psychiatric Epidemiology* 7, no. 2 (1972): 109–18.

12. J. M. Golding, M. Karno, and C. M. Rutter, "Symptoms of Major Depression among Mexican-Americans and Non-Hispanic Whites," *American Journal of Psychiatry* 147 (1990): 861–66; J. M. Golding and R. I. Lipton, "Depressed Mood and Major Depressive Disorder in Two Ethnic Groups," *Journal of Psychiatry Research* 24 (1990): 65–82.

13. D. R. Brown, W. W. Eaton, and L. Sussman, "Racial Differences in Prevalence of Phobic Disorders," *Journal of Nervous and Mental Disease* 178 (1990): 434–41; S. K. Hoppe, R. L. Leon, and J. P. Realini, "Depression and Anxiety among Mexican Americans in a Family Health Center," *Social Psychiatry & Psychiatric Epidemiology* 24 (1989): 63–68; M. Karno, J. M. Golding, M. A. Burnam, R. L. Hough, J. I. Escobar, K. M. Wells, and R. Boyer, "Anxiety Disorder among Mexican Americans and Non-Hispanic Whites in Los Angeles," *Journal of Nervous and Mental Disease* 177 (1989): 202–9; K. M. Lin, "Cultural Influences on the Diagnosis of Psychotic and Organic Disorders," in J. E. Mezzich, A. Kleinman, H. Fabrega, and

D. L. Parron, *Culture and Psychiatric Diagnosis* (Washington, DC: American Psychiatric Press, 1996), 49–62.

14. Health Resources and Services Administration, U.S. Department of Health and Human Services, "Women's Health USA 2004," http://mchb.hrsa.gov/whusa04/pages/intro.htm (accessed 19 January 2007).

15. Shankar Vedantam, "Patients' Diversity is Often Discounted," *Washington Post,* 26 June 2005.

16. World Health Organization, "Adults at Risk, 2003," http://www.who.int/whr/2003/chapter1/en/index3.htm (accessed 28 January 2007).

17. T. R. Sarbin and V. L. Allen, "Role Theory," in G. Lindzey and E. Aronson, eds., *Handbook of Social Psychology,* vol. 1 (Reading, MA: Addison-Wesley, 1968), 489.

18. Mihaly Csikszentmihalyi, *Flow: The Psychology of Optimal Experience* (New York: Harper & Row, 1990).

19. T. R. Sarbin and V. L. Allen, "Role Theory," in G. Lindzey and E. Aronson, eds., *Handbook of Social Psychology,* vol. 1 (Reading, MA: Addison-Wesley, 1968), 497.

20. Shankar Vedantam, "Social Network's Healing Power is Borne Out in Poorer Nations," *Washington Post,* 27 June 2005, A01.

21. Ibid.

22. Ibid.

23. M. Gittelman, "Persons with Schizophrenia in China," in *A New Paradigm of Medical Care for Disabled Persons: A Multi-Country Action-Learning Research Initiative,* report of the first meeting, Hotel Kaire, Rome (Italy) 6 to 8 April 2005. Report prepared by Dr. Wim H. van Brakel, www.aifo.it/english/proj/aifo-who/romemeeting0405/DRAFTREPORT-1-APR05.doc (accessed 20 January 2007).

24. R. Padmavati, R. Thara, T. N. Srinivasan, and R. G. McCreadie, "Spontaneous Dyskinesia and Parkinsonism in Never-Medicated, Chronically Ill Patients with Schizophrenia: 18-Month Follow-Up," *The British Journal of Psychiatry* 181 (2002): 135–37; T. Srinivasan, "The Long-Term Home-Making Functioning of Women with Schizophrenia," *Schizophrenia Research* 35, Issue 1 (1999): 97–98; R. Padmavati, S. Rajkumar, and T. N. Srinivasan, "Schizophrenic Patients Who Were Never Treated—A Study in an Indian Urban Community," *Psychological Medicine* 28 (1998): 1113–17.

25. For more information on the fascinating World Health Organization studies on schizophrenia, see the following original sources: R. Srinivasa Murthy, "Mental Health in the New Millennium: Research Strategies for India," *Indian Journal of Medical Research* (Aug. 2004); R. Thara, R. Padmavati, and T. N. Srinivasan, "Focus on Psychiatry in India," *British Journal of Psychiatry* 184 (2004): 366–73; E. Fuller Torey, *Surviving Schizophrenia: A Manual for Families, Consumers, and Providers,* 4th ed. (New York: HarperCollins Publishers, 2001); M. Hambrecht, K. Maurer, H. Häfner, and N. Sartorius, "An Analysis Based on the WHO Study on Determinants of Outcome of Severe Mental Disorders," *European Archives of Psychiatry and Clinical Neuroscience* 242, no. 1 (1992): 6–12; G. Harrison, K. Hopper, T. Craig, E. Laska et al., "Recovery from Psychotic Illness: A 15- and 25-Year International Follow-Up Study," *British Journal of Psychiatry* 178 (2001): 506–17; K. Hopper and J. Wanderling, "Revisiting the Developed versus Developing Country Distinction in Course and Outcome in Schizophrenia: Results from ISoS, the WHO Collaborative Follow-Up Project," International Study of Schizophrenia, *Schizophrenia Bulletin* 26, no. 4 (2000): 835–46; K. Hopper, G. Harrison, J. Aleksander, and N. Sartorius, *Recovery from Schizophrenia: An International Perspective* (Madison, CT: International Universities Press, Inc., 2004); A. Jablensky, N. Sartorius, G. Ernberg, M. Anker, A. Korten, J. E. Cooper, R. Day, and A. Bertelsen, "Schizophrenia: Manifestations, Incidence and Course in Different Cultures, a World Health Organization Ten Country Study," *Psychological Medicine Monograph Supplement* 20 (1992): 1–95; J. Leff, N. Sartorius, A. Jablensky, A. Korten, and G. Ernberg, "The International Pilot Study of Schizophrenia: Five-Year Follow-Up Findings," *Psychological Medicine* 22 (1992): 131–45.

26. Michel Foucault, "Essay on the Origins of Social Medicine," in *Power,* Volume 3 of *The Essential Foucault* (New York: Guilford Press, 2004).

27. Colin Saunders, lecture "Narrative Therapy and Addictions." For information about Saunders and his workshops, see http://www.narrativecuba. com/c-sanders1.htm.

28. For more information on Colin Saunders, see http://www.efap.ca/bio_colin_ sanders.htm.

29. See also the story of Melvin Grey Fox helping a schizophrenic in Lewis Mehl-Madrona, *Coyote Healing: Miracles in Native Medicine* (Rochester, VT: Bear & Company, 2003), chap. 3.

30. Bureau of Justice Statistics, U.S. Department of Justice, http://www.ojp. usdoj.gov/bjs/pubalp2.htm (accessed 21 January 2007).

31. Maureen Lux, *Medicine That Walks* (Toronto: University of Toronto Press, 2001), 3–4.

32. Mario E. Martinez, "The Process of Knowing: A Biocognitive Epistemology," *The Journal of Mind and Behavior* 22, no. 4 (2001): 407–26.

33. Michael Bamberg and Molly Andrews, eds., *Considering Counter-Narratives: Narrating, Resisting, Making Sense* (Amsterdam: John Benjamins Publishing, 2004), 351–71.

Chapter 2:
Transcending Limitations

1. Leslie Marmon Silko, *Ceremony* (New York: Viking, 1977).

2. Roy Porter, *For the Benefit of Mankind—A Medical History of Humanity* (New York: Norton, 1998), 188, 203.

3. See Maureen Lux, *Medicine That Walks* (Toronto: University of Toronto Press, 2001) for an amazing description of how the Canadian government tried to make its Native population die out between 1880 and 1940, with residential school child mortality rates as high as 80 percent and yet, they failed. The Native people of Canada are its fastest growing population today.

4. I write about this at length in *Coyote Healing: Miracles in Native Medicine* (Rochester, VT: Bear & Company, 2003).

5. Harvey A. Brenner, *Mental Illness and the Economy* (Cambridge, MA: Harvard University Press, 1973). See also Louis A. Ferman and Jeanne P. Gordus, "Mental Health and the Economy," review author Helen Ginsburg, *Industrial and Labor Relations Review* 35, no. 1 (Oct. 1981): 140–42; T. Elkeles and W. Seifert, "Unemployment and Health Impairments Longitudinal Analyses for the Federal Republic of Germany," *The European Journal of Public Health* 3, no. 1 (1993): 28–37.

6. Harvey A. Brenner, "Mortality and the National Economy," *The Lancet* 314, no. 8142 (1979): 568–73; H. A. Brenner, *Estimating the Effects of Economic Change on National Health and Social Well Being* (Washington, DC: Joint Economic Committee, U.S. Congress, U.S. Government Printing Office, 1984); H. A. Brenner, "Economic Change, Alcohol Consumption and Heart Disease Mortality in Nine Industrialized Countries," *Social Science and Medicine* 25, no. 2 (1987): 119–32; H. A. Brenner, "Political

Economy and Health," in *Society and Health*, Alvin R. Tarlov and Diana Chapman Walsh, eds. (New York: Oxford University Press, 1995), 211–46; H. A. Brenner and A. Mooney, "Unemployment and Health in the Context of Economic Change," *Social Science Medicine* 17, no.16 (1983): 1125–38.

7. Hiroaki Hayakawa, "Rationality of Liquidity Preferences and the Neoclassical Monetary Growth Model," *Journal of Macroeconomics* 4 (1983): 495–501.

8. Charles Waldegrave and Rosalyn Coventry, *Poor New Zealand: An Open Letter on Poverty* (Wellington: Platform Publishing, 1987).

9. Also see Garcia-Preto's writings about this process in Latina culture, "Latinas in the United States: Bridging Two Worlds," in M. McGoldrick, ed., *Re-Visioning Family Therapy: Race, Culture, and Gender in Clinical Practice* (New York: The Guilford Press, 1998), 330–34; Joel Crohn's writings about intercultural relationships, *Mixed Matches: How to Create Successful Interracial, Interethnic, and Interfaith Relationships* (New York: Fawcett, 1995); J. Crohn, "Intercultural Couples," in McGoldrick, ed., *Re-Visioning Family*, 295–308; and Christopher Sullivan and R. Rocco Cottone, "Culturally Based Couple Therapy and Intercultural Relationships: A Review of the Literature," *The Family Journal* 14, no. 3 (2006): 221–25.

10. Richard Bucke, *Cosmic Consciousness: A Study in the Evolution of the Human Mind* (Philadelphia: Innes & Sons, 1901; reprint, New York: Penguin Books, 1991).

11. Evelyn Underhill, *Mysticism: A Study in the Nature and Development of Spiritual Consciousness* (New York: Dover, 2002).

12. Ashok Gangadean, *Meditative Logic* (Philadelphia: Temple University Press, 2001).

13. Abraham Maslow, *Religions, Values and Peak-Experiences* (New York: Penguin Books, 1964). See also NNDB, "Abraham Maslow," http://www.nndb.com/people/166/000032070/.

14. Dean Hamer, *The God Gene: How Faith Is Hardwired into Our Genes* (New York: Doubleday, 2004). See also Jeffrey Kluger, "Is God in our Genes?" *TIME Magazine*, 17 October 2004.

15. Houston Smith, *Why Religion Matters: The Fate of the Human Spirit in an Age of Disbelief* (New York: HarperCollins, 2006).

16. Mircea Eliade, *Shamanism: Archaic Techniques of Ecstasy* (Princeton, NJ: Princeton University Press, 1951).

17. Earth Consciousness, http://www.hg29hh.freeserve.co.uk/Consciou.htm (accessed 22 March 2005).

18. Ervin Laszlo, *The Connectivity Hypothesis: Foundations of an Integral Science of Quantum, Cosmos, Life, and Consciousness* (Ithaca: State University of New York Press, 2004). For further discussion, also see Michael E. Zimmerman, "Humanity's Reactions to Gaia: Part of the Whole, or Member of the Community?" *The Trumpeter* 20, no. 1 (2004): 46–62, available online at http://www. tulane.edu/~michaelz/essays/integral_ecology/humanitys_relation_to_gaia.swf. See also Masaru Emoto's Web site, especially "Meeting Dr. Laszlo," http:// www.masaru-emoto.net/english/ediary200411.html#2004.11.24.

19. James Lovelock, *Ages of Gaia: A Biography of Our Living Earth* (New York: Bantam Books, 1991).

20. See, for example, "Vijnanavada," http://www.kheper.net/topics/Buddhism/ Vijnanavada.htm (accessed 28 January 2007).

21. Carl G. Jung, *Collected Works* (Princeton, NJ: Princeton University Press, Bollinger Series, 1974).

22. Ervin Laszlo, *The Whispering Pond* (New York: Hampton Roads Press, 1995).

23. This material comes from personal communications with William Lyon, University of Missouri at Kansas City, and from his as yet unpublished manuscript on medicine powers.

24. Frank G. Speck, *Naskapi: The Savage Hunters of the Labrador Peninsula* (Norman: University of Oklahoma Press, 1935), 138.

25. Robin Ridington, "Knowledge, Power, and the Individual in Subarctic Hunting Societies," *American Anthropologist* 90, no. 1 (Mar 1988): 98–110.

26. Gary Witherspoon, *Language and Art in the Navajo Universe* (Ann Arbor: University of Michigan Press, 1977).

27. Hank Wesselman, interview by Deepak Chopra, 2001, available at http:// www.sharedwisdom.com/deepak.htm (accessed 28 January 2007).

28. William Lyon, personal discussions via email, 2005; William Lyon, unpublished manuscript, 2005–2006.

29. Evan Harris Walker, *Physics of Consciousness: The Quantum Mind and the Meaning of Life* (New York: Perseus Publishing, 2000), 274–75.

30. Gladys A. Reichard, "Prayer: The Compulsive Word," *Monographs of the American Ethnological Society* 7 (New York: J. J. Augustin, 1944).

31. Paul Radin, "An Introductive Enquiry in the Study of Ojibwa Religion,"

Papers and Records of the Ontario Historical Society 12 (1914): 210–20.

32. Frances Densmore, "Chippewa Customs," *Bureau of American Ethnology* 86 (1929): 45.

33. Samuel Gill, *Sacred Words: A Study of Navajo Religion and Prayer* (Westport, CT: Greenwood, 1981), 185–86.

34. William Lyon, personal communication, 2006; William Lyon, unpublished manuscript, 2006.

35. William Lyon, unpublished manuscript, 2006.

36. William M. Beauchamp, "Iroquois Folk Lore" (Syracuse, NY: The Dehler Press, 1922).

37. Sam D. Gill, "Prayer as Person: The Performative Force in Navajo Prayer Acts," *History of Religions* 17, no. 2 (Nov. 1977): 143–57.

38. William Lyon, personal correspondence, 2006. See also William S. Simmons and Frank Speck, "Frank Speck and 'The Old Mohegan Indian Stone Cutter,'" *Ethnohistory* 32, no. 2 (Spring 1985): 155–63.

39. Olga Weyermeyer Johnson, *Flathead and Kootenay: The Rivers, the Tribe and the Region's Traders* (Glendale: Arthur H. Clarke, 1969), 129.

40. Frederica DeLaguna, "Under Mount Saint Elias: The History and Culture of the Yakutat Tlingit," 3 vols., *Smithsonian Contributions to Anthropology* (1972): 660.

41. Lyon, unpublished manuscript, 2006. For further examples of the need for removal of doubt, see Struthers and Eschiti, "The Experience of Indigenous Traditional Healing and Cancer," *Integrative Cancer Therapies* 3 (2004): 13–23.

42. Wade Davis, *The Clouded Leopard* (Vancouver: Douglas and McIntyre, 1999), 150.

Chapter 3:
The Maps That Define Our Reality

1. *Reader's Digest* (July 1977): 42.

2. A beautiful version of this story ("Coyote Steals Fire") is available in both the Dene language and in English, from the San Juan School District Media Center in Utah, www.sanjuan.k12.ut.us/media/mediaweb.htm.

3. Beth Israel Deaconess Medical Center, "Study Says Therapy Better than Pills in Treating Sleep-Onset Insomnia," http://www.bidmc.harvard.edu/default.asp?node_id=1000 (accessed 28 January 2007).

4. Tom E. Lovejoy, "How Much is an Elephant Worth?" *Nature* 382 (1996): 594.

5. Jean-François Lyotard, *The Different: Phrases in Dispute* (Minneapolis: University of Minnesota Press, 1988).

6. "Gödel's more famous incompleteness theorem states that for any self-consistent recursive axiomatic system powerful enough to describe the arithmetic of the natural numbers (Peano arithmetic), there are true propositions about the naturals that cannot be proved from the axioms." Wikipedia, "Kurt Gödel," http://en.wikipedia.org/wiki/Kurt_Godel (accessed 29 December 2006).

7. Stephen Pepper, *World Hypotheses* (Berkeley: University of California Press, 1942).

8. L. E. Hahn, "Stephen C. Peppper, 1891–1972," in P. B. Dematteis and L. B. McHenry, eds., *Dictionary of Literary Biography*, vol. 270 (Detroit: Gale Group, 2003), 251–66.

9. Wikipedia, "David Bohm," http://en.wikipedia.org/wiki/David_Bohm.

10. Yakir Ahronov and David Bohm, "Oscillation of an Optical Effect," *Physics Review* 115 (1959): 485.

11. F. David Peat and John Briggs, interview with David Bohm, originally published in *Omni*, January 1987 (accessed 29 December 2006 on Interviews Scientists, http://www.fdavidpeat.com/interviews/bohm.htm).

12. Wikipedia, "Scientific Reductionism," http://en.wikipedia.org/wiki/Scientific_reductionism (accessed 29 December 2006).

13. E. Davis, *Techgnosis: Myth, Magic and Mysticism in the Age of Information* (London: Serpent's Tail, 1999), 168.

14. Peat and Briggs, interview with David Bohm, 1987. For an expansion of these ideas, see David Pratt, "David Bohm and the Implicate Order," http://www.theosophy-nw.org/theosnw/science/prat-boh.htm (accessed 28 January 2007).

15. Ibid.

16. http://www.reiki-research.co.uk/refsjoe.html (accessed 28 January 2007).

17. L. Fruggeri, "Therapeutic Process as the Social Construction of Change," in S. McNamee and K. Gergen, eds., *Therapy as Social Construction* (Thousand Oaks, CA: Sage Press, 1992).

18. G. Nicolis and Ilya Prigogine, *Self-Organization in Nonequilibrium Systems: From Dissipative Structures to Order through Fluctuations* (New York: Wiley, 1977).

19. Gregory Bateson, *Mind and Nature: A Necessary Unity* (New York: E. P. Dutton, 1979).

20. Michel Foucault, *An Archaeology of Knowledge* (New York: Pantheon Books, 1972).

21. C. Antaki, *Explaining and Arguing: The Social Organization of Accounts* (London: Sage, 1994); D. Edwards and J. Potter, *Discursive Psychology* (London: Sage, 1992).

22. Timothy F. Allen, "A Summary of the Principles of Hierarchy Theory," http://www.isss.org/hierarchy.htm (accessed 28 January 2007).

23. Gregory Bateson, *Mind and Nature: A Neccesary Unity* (New York: E. A. Dutton, 1979).

24. Jay Haley, *Problem-Solving Therapy* (San Francisco: Jossey-Bass, 1987); Paul Watzlawick, John Weakland, Richard Fisch, *Change: Principles of Problem Formation and Problem Resolution* (New York: W. W. Norton, 1974).

25. Salvador Minuchen, *Families and Family Therapy* (Cambridge, MA: Harvard University Press, 1986); Salvador Minuchin, Bernice L. Rosman, and Lester Baker, *Psychosomatic Families: Anorexia Nervosa in Context* (Cambridge, MA: Harvard University Press, 1978).

26. Gregory Bateson, *Steps to an Ecology of Mind* (New York: Ballantine Books, 1972).

27. James Lovelock, *Ages of Gaia: A Biography of Our Living Earth* (New York: Bantam Books, 1991).

28. Robert Nadeau and Menas Kafatos, *The Non-Local Universe: The New Physics and Matters of the Mind* (Oxford, UK: Oxford University Press, 1999).

29. Ervin Laszlo, *The Interconnected Universe* (Singapore and London: World Scientific, 1995).

30. Gregory Bateson, "Consciousness versus Nature," *Peace News* 1622 (28 July 1967): 10.

31. Maurice Merleau-Ponty, *The Phenomenology of Perception* (New York: Routledge, 1976).

32. Gregory Bateson, *Steps to an Ecology of Mind* (New York: Ballantine, 1972).

33. R. P. Bajpai, "Biophoton and the Quantum Vision of Life," in H. P. Durr, F. A. Popp, and W. Schommers, eds., *What Is Life? Scientific Approaches; Philosophical Positions* (Newark, NJ: World Scientific, 2002).

34. Lev Beloussov, "The Formative Powers of Developing Organisms," in H. P. Durr, F. A. Popp, and W. Schommers, eds., *What Is Life? Scientific*

Approaches; Philosophical Positions (Newark, NJ: World Scientific, 2002).

35. Laszlo Patthy, "Modular Assembly of Genes and the Evolution of New Functions," *Genetica* 118 (2003): 217–31.

36. Ervin Laszlo, *The Interconnected Universe* (Singapore and London: World Scientific, 1995).

37. Russell Targ and Harold Puthoff, "Information Transmission under Conditions of Sensory Shielding," *Nature* (1974): 251, 602–7.

38. Harold Puthoff and Russell Targ, "A Perceptual Channel for Information Transfer Over Kilometer Distances: Historical Perspective and Recent Research," *Proceedings of the IEEE* 64, no. 3 (1976): 329–56.

39. Stanley Krippner, *Dream Experiments*, available at http://www.goertzel. org/dynapsyc/1996/subtle_fn.html#fn0 (accessed 22 May 2004).

40. Jacobo Grinberg-Zylberbaum, M. Delaflor, M. E. Sanchez-Arellano, M. A. Guevara, and M. Perez, "Human Communication and the Electrophysiological Activity of the Brain," *Subtle Energies* 3 (1993).

41. Ervin Laszlo, *Subtle Connections: Psi, Grof, Jung, and the Quantum Vaccuum*, 1996, http://www.goertzel.org/dynapsyc/1996/subtle.html (accessed 25 April 2004).

42. For further reading: L. Dossey, *Recovering the the Soul: A Scientific and Spiritual Search* (New York: Bantam, 1989); L. Dossey, *Healing Words: The Power of Prayer and the Practice of Medicine* (San Francisco: Harper, 1993); C. Honorton, R. Berger, M. Varvoglis et al., "Psi-Communication in the Ganzfeld: Experiments with an Automated Testing System and a Comparison with a Meta-Analysis of Earlier Studies," *Journal of Parapsychology* 54 (1990): 281–308; R. Rosenthal, "Combining Results of Independent Studies," *Psychological Bulletin* 85, no. 1 (1978): 185–93; M. Varvoglis, "Nonlocality on a Human Scale: Psi and Consciousness Research," in S. Hameroff, A. Kaszniak, and A. Scott, eds., *Toward a Science of Consciousness* (Cambridge, MA: MIT Press, 1996); M. Varvoglis, "Goal-Directed and Observer-Dependent PK: An Evaluation of the Conformance-Behavior Model and the Observation Theories," *The Journal of the American Society for Psychical Research* 80 (1986).

43. Ervin Laszlo, *Subtle Connections: Psi, Grof, Jumg, and the Quantum Vaccuum*, 1996, http://www.goertzel.org/dynapsyc/1996/subtle.html.

44. William Braud and Marilyn Schlitz, "Psychokinetic Influence on Electrodermal Activity," *Journal of Parapsychology* 47 (1983): 95–119.

45. Erving Goffman, *The Presentation of Self in Everyday Life* (New York: Doubleday Anchor, 1959), 81.

46. Erving Goffman, *Frame Analysis: An Essay on the Organization of Experience* (New York: Harper and Row, 1974).

47. Ibid., 252.

48. Erving Goffman, "Felicity's Condition," *American Journal of Sociology* 89 (1983): 1–53.

49. Ervin Laszlo, *The Connectivity Hypothesis: Foundations of an Integral Science of Quantum, Cosmos, Life, and Consciousness* (Ithaca: State University of New York Press, 2004): 18.

50. Ervin Laszlo, *The Whispering Pond* (London and New York: Element Books, 1996), 60.

51. Ibid., 68.

52. Ibid., 60.

53. S. O. O'Nuallain, "Inner versus Outer Empiricism in Consciousness Research," http://www.zynet.co.uk/imprint/Tucson/5.htm (accessed 28 January 2007).

54. Stanislav Grof, *Ancient Wisdom and Modern Science* (Albany, NY: State University of New York Press, 1998).

55. R. Roy, "Science and Whole Person Medicine: Enormous Potential in a New Relationship," *Bulletin of Science, Technology, and Society* 22, no. 5 (2002): 374–90.

Chapter 4:
Master Narratives

1. Nicole Krauss, *The History of Love: A Novel* (New York: Norton and Company, 2005), 167.

2. Ervin Laszlo, *The Systems View of the World: A Holistic Vision For Our Time* (Cresskill, NJ: The Hampton Press, 1996), 75–76.

3. Ervin Laszlo, *You Can Change the World: The Global Citizen's Handbook for Living on Planet Earth* (New York: SelectBooks, 2003).

4. Theodore Sarbin, "Steps to the Narratory Principle: An Autobiographical Essay," in D. J. Lee, ed., *Life and Story: Autobiographies for a Narrative Psychology* (Westport, CT: Praeger, 1994), 7.

5. Rom Harré and Luk van Langenhove, *Positioning Theory* (Oxford: Blackwell Scientific Publishers, 1999).

6. Michael Bamberg and Molly Andrews, eds., *Considering Counter-*

Narratives: Narrating, Resisting, Making Sense (Amsterdam: John Benjamins Publishing, 2004), 351–71.

7. John A. Bargh and Melissa Ferguson, "Beyond Behaviorism: On the Automaticity of Higher Mental Processes," *Psychological Bulletin* 126, no. 6 (2000): 925–45.

8. Claude M. Steele, "A Threat in the Air: How Stereotypes Shape the Intellectual Identities and Performance of Women and African-Americans," *American Psychologist* 52 (1997): 613–29; Claude M. Steele, "Thin Ice: 'Stereotype Threat' and Black College Students," *The Atlantic Monthly* 284, no. 2 (1999): 44–47, 50–54; Claude M. Steele and Joshua Aronson, "Stereotype Threat and the Intellectual Test Performance of African-Americans," *Journal of Personality and Social Psychology* 69 (1995): 797–811; Claytie Davis III, Joshua Aronson, and Moises Salinas, "Shades of Threat: Racial Identity as a Moderator of Stereotype Threat," *Journal of Black Psychology* 32, no. 4 (2006): 399–417.

9. Malcolm Gladwell, *Blink: The Power of Thinking without Thinking* (New York: Little, Brown and Company, 2005), 52–59.

10. Michael White and David Epston, *Narrative Means to Therapeutic Ends* (New York: Norton, 1990).

11. Elsewhere I have written about the crucial role of the trickster, who can be a psychotherapist or just a friend, in getting us to see our hidden (from us) stories. See my chapter on "Coyote, Raven & Rabbit: The Role of Tricksters," in *Creativity and Madness,* vol. 2 (Burbank, CA: AIMED Press, 2007).

12. Robert Munsch, *The Paper Bag Princess* (Toronto: Annick Press, 1980); B. Davies and R. Harré, "Positioning: The Social Construction of Selves," *Journal for the Theory of Social Behaviour* 20 (1990): 43–63.

13. Michael Bamberg and Molly Andrews, eds., *Considering Counter-Narratives: Narrating, Resisting, Making Sense* (Amsterdam: John Benjamins Publishing, 2004), 351–71.

14. Michael Bamberg and Neill Korobov, "Positioning a 'Mature' Self in Interactive Practices: How Adolescent Males Negotiate 'Physical Attraction' in Group Talk," *British Journal of Developmental Psychology* 22, no. 4 (Nov. 2004): 471–92.

15. Theodore Sarbin, ed., *Narrative Psychology: The Storied Nature of Human Conduct* (New York: Praeger, 1986).

16. Michael Bamberg and Neill Korobov, "Positioning a 'Mature' Self in Interactive Practices: How Adolescent Males Negotiate 'Physical Attraction' in Group Talk," *British Journal of Developmental Psychology* 22, no. 4 (Nov. 2004): 471–92.

17. Ibid.

18. Ibid.

19. Harry Goolishian and Harlene Anderson, "Understanding the Therapeutic Process: From Individuals and Families to Systems in Language," in F. W. Kaslow, ed., *Voices in Family Psychology* 1 (1990): 91–113.

20. An illustrated version of this story ("Coyote Steals Water Monster's Baby") is available in Dene and English from the San Juan School District Media Center www.sanjuan.k12.ut.us/media/mediaweb.htm.

21. Kurt Gödel, *On Formally Undecidable Propositions of Principia Mathematica and Related Systems*, B. Meltzer, trans. (New York: Dover Publications, 1980).

22. Werner Heisenberg, *The Physical Principles of the Quantum Theory*, Carl Eckart and F. C. Hoyt, trans. (Mineola, NY: Dover, 1949).

23. Ashok Gangadean, *Meditative Logic* (Philadelphia: Temple University Press, 2001).

24. Michael Bamberg, "'I know it may sound mean to say this, but we couldn't really care less about her anyway': Form and functions of 'slut-bashing' in male identity constructions in 15-year-olds," *Human Development* (forthcoming).

25. Erving Goffman, *Frame Analysis: An Essay on the Organization of Experience* (New York: Harper and Row, 1974), 558.

Chapter 5:
The Power of Large Groups in Shaping Identity

1. Quoted in D. Rieff, *A Bed for the Night* (New York: Simon and Schuster, 2003).

2. Harry Goolishian and Harlene Anderson, "Understanding the Therapeutic Process: From Individuals and Families to Systems in Language," in F. W. Kaslow, ed., *Voices in Family Psychology* 1 (1990): 91–113.

3. Norman Cameron, "The Paranoid Pseudo-Community," *The American Journal of Sociology* 49, no. 1 (July 1943): 32–38.

4. Jerome Bruner, "The Narrative Construction of Reality," *Critical Inquiry* 18, no. 1 (Autumn 1991): 1–21.

5. Juha Holma and Jukka Aaltonen, "The Sense of Agency and the Search for a Narrative in Acute Psychosis," *Contemporary Family Therapy* 19, no. 4 (Dec. 1997): 463–77.

6. Juha Holma and Jukka Aaltonen, "Narrative Understanding in Acute Psychosis," *Contemporary Family Therapy* 20, no. 3 (1998): 253–63.

Chapter 6:
Narrative Medicine in Action

1. R. Roy, "Science and Whole Person Medicine: Enormous Potential in a New Relationship," *Bulletin of Science, Technology, and Society* 22, no. 5 (2002): 374–90.

2. Daniel J. Siegel, *The Developing Mind: How Relationships and the Brain Interact to Shape Who We Are* (New York: Guilford Press, 1999).

3. Harlene Anderson and Harry Goolishian, "The Client is the Expert: a Not-Knowing Approach to Therapy," in S. MacNamee and K. Gergen, *Therapy as Social Construction* (Thousand Oaks, CA: Sage Publications, 1992).

4. Ibid., 27.

5. Theodore Sarbin, "Steps to the Narratory Principle: An Autobiographical Essay," in D. J. Lee, ed., *Life and Story: Autobiographies for a Narrative Psychology* (Westport, CT: Praeger, 1994), 7.

6. K. Armitage, *Akua Hawai'i: Hawai'ian Gods and Their Stories* (Honolulu: Bishop Museum Press, 2005), 3–4.

7. Martha Warren Beckwith, *The Kumulipo: A Hawai'ian Creation Chant* (Chicago: University of Chicago Press, 1951).

8. David J. Smail, "Clinical Psychology: Liberatory Practice or Discourse of Power?" *Clinical Psychology Forum* 80 (1990): 3–7. See also David J. Smail, *The Origins of Unhappiness: A New Understanding of Distress* (New York: HarperCollins, 1993).

9. R. Szerze, "An Ache in the Abdomen: Severe Stomach Pain Cramps a Young Lad's Life," *Parkhurst Exchange* 13, no. 9 (2005): 15.

10. Ibid; for more information about omphalocele and its treatment, see Texas Pediatric Surgical Associates, http://www.pedisurg.com/PtEduc/Omphalocele.htm.

11. Margaret Talbot, "The Placebo Prescription," *New York Times*, January 9, 2000, available at http://query.nytimes.com/gst/fullpage.html?res=9C01E6D71E38F93AA35752C0A9669C8B63.

12. All of this information about breath and spirit was brought to my attention by William Lyon and appears in his as yet unpublished manuscript on medicine powers. In subsequent notes I will reference the sources Lyon referred me to that I went on to read, but the inspiration for this reading came from Lyon. He is a true scholar, and his work has given me valuable material to use clinically. The information on Hopi ideas about cosmic breath originally came from Marie-Louise von Franz, "Time: Rhythm and Repose," in *Psyche and Matter* (Boston: Shambhala Publications, 1992).

13. C. M. Hudson, *Conversations with the High Priest of Coosa* (Chapel Hill: The University of North Carolina Press, 2003).

14. This quote appears in William Lyon's unpublished work and is from Matilda Coxe Evans Stevenson, one of the first American female anthropologists and an avid student of Zuni culture. For more information, see the University of San Francisco's department of anthropology Web site: http://web3.cas.usf.edu/main/depts/ANT/women/stevenson/Stevenson.htm.

15. This information appears in Lyon's unpublished work. For more information on the source and its originator, see W. H. Holmes, "In Memoriam: Matilda Coxe Stevenson," originally published in *American Anthropologist* 18 (1916): 552–59 and available at http://www.aaanet.org/gad/history/061stevensonobit.pdf.

16. This information appears in Lyon's unpublished work. The original source is Leslie Spier, "Klamath Ethnography," *Publications in American Archaeology and Ethnology*, vol. 30 (Berkeley: University of California Press, 1930).

17. This information appears in Lyon's unpublished book on medicine powers and is from anthropologist Carlos Troyer who studied the Zuni in 1913. These concepts are also discussed in Frank Hamilton Cushing, *The Mythic World of Zuni* (Albuquerque: University of New Mexico Press, 1988).

18. While I knew these words from speaking and singing the Lakota language, it took William Lyon to make me conscious of these connections. He discusses this further in his upcoming book on medicine powers.

19. Stanislav Grof, *Beyond the Brain: Birth, Death, and Transcendence in Psychotherapy* (Albany: State University of New York Press, 1985).

20. Lyon, unpublished manuscript on medicine powers and e-mail discussions, 2006. See also William E. Paden, *Interpreting the Sacred: Ways of Viewing Religion* (Boston: Beacon Press, 2003) for further discussion of these concepts and their expansion into other religions.

21. William Lyon, personal correspondence, 2006. More information on this culture is available in Heinz-Jurgen Pinnow, "On the Historical Position of Tlingit," *International Journal of American Linguistics* 30, no. 2 (Apr. 1964): 155–64.

Chapter 7:
Talking with Asthma

1. Lao-tzu, *Tao Te Ching*, chapter 27, from a translation by S. Mitchell. Available at http://acc6.its.brooklyn.cuny.edu/~phalsall/texts/taote-v3.html.
2. Arlette Farge, *Le goût de l'archive* (Paris: Seuil, 1989).
3. Max Tegmark, "The Multiverse," http://space.mit.edu/home/tegmark/index.html.

Chapter 8:
Talking with Mental Illness

1. Theodore Roethke, "In a Dark Time," *The Collected Poems of Theodore Roethke* (New York: Anchor Books, 1961); available at http://poetryfoundation.org/archive/poem.html?id=172120.
2. American Psychiatric Association, "Practice Guidelines for the Treatment of Patients with Bipolar Disorder," available at www.psych.org/psych_pract/treatg/pg/prac_guide.cfm (accessed 12 August 2004).
3. Lev S. Vygotsky, *Mind in Society: The Development of Higher Psychological Processes* (Cambridge, MA: Harvard University Press, 1978).
4. Stanley Fish, "Literature in the Reader: Affective Stylistics," *New Literary History* 2, no. 1 (Autumn 1970): 123–62.
5. Clifford Geertz, *Interpretation of Cultures* (New York: Basic Books, 2000).
6. Elaine Fantham and Erika Rummel, *The Collected Works of Erasmus* (Toronto: University of Toronto Press, 1989).
7. Robert Rieber, ed., *The Collected Works of L. S. Vygotsky,* vol. 5, *Child Psychology* (Boston: Kluwer Academic/Plenum Publishing, 1999).
8. Ibid., 169–74.
9. S. Zrehen, H. Kitano, and M. Fujito, "Learning in Psychologically Plausible Conditions: The Case of the Pet Robot," in Pfeiffer, Blumberg, Meyer, and Wilson, *From Animals to Animats 5: Proceedings of the Fifth International Conference on Simulation of Adaptive Behavior* (Cambridge, MA: MIT Press, 1998).

10. A. Champandard, *AI Game Development: Synthetic Creatures with Learning and Reactive Behavior* (New York: New Riders, 2003).

11. Williams M. Wittgenstein, *Mind and Meaning: Towards a Social Conception of Mind* (New York: Routledge, 2002), 265–74.

12. Ibid.

13. P. Eimas, E. Siqueland, P. Jusczyk, and J. Vigorito, "Speech Perception in Infants," *Science* 171 (1977): 303–6.

14. S. Baron-Cohen, M. Wyke, and C. Binnie, "Hearing Words and Seeing Colours: An Experimental Investigation of a Case of Synaesthesia," *Perception* 16 (1987): 761–67.

15. E. Paulesu, J. Harrison, S. Baron-Cohen, C. Frith, R. Frakowiac, and L. Goldstein, "An Examination of Coloured Speech Synaesthesia Using Positron Emission Tomography," *Brain* 118 (1995): 661–76.

16. S. Baron-Cohen, J. Harrison, L. Goldstein, and M. Wyke, "Coloured Speech Perception: Is Synaesthesia What Happens When Modularity Breaks Down?" *Perception* 22 (1983): 419–26.

17. Thom Hartmann, *The Edison Gene: ADHD and the Gift of the Hunter Child* (Rochester, VT: Park Street Press, 2003).

18. E. Paulesu, J. Harrison, S. Baron-Cohen, C. Frith, R. Frakowiac, and L. Goldstein, "An Examination of Coloured Speech Synaesthesia Using Positron Emission Tomography," *Brain* 118 (1995): 661–76.

19. A. Meltzoff and R. Borton, "Intermodal Matching by Human Neonates," *Nature* 282 (1979): 403–4.

20. E. Paulesu, J. Harrison, S. Baron-Cohen, C. Frith, R. Frakowiac, and L. Goldstein, "An Examination of Coloured Speech Synaesthesia Using Positron Emission Tomography," *Brain* 118 (1995): 661–76.

21. Jean Piaget, *The Origins of Intelligence in Children* (New York: International Universities Press, 1952).

22. D. Lewkowicz, "Development of Intersensory Functions in Human Infancy: Auditory Visual Interactions," in M. Weiss and P. Zelazo, eds., *Newborn Attention* (Norwood, NJ: Ablex, 1992).

23. C. Dehay, J. Bullier, and H. Kennedy, "Transient Projections Form the Fronto-Parietal and Temporal Cortex to Areas 17, 18, and 19 in the Kitten," *Experimental Brain Research* 57 (1984): 208–12; D. Maurer, "Neonatal Synesthesia: Implications for the Processing of Speech and Faces," in B. de Boyson-Bardies, D. de Schonen, P. Jusczyk, P. McNeilage, and J. Morton,

eds., *Developmental Neurocognition: Speech and Face Processing in the First Year of Life* (Dordrecht, Holland: Kluwer Academic Publishers, 1993).

24. R. Hoffman, "Developmental Changes in Human Visual Evoked Potentials to Patterned Stimuli at Different Scalp Locations," *Child Development* 49 (1978): 110–18.

25. Jerry Fodor, *The Modularity of the Mind* (Cambridge, MA: MIT/Bradford Books, 1983).

26. R. M. Barclay, trans., and G. M. Robertson, ed., *Manic-Depressive Insanity and Paranoia* (Edinburgh, Scotland: E & S Livingstone, 1921).

27. D. J. Kupfer, "Epidemiology and Clinical Course of Bipolar Disorder," in D. J. Kupfer, ed., *Bipolar Disorder: The Clinician's Reference Guide* (Montvale, NJ: Clinical Psychiatry LLC, 2004).

28. R. C. Kessler, K. A. McGonagle, S. Zhao et al., "Lifetime and 12-Month Prevalence of DSM-III-R Psychiatric Disorders in the United States," *Archives of General Psychiatry* 51 (1994): 8–19.

29. N. Craddock and I. Jones, "Genetics of Bipolar Disorder," *Journal of Medical Genetics* 36, no. 8 (1999): 585–94.

30. Ibid.

31. P. F. Sullivan, M. C. Neale, and K. S. Kendler, "Genetic Epidemiology of Major Depression: Review and Meta-Analysis," *American Journal of Psychiatry* 157 (2000): 1552–62.

32. R. S. El-Mallakh and S. N. Ghaemi, *Bipolar Depression: A Comprehensive Guide* (Washington, DC: American Psychiatric Publishing, Inc., 2006), see especially chapters 1, 7, 9 and 11.

33. Kenneth J. Gergen, *Realities and Relationships: Soundings in Social Construction* (Cambridge, MA: Harvard University Press, 1994), 276.

34. Thomas Caramagno, *The Flight of the Mind: Virginia Woolf's Art and Manic-Depressive Illness* (Berkeley: University of California Press, 1992).

35. Amy Weintraub, *Yoga for Depression: A Compassionate Guide to Relieve Suffering Through Yoga* (New York: Broadway, 2003).

36. David L. Rosenhan, "On Being Sane in Insane Places," *Science* 179 (1973): 250–58.

37. Thomas King, *The Truth About Stories: Broadcast Lectures,* a set of five audio CDs of CBC's Ideas broadcast lectures, produced by CBC Audio, available to purchase at https://www.anansi.ca/titles.cfm?pub_id=256.

38. Carolyn Kagan, "Making the Road by Walking It," Inaugural Professorial

Lecture, Manchester Metropolitan University, 30 January 2002, available at http://homepages.poptel.org.uk/mark.burton/proftalk8.htm.

Chapter 9:
Talking with Cancer

1. Dr. Seuss, available at The Quotations Page, http://www.quotationspage.com/quotes/Dr._Seuss/ (accessed 27 January 2007).

2. Alastair J. Cunningham, C. V. I. Edmonds, C. Phillips, K. I. Soots, D. Hedley, and G. A. Lockwood, "A Prospective, Longitudinal Study of the Relationship of Psychological Work to Duration of Survival in Patients with Metastatic Cancer," *Psychooncology* 9, no. 4 (2000): 323–39.

3. Michael Harner, *The Way of the Shaman: A Guide to Power and Healing* (New York: Harper & Row Publishers, 1980).

4. Donald M. Hines, *The Forgotten Tribes* (Issaquah, WA: Great Eagle Publishing, 1991).

5. For more information about Michael Harner and his work, see http://www.shamanism.org.

6. Fred Allen Wolf, *The Dreaming Universe: A Mind-Expanding Journey Into the Realm Where Psyche and Physics Meet* (New York: Touchstone, 1995).

7. Marlene Brant Castellano, "Updating Aboriginal Traditions of Knowledge," in J. G. S. Dei and B. L. Hall, eds., *Indigenous Knowledges in Global Contexts: Multiple Readings of Our World* (Toronto: University of Toronto Press, 2000), 21–26.

8. George Yancy, "Geneva Smitherman: The Social Ontology of African-American Language, the Power of Nommo, and the Dynamics of Resistance and Identity Through Language," *The Journal of Speculative Philosophy* 18 (4) (2004): 273–99.

9. For further discussion of the nature of spirits, see the works referenced at http://realmagick.com/articles/02/2-related.html (accessed 27 January 2007).

Chapter 10:
Making Meaning for Diabetes

1. Manuel Rozental, "Thoughts to Share as a Conversation," 23 April 2006, http://www.magma.ca/~brich/aboriginalframe2.html#anchor217685 (accessed 15 January 2007).

2. Elizabeth Debold, "Flow with Soul: An Interview with Dr. Mihaly Csikszentmihalyi," *What Is Enlightenment* magazine, available at http://www.wie.org/j21/csiksz.asp (accessed 27 January 2007).

3. Kathryn Coe, *The Ancestress Hypothesis* (New Brunswick, NJ: Rutgers University Press, 2003).

4. Spencer Johnson, *The One Minute Salesperson* (New York: Avon Books, 2002), 64.

5. Susan Richards Shreve and Porter Shreve, eds., *Outside the Law: Narratives on Justice in America* (Boston: Beacon Press, 1998).

Chapter 11:
Talking with the Universe

1. W. D. Ross, ed., *Aristotle in Nicomachean Ethics*, vol. I, book vii (Cary, NC: Oxford University Press, 1980).

2. Eduardo Duran, *Native American Psychology for a Post-Colonial Era* (Albany: State University of New York Press, 2000).

3. For a more ecumenical discussion of this topic, see Canadian Ecumenical Anti-racism Network, "Racial Justice Week," www.wicc.org/bulletins/RacialJusticeWeek.pdf (accessed 28 January 2007).

4. For more information about Christian versions of this concept, see Rozanne Elders, ed., *The Spirituality of Western Christendom* (Kalamazoo, MI: Cistercian Publications, 1976).

5. For more about this, see Vine Deloria, *God Is Red* (New York: Delta, 1981).

Chapter 12:
Creating a Roundtable of Healing

1. Kornelijus Platelis, "Snare for the Wind," available at http://www.efn.org/~valdas/platelis.html (accessed 27 January 2007).

2. C. Waldegrave, "The Challenges of Culture to Psychology and Postmodern Thinking," in M. McGoldrick, ed., *Re-visioning Family Therapy: Race, Culture and Gender in Clinical Practice* (New York: The Guilford Press, 1998).

3. W. Weiten, *Themes and Variations*, 3rd ed. (Pacific Grove, CA: Brook Cole, 1995); Juergen Habermas and J. J. Shapiro, trans, *Knowledge Human Interest* (Boston: Beacon Press, 1971).

4. Theodore R. Sarbin, "Contextualism: A World View for Modern P

in A. W. Lanfield, ed., *1976 Nebraska Symposium on Motivation* (Lincoln: University of Nebraska Press, 1977), 1–41; for more information, see Theodore R. Sarbin, "Steps to the Narratory Principle: An Autobiographical Essay," in D. J. Lee, ed., *Life and Story: Autobiographies for a Narrative Psychology* (Westport, CT: Praeger, 1994), 29.

5. Ibid., 7.

6. Maureen Lux, *Medicine That Walks* (Toronto: University of Toronto Press, 2001), 3–4.

7. Jon Kabat-Zinn, *Wherever You Go There You Are* (New York: Hyperion, 1994, 2005).

8. Madeleine L'Engle, *A Ring of Endless Light* (New York: Laurel Leaf, 1981).

9. Michel Foucault, *The Birth of the Clinic* (New York: Vintage, 1994).

Conclusion:
Revising Our Stories about Health Care and Healing

1. Quoted by Kirsti A. Dyer, "9-11: United in Courage and Grief," www.journeyofhearts.org/kirstimd/911_story.htm (accessed 27 January 2007).

2. See my essay entitled "Aboriginal Approaches to Healing Relational Trauma," in N. Potter, *Relational Trauma* (New York: Oxford University Press, 2007) for discussion about the importance of inserting forgiveness and compassion into the judicial system.

3. See my as yet unpublished paper on Narrative Therapy in a locked inpatient unit, available by request from me at narrativemedicine@gmail.com.

4. The classic story about this phenomenon is George Bernard Shaw's play *Pygmalion,* in which context alone changes a lower-class woman into an upper-class lady. The tale was made popular as the musical *My Fair Lady,* and later turned into a movie with Eddie Murphy and Dan Aykroyd, *Trading Places.*

‑‑‑hel Foucault, James D. Faubion, Paul Rainbow, Richard Hurley et al., ‑‑‑*rks of Foucault, 1954–1984,* vol. 3 (New York: New

story of Sexuality: An Introduction, vol. 1 (New ‑90).

ampton, "Toward a Re-definition of Indian Educa‑ ‑d J. Barman, eds., *First Nations Education in Can‑* ‑*ds* (Vancouver: University of British Columbia Press,